CUNNINGHAM'S MANUAL OF PRACTICAL ANATOMY

Volume 1

Cunningham's Manual of Practical Anatomy

CUNNINGHAM'S MANUAL OF PRACTICAL ANATOMY

Sixteenth edition

Volume 1 Upper and lower limbs

Dr Rachel Koshi MBBS, MS, PhD

Professor of Anatomy
Apollo Institute of Medical Sciences and Research
Chittoor, India

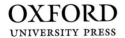

UNIVERSITY PRESS

Great Clarendon Street, Oxford, OX2 6DP,
United Kingdom

Oxford University Press is a department of the University of Oxford.
It furthers the University's objective of excellence in research, scholarship,
and education by publishing worldwide. Oxford is a registered trade mark of
Oxford University Press in the UK and in certain other countries

Thirteenth edition 1966
Fourteenth edition 1977
Fifteenth edition 1986

Impression: 7

Published in the United States of America by Oxford University Press
198 Madison Avenue, New York, NY 10016, United States of America

British Library Cataloguing in Publication Data
Data available

Library of Congress Control Number: 2016956732

ISBN 978-0-19-874936-3

Printed and bound by Thomson Press India Ltd

Oxford University Press makes no representation, express or implied, that the
drug dosages in this book are correct. Readers must therefore always check
the product information and clinical procedures with the most up-to-date
published product information and data sheets provided by the manufacturers
and the most recent codes of conduct and safety regulations. The authors and
the publishers do not accept responsibility or legal liability for any errors in the
text or for the misuse or misapplication of material in this work. Except where
otherwise stated, drug dosages and recommendations are for the non-pregnant
adult who is not breast-feeding

Links to third party websites are provided by Oxford in good faith and
for information only. Oxford disclaims any responsibility for the materials
contained in any third party website referenced in this work.

I fondly dedicate this book to the late Dr K G Koshi for his encouragement and support when I chose a career in anatomy; and to Dr Mary Jacob, under whose guidance I learned the subject and developed a love for teaching.

Oxford University Press would like to dedicate this book to the memory of the late George John Romanes, Professor of Anatomy at Edinburgh University from 1954–1984, who brought his wisdom to previous editions of *Cunningham's*.

Foreword

It gives me great pleasure to pen down the Foreword to the 16th edition of *Cunningham's Manual of Practical Anatomy*. Just as the curriculum of anatomy is incomplete without dissection, so also learning by dissection is incomplete without a manual.

Cunningham's Manual of Practical Anatomy is one of the oldest dissectors, the first edition of which was published as early as 1893. Since then, the manual has been an inseparable companion to students during dissection.

I remember my days as a first MBBS student, the only dissector known in those days was *Cunningham's* manual. The manual helped me to dissect scientifically, step by step, explore the body, see all structures as mentioned, and admire God's highest creation—the human body—so perfectly. As a postgraduate student I marvelled at the manual and learnt details of structures, in a way as if I had my teacher with me telling me what to do next. The clearly defined steps of dissection, and the comprehensive revision tables at the end, helped me personally to develop a liking for dissection and the subject of anatomy.

Today, as a Professor and Head of Anatomy, teaching anatomy for more than 30 years, I find *Cunningham's* manual extremely useful to all the students dissecting and learning anatomy.

With the explosion of knowledge and ongoing curricular changes, the manual has been revised at frequent intervals.

The 16th edition is more student friendly. The language is simplified, so that the book can be comprehended by one and all. The objectives are well defined. The clinical application notes at the end of each chapter are an academic feast to the learners. The lucidly enumerated steps of dissection make a student explore various structures, the layout, and relations and compare them with the simplified labelled illustrations in the manual. This helps in sequential dissection in a scientific way and for knowledge retention. The text also includes multiple-choice questions for self-assessment and holistic comprehension.

Keeping the concept of 'Adult Learning Principles' in mind, i.e. adults learn when they 'DO', and with a global movement towards 'Competency - based Curriculum', students learn anatomy when they dissect; *Cunningham's* manual will help students to dissect on their own, at their own speed and time, and become competent doctors, who can cater to the needs of the society in a much better way.

I recommend this invaluable manual to all the learners who want to master the subject of anatomy.

Dr Pritha S Bhuiyan
Professor and Head, Department of Anatomy
Professor and Coordinator, Department of Medical Education
Seth GS Medical College and KEM Hospital, Parel, Mumbai

Preface to the sixteenth edition

Cunningham's Manual of Practical Anatomy has been the most widely used dissection manual in India for many decades. This edition is extensively revised to meet the needs of the present-day medical student.

Firstly, at the start of each chapter and at the beginning of the description of a region, introductory remarks have been added in order to provide context to the whole human body and to the practice of medicine. In order to appreciate the 'big picture', Chapter 1 (General introduction) has been expanded and supplemented by new artwork. Throughout all three volumes, all anatomical terms are updated and explained using the latest terminology, and the language has been modernized.

Dissection forms an integral part of learning anatomy, and the practice of dissection enables students to retain and recall anatomical details learnt in the first year of medical school during their clinical practice. To make the dissection process easier and more meaningful, in this edition, each dissection is presented with a heading, and a list of objectives to be accomplished. The details of dissections have been retained from the earlier edition but are presented as numbered, stepwise easy-to-follow instructions that help students navigate their way through the tissues of the body, and to isolate, define, and study important anatomical structures.

This manual contains a number of old and new features that enable students to integrate the anatomy learnt in the dissection hall with clinical practice. Each region has images of living anatomy to help students identify on the skin surface bony or soft tissue landmarks that lie beneath. Numerous X-rays and magnetic resonance imaging further enable the student to visualize internal structures in the living. Matters of clinical importance, when mentioned in the text, are highlighted.

A brand new feature of this edition is the presentation of one or more clinical application notes at the end of each chapter. Some of these notes focus attention on the anatomical basis of commonly used physical diagnostic tests such as palpation of the arterial pulse or measurement of blood pressure. Others deal with the underlying anatomy of clinical findings in diseases such as breast cancer or the cervical rib syndrome. Common joint injuries to the knee and other limb joints are discussed with reference to the intra- and periarticular structures described and dissected. Effects of some common nerve injuries along the course of the nerve are described in a clinical context. Many clinical application notes are in a Q&A format that challenges the student to brainstorm the material covered in the chapter. Multiple-choice questions on each section are included at the end to help students assess their preparedness for the university examination.

It is hoped that this new edition respects the legacy of Cunningham in producing a text and manual that is accurate, student friendly, comprehensive, and interesting, and that it will serve the community of students who are beginning their career in medicine to gain knowledge and appreciation of the anatomy of the human body.

Dr Rachel Koshi

Contributors

Dr J Suganthy, Professor of Anatomy, Christian Medical College, Vellore, India.
Dr Suganthy wrote the MCQs, reviewed manuscripts, and provided help and advice with the artwork, and most importantly gave much moral support.

Dr Aparna Irodi, Professor, Department of Radiology, Christian Medical College and Hospital, Vellore, India.
Dr Irodi kindly researched, identified, and contributed the radiology images.

Acknowledgements

Dr Koshi would like to thank the following:

Dr Vernon Lee, Professor of Orthopedics, Christian Medical College, Vellore, India.
Dr Lee kindly critically reviewed the orthopaedic cases.

Dr Ivan James Prithishkumar, Professor of Anatomy, Christian Medical College, Vellore, India.
Dr Prithishkumar kindly reviewed the text as a critical reader, providing assistance on artwork and clinical application materials.

Radiology Department, Christian Medical College, Vellore, India.
The Radiology Department kindly provided the radiology images.

Reviewers

Oxford University Press would like to thank all those who reviewed the text and provided valuable feedback:

Dr TS Roy, MD, PhD, Professor and Head, Department of Anatomy, All India Institute of Medical Sciences, New Delhi 110029.

Dr Aastha, Associate Professor, Department of Anatomy, Christian Medical College & Hospital, Ludhiana, India.

Dr Aby S Charles, Senior Resident, Department of Anatomy, Christian Medical College, Vellore, India.

Dr Padmavathi G, Professor of Anatomy, Apollo Institute of Medical Sciences and Research, Chittoor, India.

Dr Sunil Jonathan Holla, Professor of Anatomy, Christian Medical College, Vellore, India.

Dr Sunita Kalra, Professor of Anatomy, University College of Medical Sciences, Delhi, India.

Dr Sabita Mishra, Professor of Anatomy, Maulana Azad Medical College, Delhi, India.

Dr Bertha AD Rathinam, Professor and Head, Department of Anatomy, India Institute of Medical Sciences Bhopal, Madhya Pradesh, India.

Dr Nachiket Shankar, Associate Professor of Anatomy, St John's Medical College, Bangalore, India.

Contents

PART 1
Introduction

1

CHAPTER 1
General introduction

Human anatomy is the study of the structure of the human body. For descriptive purposes, the human body is divided into regions: head, neck, trunk, and limbs. The trunk is subdivided into the chest or thorax and the abdomen. The abdomen is further subdivided into the abdomen proper and the pelvis. As you dissect the body, region by region, you will acquire first-hand knowledge of the relative positions of structures in the body. But before you begin, you need a vocabulary to define the positions of each anatomical structure, and also an elementary knowledge of the kinds of structures you will encounter.

Terms of position

The body usually lies horizontally on a table during dissection, but the dissector must remember that terms describing positions are always used as though the body is in the **anatomical position**. In this position, the person is standing upright, with upper limbs by the sides and palms directed forwards, and eyes looking straight ahead.

Descriptive terms are used to indicate the position of structures as if the body were in the anatomical position [Fig. 1.1]. **Superior** or **cephalic** refers to the position of a part that is nearer the head, while **inferior** means nearer the feet. **Caudal** (towards the tail) can replace inferior in the trunk. **Anterior** means nearer the front of the body, and **posterior** means nearer the back. **Ventral** and **dorsal** may be used instead of anterior and posterior in the trunk and have the advantage of also being appropriate for four-legged animals (*venter* = belly; *dorsum* = back). In the hand, **dorsal** commonly replaces

posterior, and **palmar** replaces anterior. In the foot, the corresponding surfaces are superior and inferior in the anatomical position, but these terms are usually replaced by **dorsal** (**dorsum** of the foot) and **plantar** (*planta* = the sole).

Median means in the middle. Thus, the **median plane** is an imaginary plane that divides the body into two equal halves, right and left. Where the median plane meets the anterior and posterior surfaces of the body are the **anterior** and **posterior median lines**. A structure is said to be median when it is bisected by the median plane. **Medial** means nearer the median plane, and **lateral** means further away from that plane. The presence of two bones, one lateral and the other medial, in the forearm (radius and ulna) and leg (fibula and tibia) have resulted in the terms **ulnar** or **radial** side of the forearm, and **tibial** or **fibular** side of the leg. The words outer and inner, or their equivalents **external** and **internal**, are used only in the sense of nearer the surface or further away from it in any direction; they are not synonymous with medial and lateral. **Superficial**, meaning nearer the skin, and **deep**, meaning further from it, are the terms most usually used when direction is of no importance. When describing the surfaces of a hollow organ, **external** refers to the outer surface, and **internal** to the inner surface.

A **sagittal plane** may pass through any part of the body, parallel to the median plane. A **coronal plane** is a vertical plane at right angle to the median plane. A transverse plane is a horizontal plane (perpendicular to both the above). All other planes are oblique planes.

Proximal (nearer to) and **distal** (further from) indicate the relative distances of structures from the root of that structure, e.g. the elbow is

4

Terms of position

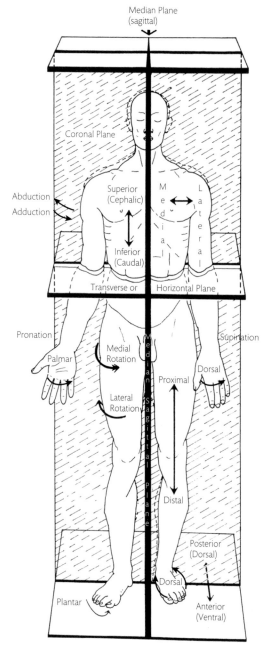

Fig. 1.1 Diagram illustrating some anatomical terms of position and movement.

The terms **superolateral** and **inferomedial**, or **anteroinferior** and **posterosuperior**, or any other combination of the standard terms, may be used to show intermediate positions.

Terms of movement

Movements take place at joints and may occur in any plane, but are usually described in the sagittal and coronal planes [Fig. 1.1]. Movements of the trunk in the sagittal plane are **flexion** (bending anteriorly) and **extension** (straightening or bending posteriorly). In the limbs, flexion is the movement which carries the limb anteriorly and folds it; extension is the movement which carries it posteriorly and straightens it. (Note flexion and extension for the knee joint do not follow this rule. Flexion of the knee folds the limb but results in the leg being carried posteriorly.) At the ankle, the terms used are **plantar flexion** (movement towards the sole) and **dorsiflexion** (movement towards the dorsum). Movements of the trunk in the coronal plane (i.e. side-to-side movement) are known as **lateral flexion**. Movement of the limb away from the median plane is **abduction**, and movement towards the median plane is **adduction**. In keeping with this definition, at the wrist, abduction refers to movement of the hand away from the median plane towards the radial (thumb) side. Abduction of the wrist is also referred to as **radial deviation**. Similarly, adduction of the wrist is also referred to as **ulnar deviation**. In the fingers and toes, abduction means the spreading apart of, and adduction the drawing together of, the digits. In the hand, this movement is in reference to the line of the middle finger. In the foot, it is in reference to the line of the second toe. The thumb lies at right angles to the fingers. Hence, abduction and adduction carry the thumb anteriorly and posteriorly, respectively.

Rotation is the term applied to the movement in which a part of the body is turned around its own longitudinal axis. In the limbs, lateral and medial rotation refers to the direction of movement of the anterior surface. (When the front of the arm or thigh is turned laterally, it is lateral rotation, and, when turned medially, it is medial rotation.) A special movement in the forearm is the rotation of the radius on the stationary ulna. This movement is **pronation**. The hand moves with the radius and is turned so that the palm faces posteriorly. The opposite movement is **supination**, and it turns the hand back to the anatom-

proximal to the wrist but distal to the shoulder. **Middle**, or its Latin equivalent *medius*, is used to indicate a position between superior and inferior or between anterior and posterior. **Intermediate** is used to indicate a position between lateral and medial.

ical position. Inversion and eversion are movements specific to the foot. Inversion turns the sole of the foot medially; and eversion turns the sole laterally.

Introduction to tissues of the body

This section contains a brief account of the structures you will come across as you dissect. Starting from the outermost covering—the skin—and working inwards into the tissue, you will encounter connective tissue arranged as superficial and deep fasciae, blood vessels, nerves, muscles and tendons, and joints and bones. A brief description of the lymphatic system is included, even though you may not encounter this in dissection.

The **skin** consists of a superficial layer of avascular, stratified squamous epithelium, the **epidermis**, and a deeper vascular, dense fibrous tissue layer, the **dermis**. The dermis sends small peg-like protrusions into the epidermis. These protrusions help to bind the epidermis to the dermis by increasing the area of contact between them. The skin is separated from the deeper structures (muscles and bones) by two layers of connective tissue, the superficial and deep fasciae [Fig. 1.2].

Superficial fascia

This fibrous mesh contains fat and connects the dermis to the underlying sheet of the deep fascia. It is particularly dense in the scalp, back of the neck, palms of the hands, and soles of the feet, and binds the skin firmly to the deep fascia in these situations. In other parts of the body, it is loose and elastic, and allows the skin to move freely.

The thickness of the superficial fascia varies with the amount of fat in it. It is thinnest in the eyelids, the nipples and areolae of the breasts, and in some parts of the external genitalia where there is no fat. In a well-nourished body, the **fat** in the superficial fascia rounds off the contours. Its distribution and amount vary in the sexes. The smoother outline of a woman's figure due to the greater amount of subcutaneous fat is a secondary sex characteristic. The superficial fascia also contains small arteries, lymph vessels, and nerves.

Deep fascia

The **deep fascia** is the dense, inelastic membrane which separates the superficial fascia from the underlying structures. It surrounds the muscles and the vessels and nerves which lie between them. The deep fascia sends fibrous partitions, or **septa**, between the muscles to the periosteum of the bones. It forms a major source of attachment for many muscles. The deep fascia also forms tunnels within which the muscles of a group can slide independently of each other. Such **intermuscular septa** are better developed between adjacent muscles having different actions [Fig. 1.2]. In the wrists and ankles, the deep fascia is thickened to form **retinacula** which hold the tendons in place, [see Fig. 1.6].

5

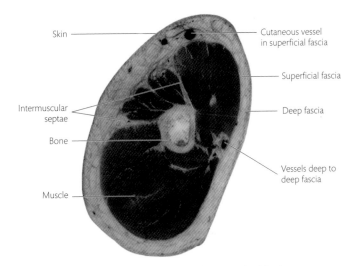

Skin — Cutaneous vessel in superficial fascia

Superficial fascia

Intermuscular septae — Deep fascia

Bone

Vessels deep to deep fascia

Muscle

Fig. 1.2 Cross-section through the arm showing the relationship of the skin, superficial fascia, cutaneous vessels and nerves, deep fascia, muscles, intermuscular septa, and bone to each other.

Image courtesy of Visible Human Project of the US National Library of Medicine.

Blood vessels

The **blood vessels** you will see and identify in dissection are the **arteries** and **veins**. For the sake of completion, a note is added about the capillaries which lie between the smallest of the arteries—the **arterioles**—and the smallest of the veins—the **venules**.

Arteries

Arteries are blood vessels which carry blood from the heart to the tissues. The largest artery in the body is the aorta which begins at the heart and is approximately 2.5 cm in diameter. It gives rise to a series of branches which vary in size with the volume of tissue each has to supply. These branch and re-branch, often unequally, and become successively smaller. The smallest arterial vessels (<0.1 mm in diameter) are known as **arterioles**. They transmit blood into the capillaries.

In many tissues, small arteries unite with one another to form tubular loops called **anastomoses**. Such anastomoses occur especially around the joints of the limbs, in the gastrointestinal tract, and at the base of the brain. When one of the arteries taking part in the anastomosis is blocked, the remaining arteries enlarge gradually to produce a **collateral circulation** and maintain blood flow to the tissue. In some tissues, the degree of anastomosis between adjacent arteries may be so minimal that blockage of one vessel cannot be compensated for by the others. Arteries which are solely responsible for perfusion of a segment of tissue are called **end arteries**. When an end artery is blocked, the tissue supplied by it dies (for lack of collateral circulation). End arteries are found in the eye, brain, lungs, kidneys, and spleen. The **nutrient artery** is an artery supplying the shaft of a long bone and is usually a branch of the main artery of the region.

Blood capillaries

These microscopic tubes form a network of channels connecting the arterioles and venules. The capillary wall consists of a single layer of flattened **endothelial cells**, through which substances are exchanged between the blood and tissues. The capillaries may be bypassed by **arteriovenous anastomoses** which are direct communications between the smaller arteries and veins. Arterioles, capillaries, and venules constitute the microcirculatory units and are not seen by the naked eye.

Veins

Veins are blood vessels that carry blood to the heart. Blood flow in the veins is sluggish, and venous return to the heart is aided by: (1) the pressure applied on veins by contracting leg muscles; and (2) the suction forces generated by the fall in intrathoracic pressure during inspiration. **Valves** in the veins prevent backflow of blood. The positions of the valves in the superficial veins can be seen as localized swellings along their course when the veins are distended with blood. Communications between superficial and deep veins permit the superficial veins to drain into deep veins. Whenever possible, you should slit open the veins in the different parts of the body to see the position and structure of the valves.

Lymph vessels

The lymph is a clear fluid formed in the interstitial tissue spaces. The lymph is transported centrally to the large veins in the neck by lymph capillaries.

Lymph capillaries, or **lymphatics**, have a structure similar to that of blood capillaries but are wider and less regular in shape. They are more permeable to particulate matter and cells than blood capillaries. **Lymph nodes** are firm, gland-like structures which filter the lymph. They vary in size, from a pinhead to a large bean, and lie along the path of lymph vessels. Small lymph vessels unite to form larger lymph vessels, many of which converge on a lymph node. The lymph passes through the node and leaves it in a vessel which usually drains into a secondary, and through it into a tertiary, lymph node. Thus, the lymph drains through a series of lymph nodes and is gathered into larger lymph vessels which enters a great vein at the root of the neck. The vessels which carry the lymph to a node are called **afferent vessels**; those that carry it away from a node are **efferent lymph vessels** (*ad* = to; *ex* = from; *fero* = carry).

In the limbs, the lymph nodes are largest and most numerous in the armpit or axilla and groin. They are usually found in groups which are linked to each other by lymph vessels.

The lymph vessels in the superficial fascia drain the lymph capillary plexuses of the skin. They converge directly on the important groups of lymph nodes situated mainly in the axilla, the groin [see Figs. 3.12, 13.8], and the neck. In the deeper tissue, most lymph vessels and nodes are situated along the deep veins.

Lymph vessels are not demonstrated by dissection but are described because of the importance of this system in clinical practice. Lymph vessels and nodes react to infection, and the vessels form a route for the spread of infection and malignancies.

Nerves

Nerves appear as whitish cords. They are made up of large numbers of fine filaments, the **nerve fibres**, which are of variable diameter, and are bound together in bundles by fibrous tissue. The fibrous tissue forms a delicate sheath—the **endoneurium**—around each nerve fibre. Bundles of nerve fibres are enclosed in a cellular and fibrous sheath—the **perineurium**. And a collection of nerve bundles are enclosed in a dense, fibrous layer—the **epineurium**.

Each nerve is the axonal process of a nerve cell. (The cell body is located either within the spinal cord or near it in the dorsal root ganglion.) The nerve is enclosed in a series of cells—the **Schwann cells**—which are arranged end-to-end on the nerve. In a large-diameter nerve fibre, each Schwann cell forms one segment of a discontinuous, laminated fatty sheath—the **myelin sheath**. Such nerves are referred to as **myelinated nerves** and are white in colour. The gaps between the segments of myelin are known as **nodes**. Thinner nerves are simply embedded in the Schwann cells. They are grey in colour and are called **non-myelinated nerves**.

Nerve fibres transmit **nerve impulses** either to or from the central nervous system. The fibres which carry impulses from the central nervous system are called **efferent nerves**. They innervate muscles and are also called **motor nerves**. Nerves which carry impulses to the central nervous system are **afferent nerves**. They transmit information from the skin and deeper tissues to the central nervous system and are the **sensory nerves**.

Nerves are described as branching and uniting with one another. However, in reality, there is usually no division of the nerve fibre at the point of branching, and never any fusion of individual nerve fibres. At points described as branching of a nerve, nerve fibres from the parent stem pass into two or more separate bundles. At points where two nerves seemingly unite, two or more bundles merge into a single one. However, an individual nerve fibre would branch near its termination and may also give off branches (**collaterals**) at any point.

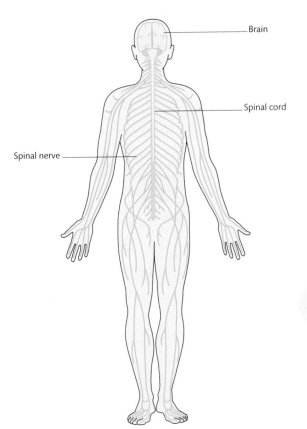

Fig. 1.3 Schematic diagram showing spinal nerves.

Reproduced with permission from Drake, R. L. and Vogl, W., Mitchell, A. W. M. Gray's Anatomy for Students. Copyright © 2005 Elsevier.

Nerves may be classified as: (1) **cranial nerves** when they are attached to the brain (cranial nerves emerge from the skull or cranium); and (2) **spinal nerves** when they arise from the spinal cord. Spinal nerves emerge from the vertebral column through the intervertebral foramina [Fig. 1.3].

Spinal nerves

There are 31 pairs of spinal nerves, named after the groups of vertebrae between which they emerge—eight of the 31 pairs are cervical, 12 thoracic, five lumbar, five sacral, and one coccygeal. All, except the cervical nerves, emerge caudal to the corresponding vertebrae. The first seven cervical nerves emerge cranial to the corresponding vertebrae. The eighth emerges between the seventh cervical and first thoracic vertebrae.

Spinal nerves are attached to the spinal cord by the ventral and dorsal roots [Fig. 1.4]. The **ventral root** consists of bundles of efferent fibres which arise from nerve cells in the spinal

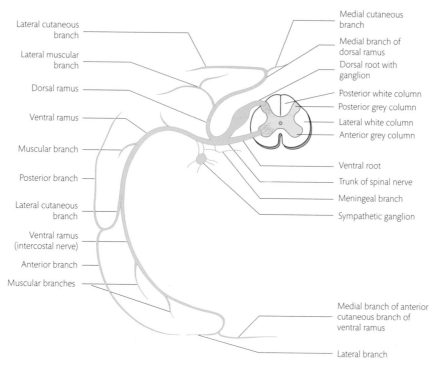

Lateral cutaneous branch

Lateral muscular branch

Dorsal ramus

Ventral ramus

Muscular branch

Posterior branch

Lateral cutaneous branch

Ventral ramus (intercostal nerve)

Anterior branch

Muscular branches

Medial cutaneous branch

Medial branch of dorsal ramus

Dorsal root with ganglion

Posterior white column

Posterior grey column

Lateral white column

Anterior grey column

Ventral root

Trunk of spinal nerve

Meningeal branch

Sympathetic ganglion

Medial branch of anterior cutaneous branch of ventral ramus

Lateral branch

Fig. 1.4 Diagram of a typical spinal nerve.

medulla. The **dorsal root** consists of bundles of afferent fibres and a swelling formed by nerve cells—the **dorsal root** or **spinal ganglion**. The fibres in the dorsal root are processes of the cells in the spinal ganglion.

The ventral and dorsal roots unite in the intervertebral foramen and form the **trunk** of the spinal nerve. The trunk is short and consists of a mixture of efferent and afferent fibres. It divides into a **ventral** and **dorsal ramus** as it emerges from the intervertebral foramen. (Do not confuse the rami (branches), into which the trunk of the spinal nerve divides, with the roots which form it.) Both ventral and dorsal rami contain efferent and afferent fibres.

The small **dorsal ramus** passes backwards into the muscle on either side of the vertebral column (erector spinae). Here it divides into lateral and medial branches which supply the muscle, and one of them sends a branch to the overlying skin. These cutaneous branches of the dorsal rami form a row of nerves on each side of the midline of the back [see Fig. 4.4].

The large **ventral rami** run laterally from the spinal trunk. In the thoracic region, the thoracic ventral rami run along the lower border of the corresponding ribs. They form the intercostal (between ribs) and subcostal (below rib) nerves (*costa* = a rib). Each ventral ramus supplies the muscle in which it lies and gives off lateral and anterior cutaneous branches. The lateral and anterior cutaneous branches, together with the cutaneous branch of the dorsal ramus, supply a strip of skin from the posterior median line to the anterior median line. The strip of skin supplied by a single spinal nerve is known as a **dermatome** [see Fig. 3.6]. In practice, no area of skin is supplied solely by a single spinal nerve, because adjacent dermatomes overlap. The total mass of muscle supplied by a single spinal nerve is a **myotome**. It should be noted that muscles receive afferent, as well as efferent nerve fibres from the spinal nerves.

The ventral rami of the cervical, first thoracic, lumbar, sacral, and coccygeal nerves unite and divide repeatedly to form **nerve plexuses**. The ventral rami of the upper cervical nerves form the cervical plexus. The ventral rami of the lower cervical and first thoracic nerves form the brachial plexus which supplies the upper limb. The ventral rami of the lumbar, sacral, and coccygeal ventral rami form plexuses of the same name. The lumbar and sacral plexuses are mainly concerned with the nerve supply of the lower limb.

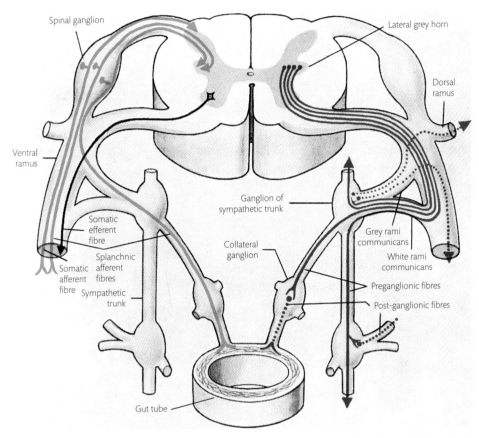

Fig. 1.5 Schematic representation of the relationship of the sympathetic system to spinal nerves and the spinal cord. Sympathetic efferent fibres (pre- and post-ganglionic, red) are shown on the right side; a somatic efferent fibre (black) and somatic and visceral afferent fibres (blue) on the left.

Autonomic nervous system

The sympathetic part of the autonomic nervous system is closely associated with the spinal nerves. Paired sympathetic trunks extend from the base of the skull to the coccyx, one on each side of the vertebral column. They are formed by a row of ganglia (groups of nerve cells) united by nerve fibres.

In the thoracic and upper two or three lumbar segments, fine, myelinated fibres run from the ventral ramus to the sympathetic trunk. These are the **white ramus communicans** [Fig. 1.5]. Fibres in the white ramus communicans have their cell bodies in the spinal cord. They traverse the ventral root and enter the ventral rami. Within the sympathetic trunk, the fibres of the white ramus communicans run longitudinally, up and down. They end on the nerve cells in the ganglia throughout the length of the sympathetic trunk.

Each ventral ramus receives a slender bundle of non-myelinated nerve fibres (the **grey ramus communicans**) from the corresponding ganglion

of the **sympathetic trunk** [Fig. 1.5]. The nerve fibres in the grey ramus communicans arise from the cells in a sympathetic ganglion. These fibres enter the ventral ramus and are distributed through all its branches. They also enter the branches of the dorsal ramus by coursing back in the ventral ramus. The **sympathetic nerves** innervate smooth muscles in the wall of the blood vessels and those associated with hair follicles and sweat glands. Thus, each spinal nerve carries efferent fibres to these involuntary structures, in addition to efferents to the muscles which are under voluntary control.

Through these nerves, the central nervous system controls the activity of the sympathetic part of the autonomic nervous system. It is important to note that the nerve fibres which connect the central nervous system to the sympathetic nervous system (white rami communicans) are found only in the thoracic and upper two to three lumbar spinal nerves.

Fibres of the white rami communicantes which end in the ganglia of the sympathetic trunk are known as **preganglionic nerve fibres**. Fibres of the grey rami communicantes which arise from the cells of the ganglia are known as **post-ganglionic nerve fibres**.

In addition to the grey rami communicantes to the spinal nerves, the sympathetic trunk distributes nerve fibres through branches which pass on to the arteries of the viscera [Fig. 1.5].

Parasympathetic nerves arise from the second, third, and fourth sacral segments of the spinal cord. They leave the spinal medulla through the ventral root and are distributed through branches of the ventral rami in these segments.

From the previous description, it should be clear that branches of nerves to the skin (cutaneous branches) are not entirely sensory but also contain sympathetic efferents. Similarly, branches to muscles are not entirely efferent but also contain sensory and sympathetic fibres. Thus, the signs of nerve injury are not simply paralysis of muscle and loss of sensation, but also loss of sweating, blood vessel control, and loss of control over smooth muscles associated with hair follicles.

Skeletal muscles

The right side of Fig. 1.6 shows some of the skeletal muscles of the body. Skeletal muscles produce movements at joints when they contract by approximating the bones (or other structures) to which they are attached. Each muscle has at least two attachments, one at each end, and in general crosses at least one joint. The action of a muscle on the joint can be worked out from its attachments and its relation to the joint. ⊃ Skeletal muscles are innervated by motor nerves. Damage to the nerve supplying the muscle results in denervation of the muscle and loss or weakness of muscle strength, i.e. paralysis. Muscles are most often used in groups, even in apparently simple movements, so that paralysis of a single muscle may not be noticed, except for a degree of weakness of the movements in which the muscle plays a part. Conducting a neurological examination on a patient suspected of having a nerve injury requires the testing of muscles supplied by the nerve.

Muscles contract in two different ways to meet the demands placed on them: (1) **isometric contraction** is when the length of the muscle remains the same, but the muscle undergoes a change in tension; and (2) **isotonic contraction** is when

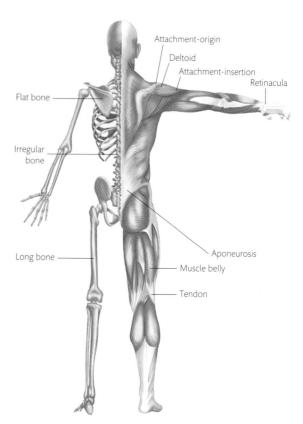

Fig. 1.6 General features of skeletal muscles and bones.

the tension of the muscle remains the same, but the muscle undergoes a change in length. Isometric contraction—without movements—occurs in all anti-gravity muscles when the person is standing still. The tension developed in a muscle is equal to the load against which it is acting, and it keeps the body steady, without any change in length. Another example is the tension developed in the shoulder muscle (deltoid) when the arm is held outstretched. There are two types of isotonic contraction: **concentric** and **eccentric**. In the simplest of terms, **concentric action** is when a muscle shortens to produce a movement. In this situation, the tension developed in the muscle is greater than the load on it. On the other hand, **eccentric action** is when the tension developed in a muscle is less than the load acting against it, and the muscle lengthens to allow the movement to occur. (The muscle stretches gradually to control the speed and force of a movement that is opposite to the one produced when shortening.) For example, the deltoid muscle which passes over

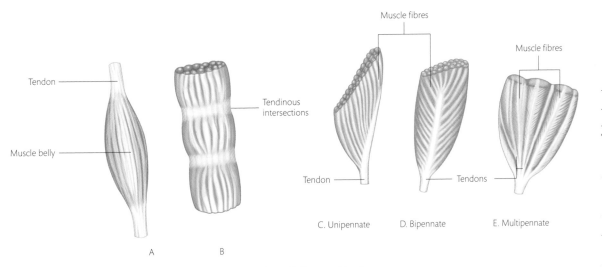

Fig. 1.7 Schematic diagram showing various arrangements of muscle fibres and tendons.

the shoulder acts to bring about abduction of the arm from the side of the body. This is its normal action. When the outstretched arm is lowered to the side, the deltoid lengthens under tension, so as to control the descent of the arm, a situation different to letting the arm fall passively against gravity. To test this, place your left hand over your right deltoid muscle, i.e. on the lateral surface of the shoulder below its tip [Fig. 1.6]. Now abduct the arm till it is horizontal, and feel the deltoid muscle hardening as it contracts (concentric action). Note that, as long as you hold the arm in this position, the deltoid remains contracted and hard (isometric contraction). Now slowly lower the arm towards the side, and note that the deltoid remains contracted throughout the action (eccentric action).

When a muscle shortens, one or both of its ends may move, but it is usual to consider one end (**the origin**) as fixed, and the other (**the insertion**) as mobile. The attachment which moves is determined by other forces in action at the time and is not an intrinsic property of the individual muscle. Thus, muscles passing from the leg into the foot will move the foot (keeping the leg steady) when the foot is off the ground, but will move the leg on the foot when the foot is on the ground. Similarly, muscles which are used to pull downwards on a rope can also be used to climb up it.

The fleshy part of a muscle (the **muscle belly**) is composed of bundles of **muscle fibres** held together by fibrous tissue within which they slide during contraction. The ends of the muscle fibres are attached to bone through fibrous tissue. At times, the fibrous tissue is so short that the belly appears to be attached directly to bone. More usually, the fibrous tissue forms long, inelastic cords known as tendons, or thin, wide sheets called **aponeuroses**, depending on the arrangement of the muscle fibres [Figs. 1.6, 1.7]. **Tendons** usually extend over the surface, or into the substance, of the muscle and thus increase the surface area for its attachment. Tendons also enable a muscle to: (a) act at a considerable distance from the muscle belly, e.g. muscles of the forearm that act on the fingers; and (b) change the direction of its pull by passing round a fibrous or bony pulley. In certain situations, bones called **sesamoid bones** develop within a tendon. Tendons which are compressed against a bony surface, e.g. the ball of the big toe, are protected by small, cartilage-covered sesamoid bones. The sesamoid bone slides on, and articulates with, the surface under pressure and prevents occlusion of blood supply to the tendon during compression.

Where two flat sheets of muscle meet each other, they usually become tendinous, and their fibres interlock (interdigitate) to form a linear tendinous strip (**raphe**) uniting the muscles. Such raphes, unlike tendons or ligaments, can be stretched along their length by the separation of their interdigitating fibres, even though the muscles forming them cannot be pulled apart. The flat muscles of the two sides of the abdominal wall meet in the anterior median plane, forming the largest raphe in the body—the linea alba. The linea alba stretches freely in extension of the trunk but still holds the muscles together.

The strength of a muscle depends on the number and diameter of its fibres. In some muscles, the number of fibres per unit volume of muscle is increased by the oblique arrangement of fibres to the tendon—like the barbs of a feather. The dorsal interossei of the hand have obliquely running fibres which converge on a central tendon. Muscles with this arrangement of fibres are termed **bipennate muscles** [Fig. 1.7] (*pennate* = feather). **Multipennate muscles**, like the deltoid and subscapularis, have a series of such intramuscular tendons. The obliquity reduces the strength of each muscle fibre, but this loss is compensated for by the increase in number of muscle fibres. The diameter and power of individual muscle fibres are increased by exercise which causes an increase in the number of contractile elements (myofibrils) in each fibre.

Muscle fibres can only contract to 40% of their fully stretched length. Thus, the short fibres of pennate muscles are more suitable where power, rather than range of contraction, is required. As there is a limitation to how much a muscle can contract, long muscles which cross several joints may be unable to shorten sufficiently to produce the full range of movement at all joints. This is known as **active insufficiency** of a muscle and is exemplified by the fact that the fingers cannot be fully flexed when the wrist is flexed. Ascertain this on your own wrist and fingers. In the same way, opposing muscles may be unable to stretch sufficiently to allow a movement to take place. This is known as **passive insufficiency**. A third set of muscles maybe is used to fix a joint (keep it steady), so that muscles producing movement can act effectively. These muscles are called fixators or **synergists**.

Muscles that are attached close to the joint on which they act have little mechanical advantage over the joint (which is the fulcrum), but great advantage in speed and range of movement of the bones (which are the levers) (example: attachment and action of the biceps brachii on the elbow joint). In cases where muscles are clustered round a joint, they are less capable of movement but help in maintaining stability in all positions. These muscles act as ligaments of variable length and tension, in place of the usual ligaments which would restrict movement. The rotator cuff muscles

of the shoulder joint are a good example of such muscles. They stabilize the shoulder but play little part in bringing about movements.

The manner in which a muscle acts on a joint depends on its relation to the joint. It should be remembered, however, that any muscle may act concentrically, isometrically, or eccentrically.

Muscles are supplied by numerous arteries and veins. The main artery and the motor nerve enter the muscle at a distinct **neurovascular hilum** (numerous smaller arteries enter elsewhere). Motor nerves entering the muscles carry impulses which cause the muscle to contract, and also sensory impulses from the muscle and tendon on the amount of tension and degree of contraction of the muscle. In addition, nerves transmit sympathetics to the blood vessels in the muscle. It is possible to stimulate contraction in individual muscles by applying an electrical impulse to the skin overlying the neurovascular hilum. ➲ Electromyography is a diagnostic procedure based on this principle. It is used to assess the integrity of the motor nerve and muscle. A denervated, but otherwise healthy, muscle will contract when an electrical stimulus is applied to it. A dystrophic muscle, on the other hand, will not contract on external stimulation.

Muscles are often classified in groups by the principal action they have on a particular joint, e.g. flexors, extensors, abductors, adductors. Although this classification is commonly used, it should be noted that it is not satisfactory because a single muscle may be a flexor of one joint and an extensor of another, e.g. rectus femoris.

The terms flexor and extensor are also used to designate groups of limb muscles which develop, respectively, from the ventral and dorsal sheets of primitive muscles (irrespective of the actual functions of the individual muscles). The anterior divisions of the ventral rami of the spinal nerves supply these 'flexor' muscles. The posterior divisions supply the 'extensors'.

Bursae and synovial sheaths

Where two adjacent structures, like muscle, tendon, skin, or bone, slide over each other, a synovial sac is often found between them to reduce friction. This synovial sac is called a **bursa**. The **bursa** is a closed sac lined with a smooth synovial membrane, which secretes a small amount of viscous fluid into the sac. When there is irritation or infection of the bursa, the secretion is increased, and the bursa

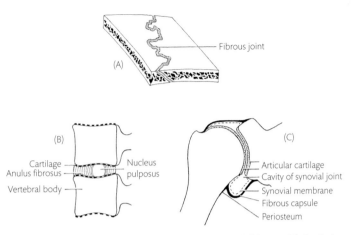

Fig. 1.8 Diagrams showing the three types of joints. (A) Fibrous joint between two skull bones. (B) Cartilaginous joint between two adjacent vertebrae (the anulus fibrosus and nucleus pulposus are parts of the intervertebral disc). (C) Synovial joint between the scapula and humerus—shoulder joint.

becomes swollen, and tender. Similar **synovial sheaths** enclose tendons where the range of movement is considerable, like in the fingers.

Joints

A joint is where two or more bones come together and articulate with each other. One way of classifying joints is according to the substance that occupies the space between the bones [Fig. 1.8]. Joints where the adjacent bones are united by a thin layer of dense fibrous tissue are **fibrous joints**. Joints where the adjacent bones are united by fibrocartilage or hyaline cartilage are **cartilaginous joints**, e.g. the discs between the bodies of the vertebrae. Fibrous and cartilaginous joints are joints where no or little movement is possible. Joints with the maximum amount of movement between the bones are **synovial joints**. In synovial joints, the articulating surfaces of the bones are covered with firm, slippery **articular cartilage**, and they slide on each other within a narrow joint cavity containing lubricant **synovial fluid** [Fig. 1.9]. Outside the cavity, the bones are held together by a tubular sheath of fibrous tissue (the **fibrous capsule** or **fibrous membrane**), which is sufficiently loose to permit movement. The fibrous capsule may be strengthened by ligaments, which are strong bands of inelastic fibrous tissue connecting bones at joints. Ligaments are often found in situations where they will not interfere with movement. For example, at the elbow joint, strong collateral ligaments are found on the medial and lateral sides. They lie approximately as radii of the arc of movement and

thus remain tight in all positions, effectively holding the bones together. (In contrast, the anterior and posterior parts of the capsule of the elbow joint are thin and loose to allow easy movement.) Some ligaments, like the iliofemoral ligament of the hip joint, act to limit excessive movement. Ligaments are often named for their position. For example, the ligaments on the side of the elbow joint are called medial and lateral collateral ligaments, or radial and ulnar collateral ligaments of the elbow joint, as they lie on the radial and ulnar sides of the elbow. The **synovial membrane** lines the inner surface of the fibrous capsule, the intracapsular non-articular parts of the bone, and intracapsular tendons and ligaments when present [Fig. 1.9].

The joint surfaces of the bones at synovial joints are of many different shapes to allow particular movements and prevent others. Based on the shape of the articulating surface, synovial joints are further subclassified [Fig. 1.10]. In a **plane synovial joint**, the surfaces of the bones are flat, permitting only slight gliding movements (example: some of the joints between the bones of the hand and foot). The function of these joints is to provide some resilience to an otherwise rigid structure. More usually, the surfaces of the articulating bones are curved. The **ball-and-socket** type of joint, e.g. shoulder and hip joints, allows the greatest amount of movement. In this type of joint, the spherical end of one bone fits into a cup-shaped recess in the other. In the shoulder, the hemispherical head of the humerus fits into the shallow glenoid fossa of the scapula. In the hip, the nearly spherical head of the femur

14

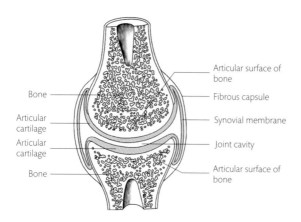

Fig. 1.9 Schematic section through a synovial joint.

Labels in figure:
Bone
Articular cartilage
Articular cartilage
Bone
Articular surface of bone
Fibrous capsule
Synovial membrane
Joint cavity
Articular surface of bone

fits deep into the cup-shaped acetabulum of the hip bone. Where the cup is shallow, e.g. the shoulder joint, the range of movements is great, but the stability is less, when compared to joints having a deep cup, e.g. the hip joint. Three types of joints allow movements in only two directions, at right angles to each other—usually flexion and extension, abduction and adduction (but no rotation): (1) **condyloid joints**; (2) **ellipsoid joints**; and (3) **saddle joints**. **Condyloid joints**, like the joints of the knuckles where the fingers meet the hand, have a bony configuration similar to the ball-and-socket type of joint, but rotation is limited by the ligaments. **Ellipsoid joints**, like the wrist joint, are also like a ball-and-socket joint, but the radius of curvature of the surfaces is long in the transverse direction and short in the anteroposterior direction, and as such rotation is not possible. **Saddle joints**, like that of the carpometacarpal joint of the

thumb, have an articular surface that is concave in one direction and convex at right angles to this—the convex surface of one bone fitting the concave surface of the other. Here again, flexion and extension and abduction and adduction are possible.

Two types of joints allow movement around only one axis: (1) in **hinge joints**, e.g. the interphalangeal joints of the fingers and the ankle joint, the configuration of the bones and the arrangement of the ligaments prevent all other movements, except those of flexion and extension; and (2) in the **pivot joints**, e.g. the proximal radio-ulnar joint, a cylindrical bone (the radius) rotates within a ring formed by another bone (the ulna) and the annular ligament [see Fig. 9.6]. At such a joint, only rotation is possible.

In joints where considerable movement is required in many different directions, e.g. the shoulder joint, the fibrous capsule is thin and lax throughout. The joint is supported by muscles which closely surround the joint and are able to stretch or tighten in any position. Where extreme mobility in one direction is required, e.g. at the knuckles or knee, the appropriate part of the fibrous capsule is entirely replaced by the tendon of a muscle.

The stability and complexity of movement at a joint are sometimes increased by placing a **disc** of fibrous tissue between the bones. This disc may have different curvatures on its two surfaces and thus convert a single joint cavity into two, each having a different type of movement. The articular disc may also act as a shock absorber within the joint or assist with the spreading of the synovial fluid between the surfaces of joints [Fig. 1.10D].

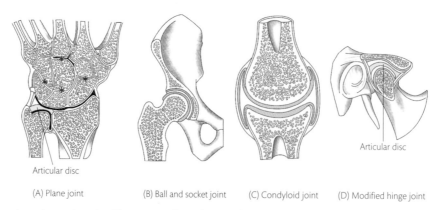

Articular disc

Articular disc

(A) Plane joint   (B) Ball and socket joint   (C) Condyloid joint   (D) Modified hinge joint

Fig. 1.10 Schematic section to show the different types of articulating surfaces in synovial joints. Asterisks indicate the articular surfaces of plane joints of the hand.

Bones

Bone is a form of connective tissue in which the intercellular substance consists of dense, white fibres embedded in a hard calcium phosphate matrix. The fibrous tissue imparts resilience to the bone, while the calcium salts resist compression forces.

Bone is found in two forms: (1) **compact bone** is dense and forms the tubular shafts of the long bones; and (2) **cancellous bone** is a lattice of bone spicules. It occurs at the ends of long bones and fills the flat and irregular bones. The spaces between the spicules are filled with a highly vascular bone marrow.

The **periosteum** is a dense layer of fibrous tissue which covers the surfaces of bones, except where they articulate with other bones. (Remember the articular surface is covered by articular cartilage.) It is continuous with muscles, tendons, ligaments, fibrous capsules of joints, intermuscular septa, and the deep fascia where a bone is.

Dry bones used in the study of anatomy have a number of important surface markings. A dry bone is smooth where: (a) it is covered, in life, by articular cartilage; (b) it gives a fleshy attachment to muscles; and (c) it is subcutaneous. It is often roughened where ligaments, aponeuroses, and tendons are attached. It has grooves lodging blood vessels, and holes (foramina) where blood vessels enter and leave the bone. Many of these features are more easily felt than seen.

It is important for the student to determine the position of each bone in the body, to be able to identify the parts of the bones which are readily visible or palpable, and to be able to identify these features on radiological images.

Bones can be classified according to their shape: (1) **long bones** of the limbs have a narrow, tubular **body** (shaft) made up of compact bone, and enlarged articular ends composed largely of cancellous bone; (2) **short bones are roughly cuboidal in shape**, e.g. bones of the wrist and foot; (3) **flat bones**, e.g. the sternum, scapula, and vault of the skull; (4) **irregular bones**, e.g. vertebrae which make up the vertebral column [Fig. 1.6]; and (5) **pneumatic bones** of the skull contain air spaces.

Bones are formed in two ways: by endochondral ossification or by intramembranous ossification.

In **endochondral ossification**, bones are preformed in cartilage—by the production of a cartilaginous model. The model consists of cartilage cells buried in a matrix and grows by the proliferation of its cells and the production of matrix [Fig. 1.11A]. This model is then replaced by bone

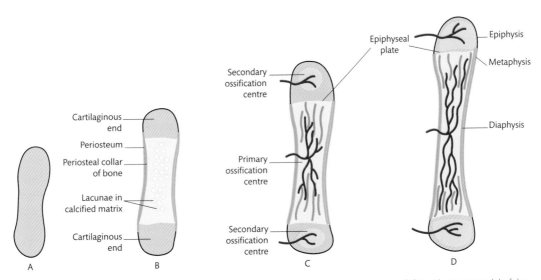

Fig. 1.11 Endochondral ossification. Diagram of the four stages in the development of a long bone. (A) Cartilaginous model of the long bone before ossification begins; 8 weeks of intrauterine life (IUL). (B) Ossification has begun in the centre where empty spaces and spicules of calcified cartilage are seen. Compact bone is laid down by the periosteum; 2–3 months of IUL. (C) Blood vessels invade the centre of the bone, and ossification of calcified cartilage begins. Later, blood vessels invade the ends of the bone which begin to ossify; childhood. (D) Most of the cartilage is replaced by bone. Growth plate is seen between the bones ossified from the primary and secondary ossification centres; adolescence-early adulthood.

by a sequence of changes that take place in the cartilaginous model:

(a) A supporting shell of bone is laid down by the periosteum on the external surface of the body of the model [Fig. 1.11B].

(b) The matrix of the cartilage deep to this becomes calcified, and the cells die, leaving empty spaces in the calcified cartilage.

(c) These spaces coalesce (join), leaving longitudinal spicules of calcified cartilage between them.

(d) This calcified cartilage is invaded by blood vessels from the surrounding shell.

(e) Bone is laid down on the spicules by the action of bone-forming cells—the **osteoblasts**. This process begins at the centre of the body of the cartilaginous model, in the part which is destined to become the centre of the shaft of the long bone. This centre (of ossification) is called the **primary ossification centre**. From the primary ossification centre, ossification spreads towards the ends which remain cartilaginous for a while after the centre has been ossified.

Secondary ossification centres develop at each end of the cartilaginous model of the long bone, and ossification in them proceeds in all directions. The bone formed at each end is separated from the ossifying body by a zone of growing cartilage called the **epiphyseal plate**. The growth cartilage serves an important function of adding new cartilage to the shaft, thus providing material for growth. As growth proceeds, the ends of the growing bone move away from the centre of the body. The external shell of bone increases in length at the same rate and results in growth in length of the long bone. When growth in length of bone is complete (in early adulthood), the growth cartilages in the long bones stop growing. Ossification from the body spreads into the growth cartilage which also becomes ossified. Fusion occurs between the bone in the body (formed from the primary ossification centre) and the bone at the ends (formed from the secondary ossification centres). This brings growth in length to a halt. After this has happened in all the bones, there is no further increase in the height of the individual.

Specific terminology is used to designate the parts of a growing long bone. The bone developed from primary ossification is termed the **diaphysis**. The **epiphysis** is the bone developed from the secondary ossification centre and lies at the end of the bone. (A bone can have more than one epiphysis at each end.) The **metaphysis** is the epiphyseal end of the diaphysis. It is the zone of active ossification [Fig. 1.11].

Growth in the diameter of the long bone is brought about by the addition of bone to the external surface of the enclosing shell. This bone is produced by a highly cellular osteogenic layer of periosteum. As the shell increases in thickness, the bone on the inner surface is removed. Thereafter, the marrow cavity increases in transverse diameter at a slightly slower rate than that of bone being added to the external surface. The process of bone removal is carried out by osteoclasts.

In short and irregular bones, ossification starts in the centre of the cartilaginous model and proceeds outwards. No external shell of bone is formed. The bone continues to grow until the adult size is reached, at which time the bone has replaced all of the cartilage, except that which persists on the articular surfaces.

The ossification centres in the bodies of the long bones (**primary ossification centres**) appear at approximately 8 weeks of intrauterine life. Those at the ends of the long bones (**secondary ossification centres**) appear much later, at or after birth. In short and irregular bones, the single ossification centre (primary centre) appears after birth [see Fig. 1.12 for ossification of hand bones]. In all cases, the ossification in the cartilage forms cancellous bone, while that formed by the periosteum is compact bone. Cancellous bone can be turned into compact bone by continuation of the ossification process.

Although most long bones have epiphyses at both ends, growth in length occurs mainly at one end. At this '**growing end**', the epiphysis usually appears earlier and fuses with the body later than that at the other end. In a growing child, injury to the growing end of a long bone is more serious than injury to the other end. Since epiphyses are visible in radiographs and are separated from the body of the bone by a clear region of growth cartilage, they have to be differentiated from fractures. It is necessary to know where epiphyses appear and till when they are normally present. The growing ends in the upper limb bones are at the shoulders and wrists, and in the lower limbs at the knees.

Bone may also be formed in connective tissue without the intervention of a cartilaginous model. This process of bone formation in connective tissue is called **membranous (intramembranous) ossification**. In this type of ossification,

(A)

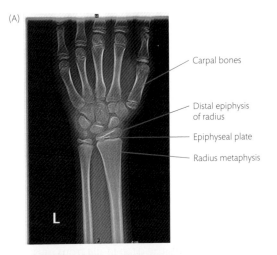

Carpal bones

Distal epiphysis of radius

Epiphyseal plate

Radius metaphysis

L

(B)

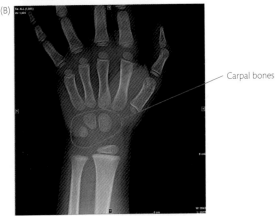

Carpal bones

Fig. 1.12 (A) X-ray of the hand of a 12-year-old child. The epiphysis at the lower end of the radius and ulna are still separated from the diaphysis by the growth cartilage. Ossification centres for all eight carpal bones have appeared. (B) X-ray of the hand of a 2-year-old child. Only three carpal bones have begun to ossify. The ossification centre for the lower end of the ulna has not yet appeared.

osteoblasts invade the fibrous membrane to form many separate spicules of bone. These spicules fuse with each other to form a lattice around the capillaries of the connective tissue. This lattice-work may persist as cancellous bone, or continued deposition of bone in the cavities of the lattice can turn it into compact bone. A periosteum with a cellular **osteogenic layer** is formed on the external surfaces of the membrane and becomes a source of bone deposition. This continuous periosteal deposition of the bone ceases at the end of growth. After that, the cellular osteogenic layer of the periosteum disappears. The outer **fibrous layer** persists and fuses with the surface of the bone. Osteogenesis from the periosteum can begin again when increased strength of a bone is required, e.g. when the weight or muscular-

ity of the individual increases. It is also the source of bone formation in regions where tendons and ligaments are attached and for much of the new bone formed at the site of healing fractures. Absorption of unnecessary bone plays an important part in bone development. In addition to increasing the size of the marrow cavity and lightening the bone, it also maintains the normal external shape of the bone throughout growth.

General instructions for dissection

In the laboratory, you will find that the cadaver for dissection is embalmed with fixatives to preserve it. The whole body has been kept moist by storing it with moist wrappings or immersing it in fluid. Be careful to ensure that the body is kept moist during the entire time you will be working on it.

For the medical student, dissection is an important way of getting a fuller understanding of the structure and function of the human body. It aids in learning simple structures like the valves in the veins, and more complex ones like the heart. Without a sound knowledge of these, the normal and abnormal circulation of the blood through the body could not be properly understood. Similarly, knowledge of the movements occurring at joints, the muscles which cause them, and the nerves innervating these muscles is essential to understand and address the effects of injury or disease in any of these elements of the musculoskeletal system.

Dissection instruments

You will require a scalpel, two pairs of forceps, preferably with rounded tips, and a strong blunt hook or seeker. In addition, you may find it useful to have a hand lens to examine small structures and a torchlight.

Organization of dissections and commonly used terms

Under the skin, the human body consists of a number of structures embedded in fibrous connective tissue which varies in density from a loose mesh to tough sheets of fibres. Dissection is the process of freeing the structures from this tissue and demonstrating them clearly.

In this manual, dissections are organized in a stepwise manner to enable you to systematically explore the region under study and learn important anatomical details. The objectives for each dissection are stated at the start to enable you to focus your attention on the particular area. Before you start dissecting, learn the meaning of the following terms.

(a) Dissect—to cut or tear apart. In the laboratory, dissecting an area requires you to separate the tissue in such a way as to expose the structure under study—muscle, vessel, nerve, etc. This can best be done by blunt dissection with a hook or forceps by isolating and pulling the structure through loose layers of connective tissue. In this way, it is possible to free organs without damaging blood vessels or nerves. Use of sharp instruments, such as scalpels or scissors, should be reserved for cutting the skin and the dense layers of the deep fascia which enclose many organs and partly conceal them.

(b) Cut or transect—to divide using a sharp instrument, usually to expose deeper lying structures.

(c) Clean—to remove fat and fascia from the surface of a muscle, or to define the edge of a muscle or to remove the connective tissue covering of a nerve or vessel.

(d) Define—to remove the connective tissue masking the border of a structure, so that the extent of the structure is more clearly seen.

(e) Retract—to pull aside or separate one structure from an adjacent structure. It is a temporary displacement done to visualize an underlying structure.

(f) Reflect—to fold back a cut structure, usually skin or transected muscle.

Removal of the skin

Remove the skin from the superficial fascia in a series of flaps which can be replaced to prevent drying of the part. It is probably better to cut through both the skin and superficial fascia and remove both of them in one layer from the underlying deep fascia by blunt dissection. The blood vessels and nerves entering the superficial fascia through the deep fascia are easily found in this way and can be traced for some distance. The alternative of searching for their minute branches in the superficial fascia is a tedious, and often unrewarding, process. The student should be aware that the distribution of cutaneous nerves is of considerable clinical importance, but this is best learnt by reference to diagrams, except in the case of the larger branches which are easily followed. In the superficial fascia, the nerves are almost always accompanied by a small artery and one or more minute veins. Larger veins are also found in the superficial fascia. They run a solitary course to pierce the deep fascia and drain into the deep veins. At such junctions, these superficial veins contain valves which prevent the reflux of blood from the deep veins.

Deep dissection

When the deep fascia has been uncovered and examined, proceed to remove it. This is made difficult because it sends fibrous sheets between the muscles, enclosing each in a separate compartment. Where a number of muscles arise together, the walls of these compartments also give origin to the muscle fibres. They thus form a tendinous sheet which appears to bind together adjacent muscles. In other places, it is relatively easy to strip the deep fascia from muscles, because only delicate strands pass between the individual bundles of muscle fibres. It is important to follow each muscle to its attachments and to define these accurately, for it is only in this way that the action of a muscle can be determined.

As each muscle is exposed and lifted from its bed, look for the neurovascular bundle entering it. Follow the structures in the neurovascular bundle back to the main nerve trunk and vessel from which they arise. In many situations, the arteries are accompanied by tributaries of the main vein which often obscure the artery and nerve. In these cases, it is advisable to remove the vein, so that a clearer view of the artery and nerve can be obtained. In any case, it will be found that there are usually multiple venous channels and that their arrangement is much less standard than that of the arteries. The arteries are less constant in their arrangement than the nerves.

Variations

We all know that the external appearance of individuals varies greatly. The same type of variation exists in the size, position, and shape of the internal organs among different individuals. Therefore, no single account of the structure of the body exactly fits every individual, and students must expect to find variations from the descriptions given in this book. For this reason, students should take every opportunity to look at the other bodies being dissected at the same time. Some of the variations are of considerable clinical importance, e.g. differences in the anastomotic arrangement between the arteries at the base of the brain, while others have little significance, e.g. an extra belly of a particular muscle or the marked difference in the arrangement of the superficial veins, even on the two sides of the same body. Congenital anomalies, variations that arise from defects in intra-uterine development, are not commonly seen in the dissection hall. Many of these are so severe that they lead to early death. Other congenital anomalies may be present throughout life without any overt sign. The student should understand the main processes of development and the effects of its abnormalities on the structure and function of the various systems.

Anatomy of the living body

In the dead preserved body, the texture and appearance of the organs have been altered. The student should remember that the purpose of studying formalin-fixed cadavers is just a tool to help visualize the living body in action, so that the effects of injury or disease can be appreciated and abnormalities can be recognized. Dissection is only a means to the end of a fuller understanding of function. In addition to studying the body by dissection, the living body should be observed and palpated.

Special radiological techniques

An increasing number of techniques are being established to visualize the internal structure of the body without surgical intervention. Of these, the oldest is the use of X-rays.

X-rays

This technique depends on the differential absorption of X-rays by the various tissues of the body on their way through it to a sensitive film (or other recording apparatus) which is blackened by development in direct proportion to the amount of X-rays reaching it. Thus, if the exposure is correct, the film is deeply blackened outside the area shaded by the body and is completely clear where a tissue intervenes which absorbs all the penetrating X-rays. Compact bone and teeth are the most absorbent tissues, while the lungs, windpipe, and intestine which contain air, are the least. Most other tissues, including those containing fluid, have an intermediate absorption per unit of thickness, except fat which has a lower level of absorption, though not as low as air.

Each point on the film (radiograph) has a density (blackness) which is directly proportional to the amount of X-rays reaching it, and hence inversely proportional to the sum of the absorptions of all the tissues which lie between the source of X-rays and that point on the radiograph. Hence, in a posteroanterior radiograph of the chest [see Fig. 2.3 in Volume 2], the lung fields are dark because the air they contain does not absorb X-rays as much as the vertebral column, the breast bone (sternum), and the tissues lying between the two lungs. Also, the absorption by the ribs, added to the absorption by the tissue in the lungs, etc., makes the ribs appear as lighter strips in the lung fields, and the fuzzy, whiter areas in the medial parts of each lung are due to absorption by the larger blood vessels (fluid-filled) in these parts of the lungs.

In examining Fig. 2.3 in Volume 2, the following points should be noted.

1. The outlines of the heart and great vessels which arise from these are obvious on the right (left side of the patient) of the median white area, because they project beyond the vertebral column and sternum into the lung fields and make a sharp contrast in absorption by comparison with that on the left where the vertebral column and sternum overlap the heart and vessels.

2. On each side, the lower part of the lung field becomes lighter.

3. Air introduced into the abdominal (peritoneal) cavity makes the lower surface of the diaphragm (a thin partition between the thorax and abdomen) and the upper surfaces of the organs immediately below it obvious, though, without that air, only the upper surface of the diaphragm would have been seen because of its contrast with the lungs. The presence of the air in the upper part of the peritoneal cavity shows that this radiograph was taken with the patient in the erect position.

If the intensity of the X-rays or the length of exposure had been increased, the lung fields would have become darker and the breast and rib 'shadows' much less obvious, though some detail of the vertebral column would have been visible. Conversely, it is possible to show minor differences in tissue absorption, e.g. fat versus tumour, most easily with low-intensity X-rays.

Thus, radiographs show the outline of structures where there is a change in X-ray absorption but cannot show the outline of two adjacent structures which have the same X-ray density. Clearly, any hollow organ, e.g. blood vessel, gut tube, etc., which can be filled with a substance which absorbs X-rays more effectively than bone, e.g. heavy metals such as barium [see Figs. 11.38, 11.65, 11.66, 17.3, all in Volume 2], or less effectively than the surrounding tissue, e.g. air, can make its outline obvious. The combination of both (double contrast) where a small amount of X-ray-opaque material is introduced into a cavity followed by air allows the first to outline the internal surface, so that irregularities are made visible by the contrast with the air [see Figs. 11.40, 11.41 in Volume 2], while use of the X-ray-opaque material alone merely produces a silhouette.

Three more recent techniques all produce pictures representing slices taken through the body at any desired level. All of these depend on special features of the tissues, and can be recorded in digital form and reproduced in any desired manner which the information permits.

Computerized tomography

Computerized tomography (CT) is a technique which uses X-rays [see Fig. 4.47 in Volume 2] and depends on the differences in absorption by different tissues—a feature which can be enhanced by the introduction of special materials like iodinated contrast media. Once a series of transverse sections have been made and the results recorded in digital form, it is possible to combine these in the computer and to construct images in a different plane (like sagittal or coronal, or even three-dimensional (3D), reconstructions), if required. By varying the timing of image acquisition following the intravenous administration of iodinated contrast media, CT images can be obtained in arterial, venous, and delayed phases. CT angiograms of different arterial systems can be easily obtained.

Ultrasound

Ultrasound (sonar) can also be used to produce electronic pictures which represent the reflection of ultrasound from surfaces where one tissue meets another. Unfortunately, ultrasound cannot be used where there is air or bone, because it is not transmitted through these, but it has the advantage that there is no evidence, unlike X-rays, of it having any damaging effects on even the most sensitive tissues. It is used therefore as a method of choice to scan the pelvis where there is the possibility of pregnancy and to determine gross abnormalities at an early stage. The method consists of passing an ultrasound transmitter and recorder over the skin and showing the computerized reflection on a cathode ray tube. The pictures produced are more difficult to read than CTs but represent sections taken through the body under the path of travel of the instrument. They are most useful when shown as a continuous recording (real-time) which can take account of movements of tissues such as the heart valves.

Magnetic resonance imaging

In magnetic resonance imaging (MRI), protons in the tissue are made to resonate in a strong magnetic field by subjecting them to an appropriate radio wavelength. Such resonations are recorded and computed, and converted electronically to pictures [see Fig. 11.56 in Volume 2]. Different areas in these pictures show different intensities depending on the amount of protons or water in the tissues—their T1 and T2 relaxation times. Imaging parameters can be adjusted to obtain different pulse sequences (like T1-weighted, T2-weighted, fluid-attenuated inversion recovery (FLAIR), etc.) with varying image contrast. MRI has better soft tissue contrast than CT scans and does not use harmful ionizing radiation like CT. By using magnetic resonance (MR) spectroscopy, it is possible to assess the biochemical composition and metabolism of the tissue. Specific parts of the brain that are activated when performing certain tasks can be mapped by using functional MRI. MR angiography images can be obtained with or without the use of contrast media (gadolinium-based agents). The main disadvantages of MRI are the limited availability, the expense involved, and the longer time taken in image acquisition.

PART 2

The upper limb

21

CHAPTER 2

Introduction to the upper limb

Introduction

There are four parts to the upper limb: the shoulder, the arm or brachium, the forearm or antebrachium, and the hand.

The term **shoulder** includes a number of smaller regions: the shoulder joint, the axilla or armpit, the scapular region around the shoulder blade, and the pectoral or breast region on the front of the chest. The scapula (or shoulder blade) and the clavicle (or collarbone) are the bones of the shoulder girdle [see Figs. 3.4, 4.2, 4.3]. The scapula and clavicle articulate with each other at the acromioclavicular joint, but the only articulation between the shoulder girdle with the rest of the skeleton is the articulation of the clavicle with the upper end of the sternum at the sternoclavicular joint. The mobile scapula is otherwise held in position entirely by muscles.

The **arm** is the part of the upper limb between the shoulder and the elbow. The arm bone is the humerus, and it articulates with the scapula at the shoulder joint, and with the radius and ulna at the elbow joint.

The **forearm** extends from the elbow to the wrist. Its bones—the radius and ulna—articulate with the humerus at the elbow joint, as mentioned above, with each other at the radio-ulnar joints, and distally the radius (but not the ulna) articulates with the carpal bones at the radiocarpal joint. In the anatomical position (supine position of the forearm), the bones are parallel, and the radius is lateral to the ulna. When the palm of the hand faces posteriorly (prone position of the forearm), the distal end of the radius has rotated around the distal end of the ulna, so that the radius lies obliquely across the ulna. These movements are called **pronation** and **supination** respectively.

The **hand** consists of the wrist or carpus, the hand proper or metacarpus, and the digits (thumb and fingers). The eight small wrist, or carpal, bones are arranged in two rows (proximal and distal), each consisting of four bones. The carpal bones articulate: (a) with one another at the intercarpal joints; (b) proximally, with the radius at the radiocarpal joint; and (c) distally, with the metacarpal bones at the carpometacarpal joints. The articulation of the carpal bones with the radius accounts for the movement of the hand with the radius in pronation and supination. The small movements that occur at each of these joints add up to allow a considerable range of movement. Posteriorly, the carpal bones are close to the skin, but anteriorly they are covered by muscles of the ball of the thumb (**thenar eminence**) and of the little finger (**hypothenar eminence**), and, between these, by the long tendons entering the hand from the forearm.

The hand proper has five metacarpal bones numbered 1 to 5, beginning from the thumb side. Proximally, the base of the metacarpal bones articulates with the distal row of carpal bones (carpometacarpal joints), and the second to fifth metacarpal bones also articulate with each other (intermetacarpal joints) [see Fig. 9.8A]. Distally, each metacarpal bone articulates with the proximal phalanx of the corresponding digit.

The **digits** are: the thumb or pollex, the forefinger or index, the middle finger or digitus medius, the ring finger or annularis, and the little finger or minimus. Each finger has three phalanges—the thumb has only two. The proximal phalanx of each finger articulates with the corresponding metacarpal head at the metacarpophalangeal joint. The phalanges articulate with one another at the proximal and distal interphalangeal joints.

CHAPTER 3
The pectoral region and axilla

Introduction

Muscles covering the front of the chest and holding the free upper limb to the torso, and their vessels and nerves constitute the **pectoral region**. The pyramidal space between the upper part of the thorax and the arm is the **axilla**.

Adjacency of the thorax, neck, and upper limb

The walls of the thorax form a conical structure which is flattened anteroposteriorly. It has an apex superiorly that is cut obliquely to form the **superior aperture of the thorax**. This is continuous above with the root of the neck and has, as its margins, the first thoracic vertebra, the first ribs, and the upper part of the sternum (manubrium). The upper limb is attached to the trunk by muscles and bones which spread out from the proximal part of the limb to the anterior and posterior surfaces of the thorax.

Overview of the axilla

The axilla is a four-sided pyramidal space between: (1) the upper limb; (2) the muscles connecting the upper limb to the front of the thorax; (3) the muscles connecting the upper limb to the back of the thorax; and (4) the lateral wall of the thorax. When the arm is by the side, the axilla is a narrow space. When the arm is abducted, the volume of the axilla increases, and its floor (base) rises, forming a definite 'armpit'. Also when the arm is abducted, the muscular inferior margin of its anterior wall stands out as the **anterior axillary fold**, and the inferior margin of the posterior wall stands out as the **posterior axillary fold** [Fig. 3.1].

The superior part of the axilla—the apex—lies lateral to the first rib and is continuous over its superior surface, with the superior aperture of the thorax below and the root of the neck above. This continuity permits blood vessels from the thorax and nerves from the neck to enter the axilla on their way to the upper limb. (These vessels and nerves pass over the superior surface of the first rib behind the clavicle [Fig. 3.2]).

Bones of the pectoral region and axilla

The clavicle extends laterally from its articulation with the sternum (sternoclavicular joint) to its articulation with the scapula (acromioclavicular joint) on the superior surface of the shoulder [Fig. 3.3].

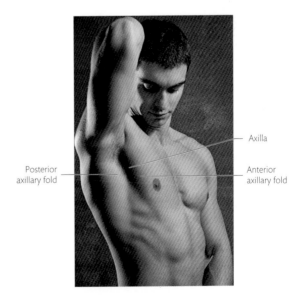

Fig. 3.1 A pyramidal-shaped hollow, the axilla, is clearly seen between the chest wall and the arm. The anterior and posterior axillary folds are seen bounding the floor of the axilla.

Copyright maxriesgo/Shutterstock.

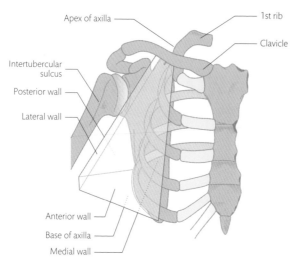

Apex of axilla
1st rib
Clavicle
Intertubercular sulcus
Posterior wall
Lateral wall
Anterior wall
Base of axilla
Medial wall

Fig. 3.2 Schematic drawing of the axilla, showing the base, apex, and four walls in relation to the bones of the thorax, pectoral girdle, and arm.

The sternoclavicular joint is the only articulation of an upper limb bone with a bone of the trunk. Thus, the clavicle acts as a support which transmits forces from the upper limb to the trunk and prevents the scapula, and hence the shoulder, from sagging downwards and medially under the weight of the limb. Sagging down of the upper limb is seen when the clavicle is fractured. The scapula lies posterior to the axilla and is almost entirely covered by muscles. Movements of the scapula are limited only by its articulation with the clavicle and, through it, with the sternoclavicular joint around which these movements are forced to take place. The scapula slides freely on the thoracic wall in the absence of bony articulations between it and the wall. The muscles of the scapula either attach the scapula to the humerus or hold it against the thorax.

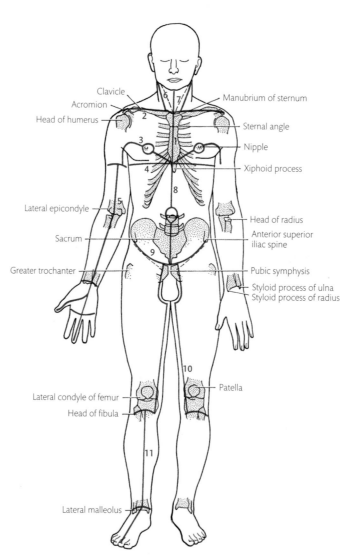

Clavicle
Acromion
Head of humerus
Manubrium of sternum
Sternal angle
Nipple
Xiphoid process
Lateral epicondyle
Head of radius
Sacrum
Anterior superior iliac spine
Greater trochanter
Pubic symphysis
Styloid process of ulna
Styloid process of radius
Patella
Lateral condyle of femur
Head of fibula
Lateral malleolus

Fig. 3.3 Landmarks and incisions. Left forearm pronated, right forearm supinated.

Surface anatomy of the pectoral region and axilla

All points mentioned in this section should be confirmed on the living body and on specimens of the bones.

The **clavicle** (collar bone) is palpable throughout its length. It follows a slight curve which is convex forwards in its medial two-thirds and concave forwards in its lateral one-third [Fig. 3.4]. Draw a finger along your clavicle, and note that its ends project above the acromion of the scapula laterally and the manubrium of the sternum medially. Thus, the positions of these joints are easily identified, though the medial end of the clavicle is somewhat obscured by the attachment of the sternocleidomastoid muscle.

Between the medial ends of the clavicles, feel the **jugular notch** on the superior margin of the manubrium [Fig. 3.5]. Draw a finger downwards from this notch in the median plane till a blunt transverse ridge is felt on the sternum. This bony landmark is the **sternal angle**, a joint between the manubrium and the body of the sternum. At this level, the **cartilage of the second rib** articulates with the side of the sternum. The

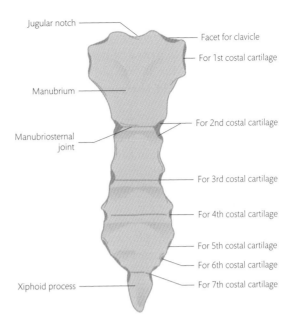

Fig. 3.5 Sternum (anterior view).

second rib may be identified in this way, even in obese subjects, for the sternal angle is always readily palpable. The other ribs are identified by counting down from the second rib. The anterior part of the first rib is hidden by the medial part of the

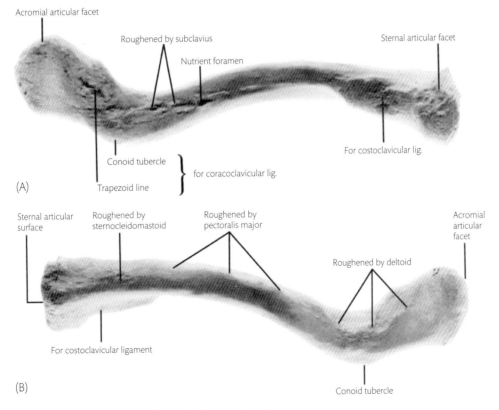

Fig. 3.4 (A) Right clavicle, inferior surface. (B) Right clavicle, superior surface.

clavicle. Immediately inferior to the lower end of the body of the sternum is a small median depression, the **epigastric fossa** which overlies the **xiphoid process**—the lowest piece of the sternum. The **cartilages of the seventh ribs** lie on either side of this fossa.

The **nipple** is very variable in position, even in the male, but usually lies over the fourth intercostal space, near the junction of the ribs with their cartilages. It is just medial to a vertical line passing through the middle of the clavicle (the **midclavicular line**).

The **infraclavicular fossa** is a depression inferior to the junction of the lateral and middle thirds of the clavicle. The pectoralis major muscle on the front of the chest lies medial to the fossa, and the deltoid muscle, which clasps the shoulder, is lateral to it. The **coracoid process** of the scapula can be felt just lateral to the fossa and under cover of the deltoid muscle, 2–3 cm below the clavicle.

Follow the clavicle laterally to its articulation with the **acromion**—a subcutaneous, flattened piece of the bone about 2.5 cm wide, on the top of the shoulder. The **acromioclavicular joint** can be felt as a slight dip, for the clavicle projects slightly above the level of the acromion (*acron* = summit; *omos* = shoulder).

Raise the arm from the side, i.e. abduct it, and identify the hollow of the **axilla**, the anterior axillary fold (containing the pectoralis major muscle), and the posterior axillary fold (containing the latissimus dorsi and teres major muscles) [Fig. 3.1]. The teres major is a thick, rounded muscle which connects the inferior angle of the scapula to the humerus and can be felt in the posterior axillary fold when the arm is raised above the head. The latissimus dorsi muscle extends from the lower part of the back to the humerus. It can be made to stand out by depressing the horizontal arm against resistance.

With the arm by the side, push your fingers into the axilla. The anterior and posterior walls are soft and fleshy, but the lateral margin of the scapula can be felt in the posterior wall. The medial wall is formed by the ribs covered by a sheet-like muscle—the serratus anterior. In the lateral angle, the biceps brachii and coracobrachialis muscles lie parallel to the humerus. Some of the large nerves in the axilla can be rolled between the fingers and the humerus, and the axillary artery can be felt pulsating. By pushing the fingers up into the axilla, the head

of the humerus can be felt laterally and the lateral border of the first rib medially.

Pectoral region

Cutaneous nerves

The skin on the anterior and lateral surfaces of the thorax is supplied by:

1. The supraclavicular nerves from the cervical plexus—principally the fourth cervical ventral ramus.
2. The anterior and lateral cutaneous branches of the ventral rami of the second to eleventh thoracic nerves (intercostal nerves) [Fig. 3.6].

The **supraclavicular nerves** [Fig. 3.7] arise in the neck from the third and fourth cervical nerves (C3, C4). Diverging as they descend, the nerves

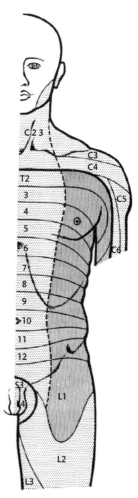

Fig. 3.6 Dermatomal pattern on the front of the trunk. The areas of skin supplied by ventral rami are illustrated.

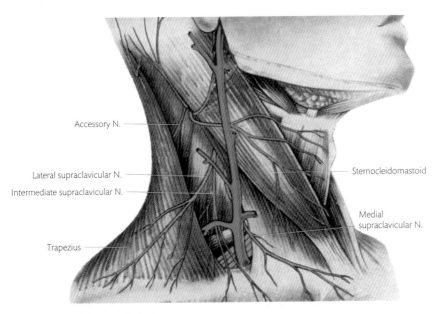

Fig. 3.7 Course and distribution of the supraclavicular nerves.

Accessory N.

Lateral supraclavicular N.

Intermediate supraclavicular N.

Trapezius

Sternocleidomastoid

Medial
supraclavicular N.

pierce the deep fascia in the neck. They cross the clavicle to supply the skin on the front of the chest and shoulder [see Figs. 5.8, 5.9] down to a horizontal line at the level of the second costal cartilage. They are named, according to their positions: medial, intermediate, and lateral.

The **anterior cutaneous branches of the intercostal nerves** (except the first and occasionally the second) emerge from the intercostal spaces near the lateral border of the sternum, pierce the pectoralis major, and supply the skin from the anterior median line almost to a vertical line through the middle of the clavicle (mid-clavicular line) [see the course of the ventral rami in Fig. 1.5]. They are accompanied by perforating branches of the internal thoracic artery, an artery which lies immediately deep to the costal cartilages. In the female, these arterial branches are enlarged in the second to fourth spaces to supply the mammary gland. The arteries have lymph vessels running with them from the skin of the anterior thoracic wall and the medial part of the mammary gland (breast) to **parasternal** nodes which lie beside the internal thoracic artery.

The **lateral cutaneous branches of the intercostal nerves** pierce the deep fascia along the mid-axillary line. Each nerve divides and enters the superficial fascia as anterior and posterior branches. The nerves pierce, or pass between, the digitations of the serratus anterior but play no part in supplying this muscle, the pectoral muscles, or the

latissimus dorsi over which they run. They supply the part of the skin between the parts supplied by the anterior cutaneous branches (midline in front to the mid-clavicular line) and the dorsal ramus (midline of the back to approximately 10 cm from the midline).

There are usually no lateral or anterior cutaneous branches from the first intercostal nerve. The lateral cutaneous branch of the second intercostal nerve is the **intercostobrachial nerve**. It emerges as a large single branch and communicates with the medial cutaneous nerve of the arm and the lateral cutaneous branch of the third intercostal nerve. Together, these three nerves supply the skin of the medial side of the arm and the floor of the axilla.

Dissection 3.1 describes how to reflect the skin of the front and side of chest.

The breast

The mamma or breast is made up of: (1) the mammary gland; (2) the fatty superficial fascia in which it is embedded; and (3) the overlying skin with the nipple and the surrounding pigmented skin—the **areola** [Fig. 3.8].

In the male, the mammary gland is rudimentary; the nipple is small, and the areola is commonly surrounded by fine hairs. In the non-lactating female, the breast consists mainly of the fatty tissue of the superficial fascia, in which are enclosed 15 to 20 lobes of rudimentary glandular tissue. These glands radiate outwards from the

DISSECTION 3.1 Skin reflection of the front and side of the chest

Objectives

I. To reflect the skin on the front and side of the chest. II. To examine the superficial fascia. III. To find the cutaneous vessels and nerves.

Instructions

1. Make the skin incisions 1–4, shown in Fig. 3.3. Make sure to carry incision 4 backwards as far as the posterior axillary fold.

2. Cut through the superficial fascia in incisions 1, 3, and 4.

3. Start from the midline (incision 1). Reflect the flaps of skin and the superficial fascia laterally by blunt dissection. Do not detach them. Leave the nipple and the surrounding skin in position as a landmark.

4. As the flap is separated from the skin of the neck along the clavicle, split the superficial fascia with a blunt instrument. Avoid cutting through the thin sheet

of muscle (platysma) and the supraclavicular nerves [Fig. 3.7]. The supraclavicular nerves pass anterior to the clavicle to supply the skin of the upper part of the anterior thoracic wall and the shoulder.

5. Identify the medial, intermediate, and lateral branches of the supraclavicular nerves.

6. Note the fibrous strands connecting the deep fascia to the skin, especially deep to the breast in the female.

7. Find the anterior cutaneous nerves and vessels which emerge from the anterior ends of the intercostal spaces. Follow the branches of one of these nerves medially and laterally as far as possible.

8. Find the lateral cutaneous branches which pierce the chest wall in the mid-axillary line. They emerge through the deep fascia, one inferior to the other, in a vertical line. Follow the branches of one of them anteriorly and posteriorly as far as possible.

---

nipple, giving the gland the shape of a flattened cone. Each lobe has a main **lactiferous duct** which passes to open separately on the nipple. At the base of the nipple, the duct is dilated to form a **lactiferous sinus**. The gland has no capsule, but its lobes are separated by fibrous strands of the superficial fascia which pass from the skin to the deep fascia. These fibrous strands are attached

to the gland and anchor it both to the skin and to the underlying deep fascia.

The base of the mammary gland extends from the margin of the sternum to almost the mid-axillary line, and from the second to sixth ribs. It lies largely on the pectoralis major muscle. Inferolaterally, it extends on to the costal origins of the serratus anterior and the external oblique muscle

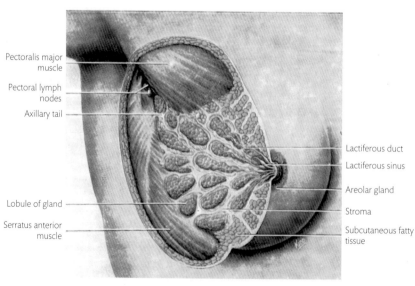

Pectoralis major muscle

Pectoral lymph nodes

Axillary tail

Lobule of gland

Serratus anterior muscle

Lactiferous duct

Lactiferous sinus

Areolar gland

Stroma

Subcutaneous fatty tissue

Fig. 3.8 Dissection of the right mammary gland.

of the abdomen. The '**axillary tail**' arises from the superolateral quadrant of the breast and passes into the axilla, up to the level of the third rib [Fig. 3.8]. The apex of the gland—the **nipple**—lies a little below the midpoint of the gland, approximately at the fourth intercostal space in the nulliparous woman. The nipple is free of fat but contains circular and longitudinal smooth muscle fibres which can erect or flatten it. The skin of the nipple and areola contains modified sweat and sebaceous glands, particularly at the outer margin of the areola. These sebaceous glands tend to enlarge in the early stages of pregnancy, and shortly thereafter there is an increase in pigmentation in both the nipple and areola which never return to their original colour. In the later stages of pregnancy, the greater part of the fat in the gland is replaced by the proliferation of its ducts and the growth of many secretory alveoli from their branching ends.

The gland receives its **blood supply** from perforating branches of the intercostal and internal thoracic arteries medially and from the lateral thoracic artery laterally.

Lymph vessels drain principally: (a) to the axillary lymph nodes—(i) along the axillary tail to the **pectoral lymph nodes**, and (ii) through the pectoralis major and clavipectoral fascia to the **apical axillary nodes** via the **infraclavicular nodes**; (b) to the **parasternal nodes** along the internal thoracic artery by passing along the branches of that artery which supply the gland; and (c) some lymph also drains to the posterior intercostal nodes. Since there is communication of lymph vessels across the median plane, there may be drainage to the opposite side, especially when some of the pathways are blocked by disease [Fig. 3.9].

Dissection 3.2 describes the dissection of the breast.

This is not usually very successful in the elderly female and should not be attempted in the male.

Deep fascia

The deep fascia covering the pectoralis major is continuous with the periosteum of the clavicle and sternum, and passes over the infraclavicular fossa and deltopectoral groove (between the pectoralis major and the deltoid) to become continuous with the fascia covering the deltoid. It curves over the inferolateral border of the pectoralis

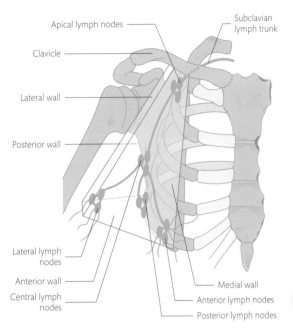

Fig. 3.9 Lymph nodes and lymph vessels of the axilla.

major to become continuous with the fascia of the axillary floor (**axillary fascia**). The axillary fascia stretches between the pectoralis major and the latissimus dorsi. When the arm is abducted, the axillary fascia rises into the axilla to form the armpit.

The **clavipectoral fascia** lies in the anterior wall of the axilla, deep to the pectoralis major. It extends from the clavicle to the axillary fascia and encloses the pectoralis minor and subclavius muscles [Fig. 3.10].

See Dissection 3.3 for instructions on dissecting the pectoral region.

DISSECTION 3.2 The breast

Objective

I. To identify the lactiferous ducts and lobes of the mammary gland.

Instructions

1. Attempt to pass a bristle through one of the ducts of the nipple.

2. Attempt to identify one of the lobes of the gland by blunt dissection.

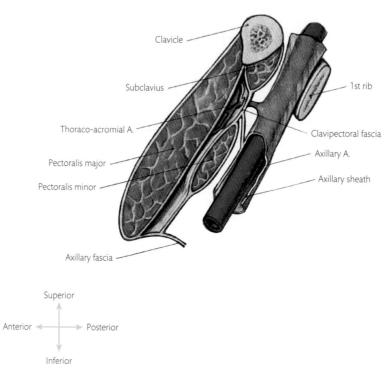

Fig. 3.10 Diagram of the clavipectoral fascia shown enclosing the subclavius and pectoralis minor and extending to the axillary fascia.

DISSECTION 3.3 Pectoral region-1

Objectives

I. To study the pectoralis major and the deltoid.   II. To identify the cephalic vein.

Instructions

1. Cut the deep fascia in the deltopectoral groove to uncover the cephalic vein passing to the infraclavicular fossa [see Fig. 3.12].

2. Occasional lymph nodes found beside the vein receive lymph from the adjacent superficial tissues and transmit it through the infraclavicular fossa to the apical nodes of the axilla [Fig. 3.9].

3. Remove the fascia from the anterior parts of the pectoralis major and the deltoid, and define the attachments of these muscles.

Pectoralis major

This powerful, fan-shaped muscle takes origin from the medial half of the front of the clavicle, the anterior surfaces of the sternum and upper six costal cartilages, and the aponeurosis of the external oblique muscle of the abdomen [Fig. 3.11]. It is inserted into the lateral lip of the intertubercular sulcus or crest on the humerus [see Fig. 5.1A]. At the insertion, the abdominal part twists under the sternocostal part to form a U-shaped tendon with it. The lowest abdominal fibres are inserted deep to the upper sternocostal fibres, while the intermediate fibres form the base of the U in the anterior axillary fold.

The clavicular part passes inferolaterally, fuses with the anterior layer of the U-shaped tendon, and extends further inferiorly on the humerus. The clavicular part lies at right angles to the abdominal and lower sternocostal parts and has different actions [Fig. 3.11].

Nerve supply: medial and lateral pectoral nerves. **Actions**: the pectoralis major adducts and medially rotates the humerus. With the arm above the head, the lowest fibres act with the latissimus dorsi to pull down the arm or raise the body, as in climbing a rope. The muscle can also return the extended humerus to the anatomical position, then continue to flex the shoulder joint with its clavicular part which passes in front of the shoulder.

Pectoralis minor

This triangular muscle originates from the third to fifth ribs, near their cartilages, and passes superolaterally to the tip of the coracoid process [Fig. 3.11].

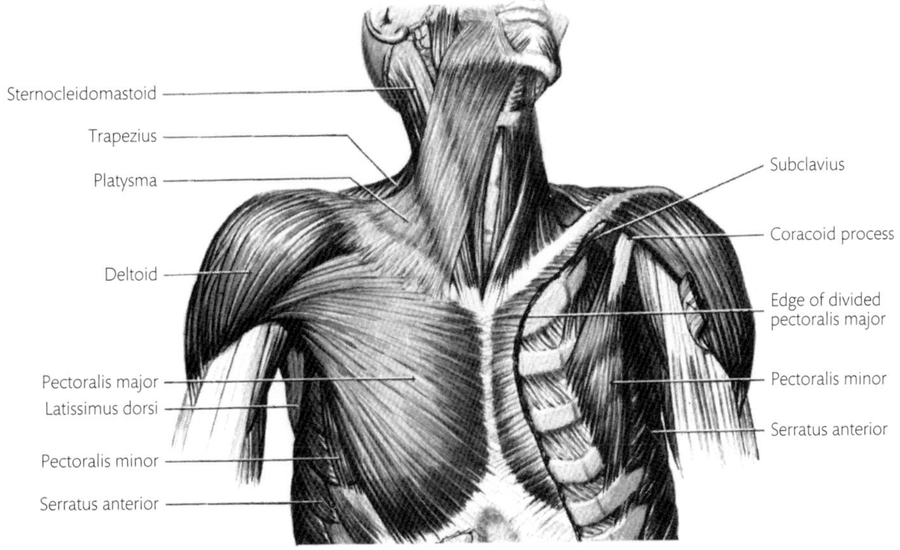
Sternocleidomastoid
Trapezius
Platysma
Deltoid
Pectoralis major
Latissimus dorsi
Pectoralis minor
Serratus anterior
Subclavius
Coracoid process
Edge of divided pectoralis major
Pectoralis minor
Serratus anterior

Fig. 3.11 Muscles of the anterior wall of the trunk. On the left side, the pectoralis major is removed to show the pectoralis minor and subclavius.

Nerve supply: medial pectoral nerve. **Actions**: it pulls the scapula (and hence the shoulder) downwards and forwards. It raises the ribs in inspiration when the scapula is fixed.

Dissection 3.4 continues the dissection of the pectoral region.

Subclavius

This small muscle arises from the adjacent parts of the upper surfaces of the first costal cartilage and rib. It passes parallel to the clavicle and is inserted into the groove on the inferior surface of the

DISSECTION 3.4 Pectoral region-2

Objectives

I. To study the pectoralis minor, subclavius, and clavipectoral fascia. II. To identify and trace the cephalic vein, thoraco-acromial artery, and medial and lateral pectoral nerves. III. To explore the continuity of the axillary vessels with the subclavian vessels.

Instructions

1. Cut across the clavicular head of the pectoralis major below the clavicle, and reflect it towards its insertion. Identify the branches of the lateral pectoral nerve and thoraco-acromial artery that pierce the clavipectoral fascia to enter the pectoralis major.
2. Cut across the remainder of the pectoralis major about 5 cm from the sternum. Reflect it laterally. Identify the branch of the medial pectoral nerve which pierces the pectoralis minor to enter the pectoralis major.
3. Note the entire sheet of the clavipectoral fascia deep to the pectoralis major, and then remove it from the pectoralis minor.
4. Trace the pectoralis minor to its attachments.
5. Follow the cephalic vein through the upper part of the clavipectoral fascia to the axillary vein, and the thoraco-acromial artery and the lateral pectoral nerve to their origins.
6. Expose the vessels and nerves superior to the pectoralis minor.
7. Cut through the anterior layer of the clavipectoral fascia immediately inferior to, and parallel with, the clavicle to expose the subclavius muscle.
8. Gently push a finger, inferior to that muscle, along the line of the axillary vessels. It will pass over the first rib, deep to the clavicle, into the root of the neck. If the finger is pressed medially between the axillary artery and vein, the firm resistance of the scalenus anterior muscle can be felt on the upper surface of the first rib between the artery and vein. (Note that the vessels felt on the first rib are the subclavian vessels.)
9. Pass a finger deep to the pectoralis minor through the lower part of the axilla. Lift it from the subjacent structures, but preserve the medial pectoral nerve which enters its deep surface.

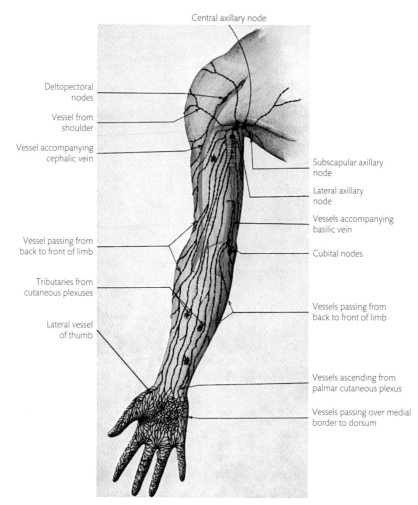

Fig. 3.12 Superficial lymph vessels and lymph nodes of the front of the upper limb.

clavicle [Figs. 3.10, 3.13]. **Nerve supply**: nerve to subclavius from the upper trunk of the brachial plexus. **Actions**: it holds the medial end of the clavicle against the articular disc of the sternoclavicular joint during movements of the shoulder girdle.

Sternoclavicular joint

The sternoclavicular joint is a synovial joint between the shallow notch at the superolateral angle of the manubrium of the sternum and the larger medial end of the clavicle. A complete articular disc intervenes

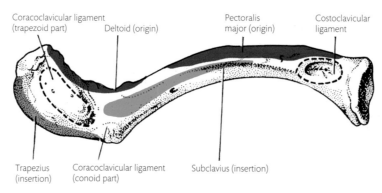

Fig. 3.13 Muscle attachments of the inferior surface of the right clavicle.

between these two articular surfaces. The joint also extends on to the superior surface of the first costal cartilage. This is the only articulation of the upper limb bones with the axial skeleton. Thus, the clavicle forms a support which maintains the scapula in position and transmits forces from the upper limb to the trunk, e.g. forces generated in falling on the outstretched hand. Functionally, the joint behaves like a ball-and-socket joint with a wide range of movements, since it has to move with each change in scapular position. It is subject to considerable force, but the bony surfaces give little intrinsic stability. For this reason, it is strengthened by powerful ligaments which are designed to prevent dislocation of the medial end of the clavicle from the shallow fossa on the sternum. The **articular capsule** is attached close to the articular margins of the bones. It is thickened anteriorly and posteriorly to form the anterior and posterior **sternoclavicular ligaments** [Fig. 3.14].

The **articular disc** is a nearly circular plate of fibrocartilage attached at its margins to the articular capsule. It divides the joint into two separate synovial cavities. Its strongest attachments are to the upper surface of the medial end of the clavicle and to the junction of the sternum and first costal cartilage. It assists the costoclavicular ligament in preventing the upward displacement of the medial end of the clavicle and acts as a shock absorber of compression forces applied from the upper limb.

DISSECTION 3.5 Sternoclavicular joint

Objectives

I. To examine the ligaments of the sternoclavicular joint.   II. To examine the articular disc of the sternoclavicular joint.

Instructions

1. Separate the subclavius from its costal attachment, and turn it laterally to expose the strong costoclavicular ligament.

2. Expose the anterior and superior surfaces of the articular capsule of the sternoclavicular joint as far as possible. Remove the anterior part of the articular capsule, and identify the articular disc between the clavicle and the sternum, but leave the clavicle in position.

The **costoclavicular ligament** is a powerful band which passes upwards and laterally from the junction of the first rib and its cartilage to a rough area on the inferior surface of the clavicle near its medial end. The **interclavicular ligament** passes between the medial ends of the two clavicles and is fused with the articular capsules and the jugular notch of the sternum [Fig. 3.14].

Dissection 3.5 explains the dissection of the sternoclavicular joint.

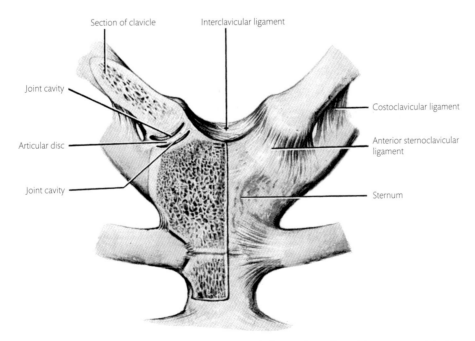

Fig. 3.14 Sternoclavicular joint. A coronal section has been made through the anterior surface of the sternum and clavicle on the right side, opening the right sternoclavicular joint.

Axilla

Boundaries and contents

Start by reviewing the overview of the axilla on page 25 and Fig. 3.2. The anterior wall of the axilla extends from the clavicle to the **anterior axillary fold**. It consists of the pectoralis major, the pectoralis minor, the subclavius, and the fascia enclosing them [Fig. 3.11]. The posterior wall consists of the lateral part of the costal surface of the scapula, covered by the subscapularis superiorly, and the teres major muscle with the latissimus dorsi winding round its lower border inferiorly. Identify these muscles, using Fig. 3.15. The **anterior** and **posterior axillary folds** are formed by the lower borders of the pectoralis major and the latissimus dorsi,

respectively. The convex medial wall is formed by the lateral wall of the thorax (the first five ribs and intercostal spaces) covered by the serratus anterior. The narrow lateral boundary is formed by the humerus covered by the upper parts of the biceps and coracobrachialis muscles.

The **apex** of the axilla is bounded by the clavicle, first rib, and upper border of the scapula. It is continuous medially with the superior aperture of the thorax and the root of the neck. Through the apex, vessels from the thorax and the nerves of the brachial plexus from the neck enter the axilla [Fig. 3.2]. These vessels and nerves descend through the axilla to the arm and form the contents of the axilla, together with the axillary lymph nodes and loose fatty tissue.

See Dissection 3.6 which begins the dissection of the axilla.

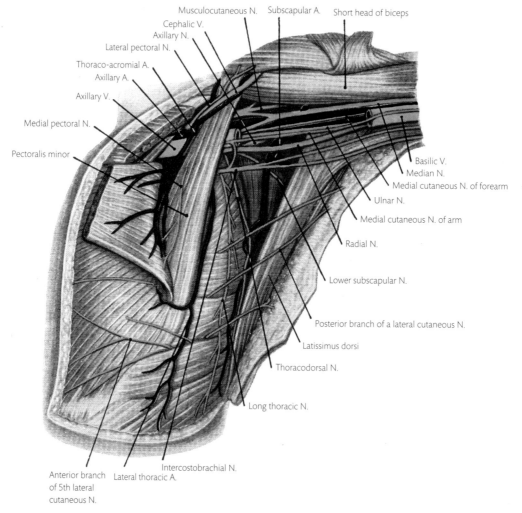

Fig. 3.15 Contents of the axilla exposed by reflection of the pectoralis major and removal of fat, the fascia, and lymph nodes. Part of the axillary vein has been removed to display the medial cutaneous nerve of the forearm and the ulnar nerve.

Objectives

I. To remove the loose connective tissue and fat of the axilla.
II. To remove the fascia overlying the lateral wall of the axilla.   III. To identify and trace the axillary artery, axillary vein, musculocutaneous nerve, median nerve, ulnar nerve, medial cutaneous nerve of the arm and forearm, intercostobrachial nerve, lateral cutaneous branches of upper intercostal nerves, lateral thoracic artery, and long thoracic nerve.

Instructions

1. Remove the loose connective tissue, fat, and lymph nodes in the axilla to expose its contents. Only a few of the large number of lymph nodes will be seen, unless they are enlarged by disease, so it is not worth trying to dissect them, though they will be felt as slightly firmer structures among the fat. Lymph vessels will not be seen.

2. Expose the coracobrachialis and short head of the biceps muscles which arise from the tip of the coracoid process.

3. Find the **axillary artery** and the **median nerve** medial to these muscles and the **musculocutaneous nerve** entering the deep surface of the coracobrachialis. Follow this nerve upwards, and find its branch to the muscle.

4. Identify the **axillary vein** medial to the axillary artery.

5. Between the axillary artery and vein, identify the **medial cutaneous nerve of the forearm** and more posteriorly the larger **ulnar nerve**.

6. Find the **medial cutaneous nerve of the arm** medial to the vein. Trace it superiorly. A branch from the **intercostobrachial nerve** usually joins it. Follow this branch upwards to the emergence of the intercostobrachial nerve from the second intercostal space in the medial axillary wall. Trace that nerve down to the axillary floor and the medial side of the arm.

7. Note again the series of lateral cutaneous branches of the third, fourth, fifth, and sixth intercostal nerves, as they emerge in a vertical line inferior to the point of emergence of the intercostobrachial nerve. Note that the nerves emerge posterior to the pectoralis major and between the digitations (attachments) of the serratus anterior on each rib.

8. Find the lateral thoracic artery and the long thoracic nerve descending on the lateral surface of the serratus anterior muscle which they supply [Fig. 3.15].

Serratus anterior

The serratus anterior arises from the outer surface of the upper eight ribs. Its fibres pass posteriorly around the lateral surface of the chest wall forming the medial wall of the axilla. On the back, the fibres run deep to the scapula and are inserted into the costal surface of the scapula along the medial border. **Nerve supply**: long thoracic nerve [Figs. 3.15, 3.16, 3.17]. **Actions**: it holds the scapula against the ribs and protracts the scapula. The lower fibres are powerful lateral rotators of the scapula.

Axillary artery

This is the main artery of the upper limb. It is a continuation of the subclavian artery at the outer border of the first rib. It passes through the apex and lateral part of the axilla to become the brachial artery at the lower border of the teres major, close to the humerus. For the purpose of description, it is divided into three parts which lie superior, posterior, and inferior to the pectoralis minor. The cords of the brachial plexus lie posterior to the first part and are arranged around the second part according

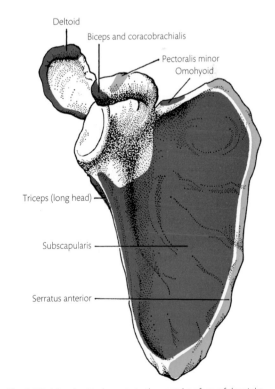

Fig. 3.16 Muscle attachments to the costal surface of the right scapula.

Labels in figure:
Deltoid
Biceps and coracobrachialis
Pectoralis minor
Omohyoid
Triceps (long head)
Subscapularis
Serratus anterior

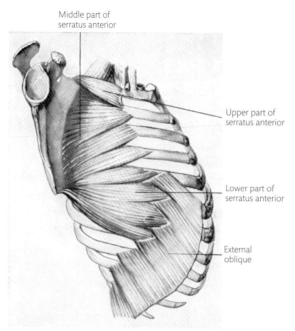

Fig. 3.17 Serratus anterior. The scapula is drawn away from the side of the chest to show the insertion into the scapula.

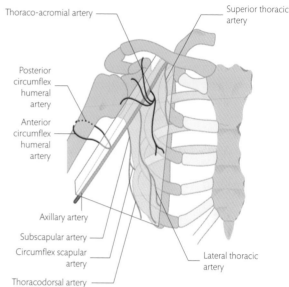

Fig. 3.18 Diagrammatic representation of the axillary artery and its branches.

to their names. The main nerves arising from the cords surround the third part.

The axillary artery supplies the structures in, and surrounding the axilla [Fig. 3.18]: (a) the **thoraco-acromial artery** arises from the second part of the axillary artery and supplies the anterior axillary wall of the axilla, including the clavicle, acromion, and anterior part of the deltoid; (b) the **superior** and **lateral thoracic arteries** supply the medial axillary wall and the lateral part of the mammary gland and surrounding structures; (c) the **subscapular artery** supplies the posterior axillary wall, including the scapula and muscles covering its posterior aspect; it gives off two branches—**circumflex scapular** and **thoraco-dorsal** arteries—which anastomose with branches from the subclavian artery; and (d) the **anterior** and **posterior circumflex humeral arteries** supply the proximal part of the humerus, the muscles covering it, and the shoulder joint.

Axillary vein

The axillary vein lies on the anteromedial aspect of the axillary artery and has the same extent. It is the continuation of the **basilic vein** and receives tributaries corresponding to the branches of the axillary artery. In addition, the axillary vein also receives the venae comitans of the brachial artery

inferiorly, and the cephalic vein superiorly. It continues as the subclavian vein at the outer border of the first rib [Fig. 3.15].

Dissection 3.7 continues the dissection of the axilla.

Axillary lymph nodes

These lymph nodes drain the lymph vessels of the upper limb and the superficial vessels of the trunk above the level of the umbilicus and iliac crest. The nodes are scattered throughout the fascia of the axilla and, for the most part, transfer lymph towards the nodes at its apex (**apical nodes**). For descriptive purposes, the axillary lymph nodes are divided into five groups, four of which lie in one angle of the axillary pyramid and drain a specific territory. The **lateral nodes** lie along the axillary vessels and drain the greater part of the upper limb. The **pectoral** or **anterior group** lies in the anteromedial angle, deep to the pectoralis major, and drains the superficial tissues of the anterior and lateral parts of the thoracic and upper abdominal walls. The **subscapular** or **posterior group** lies along the subscapular vessels and drains lymph from the corresponding region on the back. All these nodes communicate with the more centrally placed **central nodes**. The efferents of all these nodes pass to the apical group [Fig. 3.9], which also receives vessels from nodes on the cephalic vein and in the infraclavicular fossa. The efferents of the

Objectives

I. To clean the connective tissue and fascia over the axillary artery, ulnar nerve, radial nerve and its branches, axillary nerve, and subscapular artery and its branches. II. To examine the relationship of the cords of the brachial plexus to the axillary artery. III. To remove the fascia and define the posterior wall of the axilla.

Instructions

1. Expose the axillary artery and vein, and the large nerves surrounding them. If necessary, remove the smaller tributaries of the vein, in order to get a clear view of the nerves. (Since the veins follow the branches of the artery, their loss is of little significance.)

2. Identify and follow the **ulnar nerve**. It lies behind and between the axillary artery and vein.

3. Find the **median nerve** lateral to the axillary artery. Follow its lateral root to the lateral cord of the brachial plexus, and its medial root to the medial cord of the brachial plexus.

4. Identify the **radial nerve** which lies behind the artery. Trace the radial nerve proximally and distally to the lower border of the subscapularis.

5. Find the **axillary nerve** which passes posteriorly along with the posterior humeral circumflex artery.

6. Find the posterior cutaneous nerve of the arm.

7. Find muscular branches of the radial nerve to the long and medial heads of the triceps muscle.

8. Find the **subscapular artery** as it arises from the axillary artery close to the axillary nerve. Trace it and its major branches—the circumflex scapular and thoracodorsal arteries. The thoracodorsal artery runs along the chest wall parallel to the margin of the latissimus dorsi, together with the thoracodorsal nerve to that muscle. (You will study the latissimus dorsi in further detail later.) The **circumflex scapular artery** lies close to the nerve (lower subscapular nerve) entering the teres major.

9. Cut across the pectoralis minor, and follow the axillary vessels to the outer border of the first rib. Note that the medial, lateral, and posterior **cords of the brachial plexus** lie around the artery posterior to the pectoralis minor. Above the level of the pectoralis minor, all three cords of the brachial plexus lie posterior to the artery.

10. Expose the anterior surface of the subscapularis, and identify the **upper subscapular nerve(s)** entering it. Follow the **upper** and **lower subscapular** and **thoracodorsal nerves** to their origin from the posterior cord of the brachial plexus [Fig. 3.15].

apical nodes form the **subclavian lymph trunk** which usually drains into the subclavian vein.

Brachial plexus

The brachial plexus is an important nerve plexus that supplies sensory and motor innervation to the upper limb. The plexus begins in the lower part of the neck **(supraclavicular part**: roots and trunks) and passes as divisions behind the middle third of the clavicle into the apex of the axilla [Figs. 3.19, 3.20. 3.21].

Roots of the brachial plexus

The **roots** of the brachial plexus are formed by the ventral rami of the lower four cervical nerves, the greater part of the ventral ramus of the first thoracic nerve (C5 to T1). Small twigs from the ventral rami of the fourth cervical and second thoracic nerves may join the plexus.

Trunks and divisions of the brachial plexus

Three trunks—the superior, middle, and inferior trunks—arise from the roots. The ventral rami of the fifth and sixth cervical nerves unite to form the **superior trunk** [Fig. 3.21]. The seventh cervical ventral ramus continues as the **middle trunk**. The eighth cervical and first thoracic ventral rami unite to form the **inferior trunk**. A short distance above the clavicle, each of these trunks splits into an anterior and posterior division.

Cords of the brachial plexus

The three **posterior divisions** unite to form the **posterior cord** of the plexus. The posterior cord supplies the extensor muscles and the skin on the back of the limb. The three **anterior divisions** supply the flexor muscles and the skin on the front

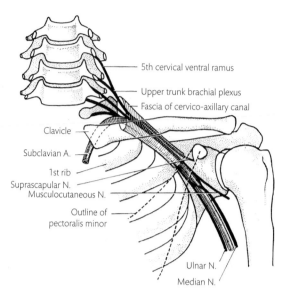

Fig. 3.19 Diagram showing the route of entry of the nerves and subclavian artery into the upper limb. The fascial sheath which binds these structures into a narrow bundle is the axillary sheath.

40

of the limb. The anterior divisions of the upper and middle trunks unite to form the **lateral cord** of the plexus, and the anterior division of the lower trunk forms the **medial cord**.

In the axilla (**infraclavicular part**), the cords first lie posterior to the first part of the axillary artery, but lower down posterior to the pectoralis minor, they surround the second part of the axillary artery in positions which correspond to their names. The plexus ends at the lower border of the pectoralis minor by dividing into a number of branches.

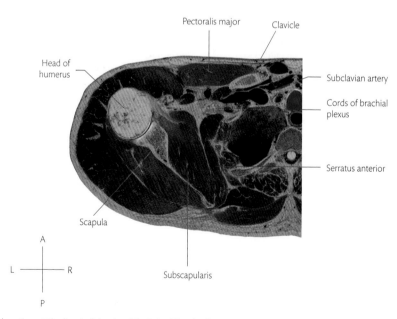

Fig. 3.20 Horizontal section at the level of the shoulder joint. The chief structures in the axilla and its walls are shown. A = anterior; P = posterior; L = left; R = right.

Image courtesy of the Visible Human Project of the US National Library of Medicine.

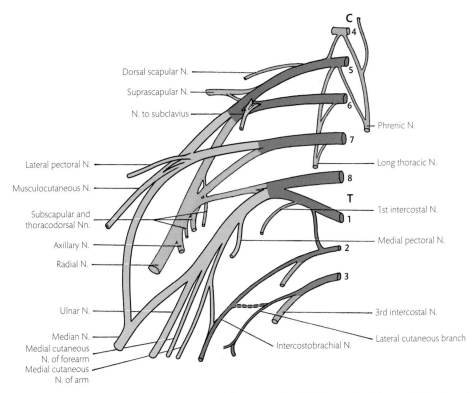

Fig. 3.21 Diagram of the right brachial plexus. Ventral divisions, light orange; dorsal divisions, yellow. C = cervical; T = thoracic.

The plexus is so arranged that each cord and the nerves which arise from it contain nerve fibres from more than one spinal (segmental) nerve. Thus, the lateral cord contains nerve fibres from the cervical (C.) nerves 5 to 7 [Fig. 3.21], the medial cord from C. 8 and thoracic (T.) 1 (and 2), and the posterior cord from C. 5 to C. 8 (and T. 1). A knowledge of these 'segmental values', or root values, is of importance in the diagnosis of injuries to the spinal nerves or to the spinal cord from which they arise.

Branches of the brachial plexus

Branches arising in the neck but distributed to the upper limb

The **dorsal scapular nerve** (C. 5) supplies the rhomboid major and minor and levator scapulae. It will be seen later on the deep surface of the rhomboid muscles.

The **suprascapular nerve** (C. 5, 6) supplies the supraspinatus and infraspinatus muscles. It runs inferolaterally behind the clavicle and crosses the superior border of the scapula to its posterior surface [Fig. 3.22].

The **nerve to subclavius** (C. 5, 6) descends in front of the plexus to supply the subclavius.

The **long thoracic nerve** (C. 5, 6, 7) arises from the posterior aspect of these ventral rami. It descends behind the brachial plexus and axillary artery and then on the lateral surface of the serratus anterior muscle which it supplies.

Branches arising in the axilla

The **lateral** and **medial pectoral nerves** pass forward from the corresponding cords of the brachial plexus. They communicate in front of the axillary artery and pass to supply the pectoral muscles in the anterior axillary wall. The lateral pectoral nerve (C. 5, 6, 7) pierces the clavipectoral fascia to enter the deep surface of the pectoralis major superior to the pectoralis minor. The medial pectoral nerve (C. 8, T. 1) supplies and pierces the pectoralis minor to enter the pectoralis major.

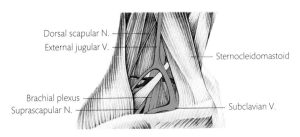

Fig. 3.22 Dissection of the lower part of the posterior triangle of the neck showing the supraclavicular part of the brachial plexus.

The **upper** and **lower subscapular nerves** (C. 5, 6) arise from the posterior cord of the brachial plexus with the thoracodorsal nerve. They supply the muscles of the posterior axillary wall. The upper supplies the subscapularis muscle; the lower supplies the lower fibres of the subscapularis and teres major.

The **thoracodorsal nerve** (C. 6, 7) passes posteroinferiorly to supply the latissimus dorsi muscle. It runs with the thoracodorsal artery on the deep surface of the muscle.

The **axillary nerve** (C. 5, 6) is a terminal branch of the posterior cord of the brachial plexus and is formed near the lower border of the subscapularis. It leaves the axilla by passing back inferior to the subscapularis.

The **musculocutaneous nerve** (C. 5, 6) arises in the axilla from the lateral cord of the brachial plexus and passes inferolaterally to supply, and then pierce, the coracobrachialis.

The **median nerve** (C. 5, 6, 7, 8; T. 1) is formed lateral to the axillary artery by one root each from the medial and lateral cords of the brachial plexus. It crosses anterior to the axillary artery and comes to lie on its medial side.

The **ulnar nerve** (C. 8; T. 1) arises from the medial cord of the brachial plexus and runs down between the axillary artery and vein.

The **radial nerve** (C. 5, 6, 7, 8; occasionally T. 1) is the other terminal branch of the posterior cord of the brachial plexus in the axilla. In the axilla, it gives off the **nerve to the long head of the triceps**—a muscle of the arm.

See Clinical Applications 3.1 and 3.2.

CLINICAL APPLICATION 3.1 Breast cancer

The following observations were made during breast examination of a 36-year-old woman with breast cancer. The right breast was firmly adherent to the underlying tissue.

Study question 1: name the tissue which lies immediately deep to the breast. What does this immobility/tethering of the breast tell you about the disease process? (Answer: deep fascia, pectoralis major, and serratus anterior. The breast being fixed to the underlying tissue means that the cancer has invaded the underlying muscle.) The skin over the upper lateral quadrant of the breast is thick and pitted, resulting in an orange-peel appearance. This appearance is caused by two factors: (a) blockage of lymph vessels by cancer cells, resulting in lymphoedema;

and (b) the fact that the subcutaneous tissue is prevented from swelling uniformly by the shortened suspensory ligaments which are also invaded by disease.

Study question 2: to what structures are the suspensory ligaments attached? (Answer: the suspensory ligaments run from the glands to the underlying deep fascia and to the overlying skin.)

Study question 3: on examination of the axilla, hard and 3 cm-sized masses were felt immediately deep to the anterior axillary fold. What are these masses likely to be, and how are they related to the disease process? (Answer: the masses are most likely enlarged anterior axillary lymph nodes, to which the cancer cells from the breast have spread.)

CLINICAL APPLICATION 3.2 Axillary lymph node dissection

Axillary lymph node dissection is a surgical procedure that is used for staging breast cancer. The surgeon explores the axilla to identify, examine, and remove lymph nodes. Axillary lymph node status on whether or not they are invaded by cancer cells, and to what extent they are involved, gives valuable information for planning treatment. Lymph drainage of the upper limb may be impeded after removal of the axillary nodes.

Study question 1: why is it common for patients who have undergone this procedure to have swelling of the upper limb? What name is given to swelling due to this cause? (Answer: the upper limb drains into the axillary

lymph nodes, which have been removed during surgery. As such, the lymph collects in the limb tissue. Such swelling is called 'lymphoedema'.) The long thoracic nerve and the thoracodorsal nerve have a long course in the axilla and may become infiltrated by cancer cells. These nerves may also be damaged during the surgery. The thoracodorsal nerve lies on the posterior wall of the axilla and enters the latissimus dorsi near its medial border. The axillary tail of the breast lies close to it.

Study question 2: what would be the result of damage to the thoracodorsal nerve? (Answer: weakened medial rotation and adduction of the arm.)

CHAPTER 4
The back

Turn the body face downwards, and examine the structures which connect the upper limb to the back of the trunk.

Surface anatomy of the back

Begin by reviewing the structure of the scapula [Figs. 4.1, 4.2, 4.3].

The **scapula** is placed against the posterolateral wall of the thorax. It lies over the second to seventh ribs and extends into the posterior wall of the axilla. It is thickly covered with muscles, but most of its outline can be felt in the living subject. Find the acromion at the top of the shoulder. Draw your finger along the bony ridge (crest of the spine of the scapula) which runs medially and slightly downwards from the acromion to the medial border of the scapula [Fig. 4.2]. Trace the medial border to the inferior angle and, if possible, to the superior angle, palpating it through the muscles that cover it. The scapula is held in position by muscles and the clavicle. It is very mobile—the scapulae move apart when the arms are folded across the chest. When the shoulders are drawn back, the medial borders of the scapulae are brought close to each other and the posterior median line.

The rib felt immediately inferior to the inferior angle of the scapula is usually the **eighth rib**, and the lower ribs may be counted from it. The twelfth rib is not palpable, unless it projects beyond the lateral margin of the back muscle—the erector spinae [Fig. 4.1].

The **iliac crest** is the curved bony ridge felt below the waist. Trace it forwards to the **anterior superior iliac spine** and backwards to the **posterior superior iliac spine**. The posterior superior iliac spine is felt in a shallow dimple in the skin above the buttock and about 5 cm from the median plane. Between the left and right dimples is the back of the **sacrum**. Usually three sacral spines can be palpated in the median plane. The **coccyx** is the slightly mobile bone felt deep between the buttocks in the median plane.

Feel the tips of the **spines of the vertebrae** in the median furrow of the back. These are the only parts of the vertebral column which are easily felt. It is difficult to identify individual spines directly, but the seventh cervical spine (**vertebra prominens**) is the uppermost spine which can be readily felt at the root of your neck. Below this, the approximate levels of other spines are as described in Table 4.1.

Above the vertebra prominens, only the **second cervical spine** can be felt easily. It is about 5 cm below the **external occipital protuberance** which is on the lower part of the back of the head where the median furrow of the neck (**nuchal groove**) meets the skull. The short cervical spines (compare with C7) are separated from the skin by a median fibrous partition—the **ligamentum nuchae**. The posterior edge of the ligamentum nuchae stretches from the external occipital protuberance to the seventh cervical spine.

The **superior nuchal line** is a curved ridge on the occipital bone of the skull, extending laterally

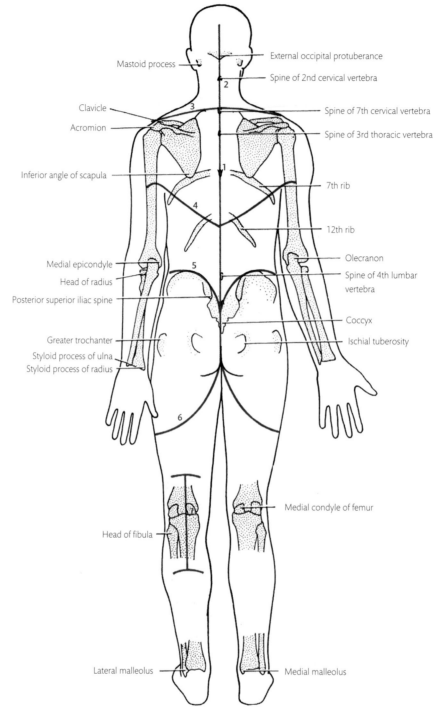

Mastoid process

External occipital protuberance

Spine of 2nd cervical vertebra

2

Clavicle

3

Spine of 7th cervical vertebra

Acromion

Spine of 3rd thoracic vertebra

Inferior angle of scapula

1

7th rib

4

12th rib

Medial epicondyle

Olecranon

5

Head of radius

Spine of 4th lumbar vertebra

Posterior superior iliac spine

Coccyx

Greater trochanter

Ischial tuberosity

Styloid process of ulna
Styloid process of radius

6

Medial condyle of femur

Head of fibula

Lateral malleolus

Medial malleolus

Fig. 4.1 Landmarks and incisions. Left forearm pronated, right forearm supinated.

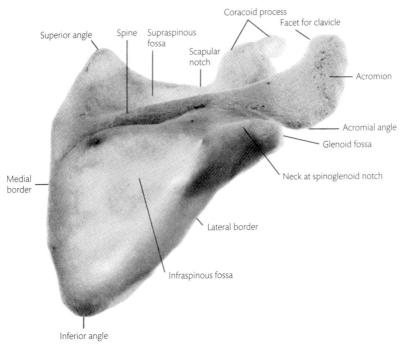

Fig. 4.2 Dorsal surface of the right scapula.

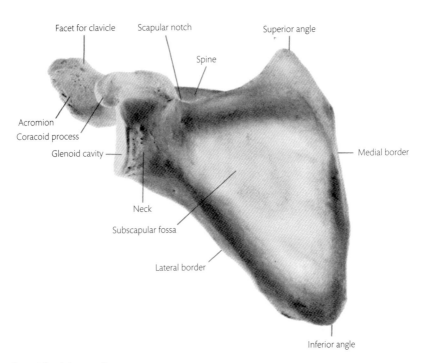

Fig. 4.3 Ventral surface of the right scapula.

Table 4.1 Vertebral levels for bony surface landmarks

Vertebral spine	Level
Third thoracic	Junction of the scapular spine and medial border
Seventh thoracic	Inferior angle of the scapula
Fourth lumbar	Highest point of the iliac crest
Second sacral	Posterior superior iliac spine

from a midline bony elevation—the external occipital protuberance.

See Dissection 4.1 for instructions on skin reflection and cutaneous nerves of the back.

DISSECTION 4.1 Skin reflection of the back

Objectives

I. To reflect the skin of the back.   II. To identify the cutaneous nerves of the back.

Instructions

1. Make the skin incisions 1, 3, 4, and 5 [Fig. 4.1].

2. Reflect the two skin flaps laterally, stripping the skin and the superficial fascia from the deep fascia by blunt dissection.

3. Find the cutaneous nerves as they pierce the deep fascia [Fig. 4.4]. This is more difficult than on the flexor surface, because of the denser connections of the superficial fascia to the deep fascia on the back.

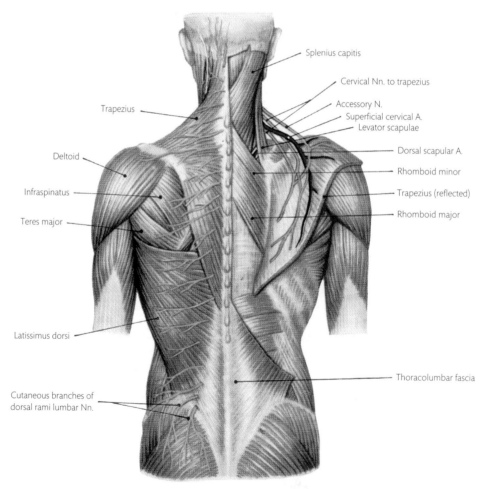

Splenius capitis
Cervical Nn. to trapezius
Accessory N.
Superficial cervical A.
Levator scapulae
Dorsal scapular A.
Rhomboid minor
Trapezius (reflected)
Rhomboid major
Trapezius
Deltoid
Infraspinatus
Teres major
Latissimus dorsi
Cutaneous branches of dorsal rami lumbar Nn.
Thoracolumbar fascia

Fig. 4.4 Dissection of muscles and nerves of the back.

Cutaneous nerves and arteries

The cutaneous nerves of the back are branches of the **dorsal rami of the spinal nerves**. Each dorsal ramus divides into a medial and a lateral branch [see Fig. 1.4]. Both of these enter and supply the erector spinae muscles. But only one continues through the erector spinae to supply the overlying skin. In the cervical and upper six or seven thoracic segments, the medial branches from the dorsal rami form the **cutaneous nerves**. They pierce the deep fascia close to the median plane. Below this level, the lateral branches form the cutaneous nerves and emerge in line with the lateral edge of the erector spinae, piercing either the latissimus dorsi (upper nerves) or the dense deep fascia (thoracolumbar fascia) of the small of the back (lower nerves). Each of these cutaneous nerves divides into a smaller medial and a larger lateral branch. In the thoracic and lumbar nerves, branches of the dorsal rami descend before entering the skin. Thus, the area of skin supplied by the dorsal ramus of each nerve lies at a lower level than that at which the spinal nerve emerges. This makes the **dermatomes** of the trunk more nearly horizontal than would be expected from the oblique course of the ventral rami.

The cutaneous branches of the dorsal rami of the upper three lumbar nerves pierce the deep fascia a short distance superior to the iliac crest and turn down to supply the skin of the gluteal region.

The **arteries** which accompany the cutaneous nerves of the back arise from the dorsal branches of the posterior intercostal and lumbar arteries.

Muscles that attach the scapula to the trunk

Two of these muscles—the **pectoralis minor** and the **serratus anterior**—have been seen already. Other muscles attaching the scapula to the trunk are the **trapezius, rhomboid major, rhomboid minor**, and **levator scapulae** [Fig. 4.4].

The latissimus dorsi will also be seen in the dissection of the back. The latissimus dorsi and pectoralis major are the only two muscles which attach the humerus to the trunk.

See Dissection 4.2.

Trapezius

The trapezius is a broad muscle placed superficially in the upper part of the back. The right and left trapezius together are shaped like a trapezium, which gives the muscle its name. It has an extensive origin from the external occipital protuberance and the superior nuchal line on the occiput, the ligamentum nuchae and seventh cervical vertebra in the neck, the spines of all 12 thoracic vertebrae, and the supraspinous ligaments. From this almost completely midline origin, the fibres run laterally and come together to be inserted into the lateral third of the clavicle, the acromion, and the crest of the spine of the scapula [Fig. 4.5]. **Nerve supply**: cranial nerve XI—the spinal accessory nerve [Fig. 4.4]. **Actions**: elevation of the shoulder, and retraction and lateral rotation of the scapula.

Latissimus dorsi

This broad sheet of muscle arises from the lower six thoracic spines and the supraspinous ligaments between them, deep to the trapezius; the thoracolumbar fascia [Fig. 4.4]; posterior part of the iliac crest; and lower three or four ribs. The fibres of the latissimus dorsi come together and wind around the inferior border of the teres major to reach its anterior surface and are inserted into the intertubercular sulcus of the humerus [see Fig. 5.1A]. **Nerve supply**: thoracodorsal nerve [see Fig. 3.15]. **Actions**: it is a powerful adductor of the humerus and a depressor of the shoulder. It is used to pull the arm down from its fully abducted position above the head, as in rope climbing. When the shoulder is flexed, it acts as an extensor of that joint. When the shoulder is fixed, it helps with retraction and medial rotation of the scapula.

Levator scapulae

The levator scapulae takes origin from the transverse processes of cervical vertebrae 1 to 4 and is inserted into the medial border of the scapula, between the superior angle and the root of the spinous process. **Nerve supply**: dorsal scapular nerve [Fig. 4.4]. **Actions**: elevation and medial rotation of the scapula.

Objectives

I. To study the muscles of the back—latissimus dorsi, trapezius, levator scapulae, rhomboid minor, rhomboid major, serratus anterior, inferior belly of the omohyoid.
II. To identify and trace the dorsal scapular nerve, the deep branch of the transverse scapular artery, and the suprascapular vessels and nerves.

Instructions

1. Remove the deep fascia from the surface of the trapezius below the spine of the seventh cervical vertebra. The upper part of the muscle will be dissected with the head and neck.

2. Expose the **latissimus dorsi** [Fig. 4.4]. This is difficult because of the varying direction of its fibres and the thinness of its upper part which has an ill-defined margin. Define its attachment to the thoracolumbar fascia and to the iliac crest. Expose the lateral border of the muscle and its slips from the lowest three or four ribs. These lower fibres interdigitate with the external oblique muscle of the abdomen.

3. Cut the **trapezius** horizontally halfway between the clavicle and the spine of the scapula, and vertically 5 cm lateral to the median plane. In the latter cut, take care not to injure the underlying rhomboid muscles, as the trapezius is thin near its origin. Reflect the lower part of the **trapezius**, and define its attachments to the thoracic vertebral spines, the medial border of the acromion, and the superior margin of the crest of the spine of the scapula.

4. Note the superficial branch of the transverse cervical vessels and the accessory nerve on the deep surface of the lateral part of the trapezius. Expose the upper part of the muscle at its attachments to the clavicle and the acromion [Fig. 4.5].

5. Define the **levator scapulae**, **rhomboid minor**, and **rhomboid major** muscles which are attached from above downwards, in that order, to the medial border of the scapula, deep to the trapezius [Fig. 4.6]. The rhomboid minor is attached where the spine of the scapula meets the medial border. Only the lower part of the levator scapulae can be seen at this time. Free this part of the muscle from the underlying fat, and identify the **dorsal scapular nerve** and the **deep branch of the transverse cervical artery**. Follow them to the deep surface of the rhomboid muscles.

6. Divide both rhomboid muscles midway between the vertebral spines and the medial border of the scapula. Reflect these muscles, and define their attachments.

7. Trace the dorsal scapular nerve and the deep branch of the transverse cervical artery deep to them.

8. Lift the medial border of the scapula from the thoracic wall. Note how easily the scapula and the underlying **serratus anterior muscle** are lifted clear because of the loose connective tissue deep to them.

9. Pass one hand between the thoracic wall and the serratus anterior. Then place the other hand in the axilla from the front, and slide it backwards between the subscapularis and the serratus anterior which is now between your hands. Define the attachment of the serratus anterior to the scapula [see Fig. 3.17].

10. Turn the latissimus dorsi downwards and note how the inferior digitations of the serratus anterior converge on the anterior surface of the inferior angle of the scapula [see Fig. 3.17].

11. Remove the fat from the suprascapular region deep to the cut edge of the trapezius, and find the inferior belly of the **omohyoid muscle**, and the **suprascapular vessels** and **nerve** passing to the superior border of the scapula at the scapular notch [Figs. 4.2, 4.3].

Rhomboid minor

The rhomboid minor arises from the lower part of the ligamentum nuchae and the spine of the first thoracic vertebra. It is inserted into the medial border of the scapula, at the root of the spine. **Nerve supply**: dorsal scapular nerve [Fig. 4.4]. **Actions**: retraction and elevation of the scapula.

Rhomboid major

The rhomboid major arises from the spines of the second to fifth thoracic vertebrae. It is inserted into the medial border of the scapula, inferior to the root of the spine. **Nerve supply**: dorsal scapular nerve [Fig. 4.4]. **Actions**: retraction, medial rotation, and elevation of the scapula.

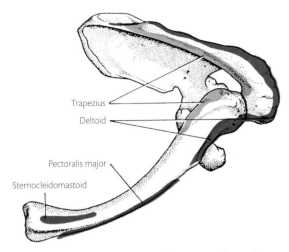

Fig. 4.5 Shoulder girdle from above, showing muscle attachments.

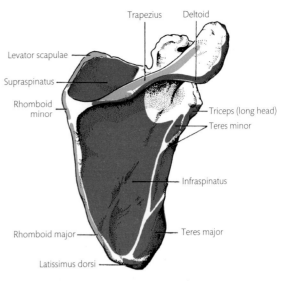

Fig. 4.6 Muscle attachments to the dorsal surface of the right scapula.

Spinal accessory nerve

The accessory, or eleventh, cranial nerve consists of cranial and spinal parts. The **spinal part** arises from the cervical spinal cord (C. 1 to 5), enters the skull, and re-emerges in the neck. It passes postero-inferiorly through the sternocleidomastoid [see Fig. 3.7] to the deep surface of the trapezius supplying both muscles.

Dorsal scapular nerve

This nerve passes posteroinferiorly in the lower part of the neck from the ventral ramus of the fifth cervical nerve. It runs deep to the lower part of the levator scapulae and the rhomboid muscles, and supplies them. It is accompanied by the deep branch of the transverse cervical artery [Fig. 4.4].

Transverse cervical artery

The **transverse cervical artery** is a branch of the thyrocervical trunk from the first part of the subclavian artery. It divides into a **superficial cervical artery** which accompanies the spinal accessory nerve deep to the trapezius, and the **dorsal scapular artery**, which accompanies the dorsal scapular nerve deep to the levator scapulae and the rhomboids [Fig. 4.4]. Both branches take part in the anastomosis around the scapula.

Movements of the scapula

The scapula is able to slide freely over the chest wall because of the loose connective tissue deep to the serratus anterior. The scapular movements are protraction, retraction, elevation, depression, and medial and lateral rotation. These movements are produced by the muscles which attach the scapula to the trunk and indirectly by the muscles passing from the trunk to the humerus when the shoulder joint is fixed. All these movements take place around the **sternoclavicular joint**, with minor adjustments at the **acromioclavicular joint**.

Protraction

This forward movement of the scapula on the chest wall is produced by the **serratus anterior** and is assisted by the pectoral muscles [Fig. 4.7B]. During protraction, all eight digitations of the serratus anterior contract with the **pectoralis minor** and the sternocostal fibres of the **pectoralis major** [see Fig. 3.17]. This movement is used in reaching forwards, punching, and pushing.

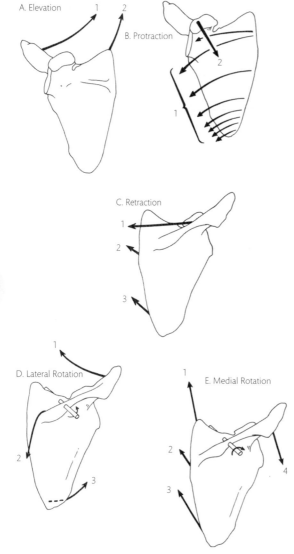

Fig. 4.7 Diagrams to show the direction of pull of muscles acting on the scapula. (A) Elevation of the scapula: 1. upper fibres of the trapezius; 2. levator scapulae. (B) Protraction of the scapula, as in punching or stretching forwards: 1. the serratus anterior pulls the scapula forwards; 2. the pectoralis minor assists. (C) Retraction of the scapula, as in drawing the shoulders back: 1. middle fibres of the trapezius; 2. rhomboid minor; 3. rhomboid major. (D) and (E) Rotation of the scapula. In these figures, the axis of movement is shown as a rod piercing the scapula. The arrow shows the direction of rotation. Lateral rotation: 1. upper fibres of the trapezius; 2. lower fibres of the trapezius; 3. lower part of the serratus anterior. Medial rotation: 1. levator scapulae; 2. rhomboid minor; 3. rhomboid major; 4. the weight of the upper limb.

Retraction

Retraction is the reverse of protraction. It draws the scapulae back towards the median plane and braces back the shoulders. It is produced by the contraction of the middle fibres of the **trapezius** which pass horizontally from the ligamentum nuchae,

and the seventh cervical and upper thoracic spines to the acromion and the lateral part of the spine of the scapula, and also by the **rhomboid muscles** passing from a similar origin to the medial border of the scapula [Fig. 4.7C].

Elevation

Elevation, as in shrugging the shoulders, is achieved by the simultaneous contraction of the **levator scapulae** and the upper fibres of the **trapezius** which descend from the skull and ligamentum nuchae to the clavicle and acromion [Fig. 4.7A].

Depression

This movement is achieved by gravity and the contraction of the pectoralis minor, the lower fibres of the pectoralis major and trapezius, and the latissimus dorsi.

Lateral rotation

Rotation takes place around a horizontal axis passing through the middle of the scapular spine and the sternoclavicular joint [Fig. 4.7D]. In **lateral rotation**, the upper fibres of the **trapezius** raise the acromion and lateral part of the clavicle, while its lower fibres depress the medial end of the spine of the scapula. Together, they laterally rotate the scapula. The lower five digitations of the **serratus anterior** converge on the inferior angle of the scapula and play a powerful part in this movement by pulling that angle laterally and forwards. Lateral rotation tilts the glenoid cavity upwards [Fig. 4.3] and is important in abduction of the upper limb above the horizontal. Normally, scapular and shoulder joint movements occur together, but, if the scapular movement is paralysed, abduction of the limb to the horizontal cannot be achieved because the weight of the limb forces the scapula into medial rotation.

Medial rotation

This is the opposite movement to lateral rotation. Gravity plays a large part in this movement, as in depression of the scapula. In addition, combined contraction of the levator scapulae, rhomboids, and latissimus dorsi produces an active movement which is assisted by the pectoral muscles [Fig. 4.7E].

When all the muscles attaching the scapula to the trunk are contracted, the scapula is fixed to form a stable base on which upper limb movements can take place. It is also used in transmitting forces from the trunk to the upper limbs, as in lifting heavy weights in the hands by straightening the flexed legs.

Muscles acting on, and movements of, the scapula

Having studied the muscles acting on the scapula and its movements, review the details of the muscles using Table 4.2. This table lists the origin, insertion, nerve supply, and action of muscles acting on the shoulder girdle. In Table 4.3, the muscles are grouped according to their actions (and the nerve supply of each muscle is repeated). This allows an easy assessment of the degree of loss of a particular movement, following the destruction of a particular nerve. (These tables show only the actions of a particular muscle when it actively shortens.)

Clinical Applications 4.1 and 4.2 demonstrate how this anatomy relates to your clinical practice.

Table 4.2 Trunk muscles acting on the shoulder girdle

Muscle	Origin	Insertion	Action	Nerve supply
Trapezius	Upper fibres: Occiput, external occipital protruberance, and superior nuchal line Ligamentum nuchae Seventh cervical spine	Clavicle, lateral third Scapula, acromion, medial edge Scapula, superior margin of spine	Elevates shoulder	Spinal accessory
	Lower fibres: Seventh cervical spine All thoracic vertebral spines	Scapula, superior margin of spine	1. Retracts scapula 2. Depresses medial part of spine of scapula	Spinal accessory
	All fibres: Occiput, external occipital protruberance, and superior nuchal line Ligamentum nuchae Seventh cervical spine All thoracic vertebral spines	Clavicle, lateral third Scapula, acromion, medial edge Scapula, superior margin of spine	Rotates scapula laterally	Spinal accessory
Serratus anterior	Upper eight ribs, anterolateral surface	Scapula, medial border	1. Protracts scapula 2. Holds scapula against ribs 3. Lower 5 digitations laterally rotate scapula	Long thoracic nerve
Pectoralis minor	Ribs 3–5, anterolateral surface	Scapula, coracoid process	1. Protracts scapula 2. Depresses shoulder	Medial pectoral nerve
Rhomboid major	Second to fifth thoracic vertebral spines	Scapula, medial border inferior to spine	1. Retracts scapula 2. Medially rotates scapula 3. Elevates scapula	Dorsal scapular nerve
Rhomboid minor	Lower ligamentum nuchae First thoracic vertebral spine	Scapula, medial border at spine	1. Retracts scapula 2. Elevates scapula	Dorsal scapular nerve
Levator scapulae	Cervical transverse processes 1–4	Scapula, medial border between superior angle and rhomboid minor	1. Elevates scapula 2. Medially rotates scapula	Dorsal scapular nerve
Subclavius	First costal cartilage	Clavicle, inferior surface	Holds clavicle to sternum	Nerve to subclavius
Pectoralis major, sternocostal*	Sternum Costal cartilages 1–6	Humerus, lateral lip of intertubercular sulcus	1. Protracts scapula 2. Depresses shoulder	Medial and lateral pectoral nerves
Latissimus dorsi*	Lower ribs Thoracolumbar fascia Iliac crest	Humerus, intertubercular sulcus	1. Depresses shoulder 2. Medially rotates scapula 3. Retracts scapula	Thoracodorsal nerve

* The sternocostal part of the pectoralis major and latissimus dorsi can act on the scapula only when the shoulder is fixed.

Table 4.3 Movements of the shoulder girdle

Movement	Muscles	Nerve supply (motor)
Elevation	Levator scapulae	Dorsal scapular, and C. 3 and 4
	Trapezius, upper part	Accessory
	Rhomboids	Dorsal scapular
Depression	Pectoralis minor	Medial pectoral
	Trapezius, lower part	Accessory
	Latissimus dorsi*	Thoracodorsal
	Pectoralis major, lower sternocostal part*	Medial pectoral
Protraction	Serratus anterior	Long thoracic
	Pectoralis minor	Medial pectoral
	Pectoralis major, sternocostal part*	Medial and lateral pectoral
Retraction	Rhomboid major and minor	Dorsal scapular
	Trapezius, middle part	Accessory
	Latissimus dorsi*	Thoracodorsal
Lateral rotation, e.g. in abduction of arm	Serratus anterior, lower 5 digitations	Long thoracic
	Trapezius, upper and lower parts	Accessory
Medial rotation	Rhomboid major and minor	Dorsal scapular
	Levator scapulae	Dorsal scapular, and C. 3 and 4
	Pectoralis major, lower sternocostal part*	Medial pectoral
	Pectoralis minor	Medial pectoral
	Latissimus dorsi*	Thoracodorsal

* These muscles can only act on the scapula through a fixed shoulder joint.

CLINICAL APPLICATION 4.1 Winging of the scapula

The long thoracic nerve descends from the brachial plexus and runs on the lateral surface of the serratus anterior before supplying that muscle. It may be affected in metastatic cancer of axillary lymph nodes and surgical resection of axillary lymph nodes. It is also vulnerable to damage by direct trauma, such as a blow to the ribs, because of its superficial location when the arm is raised in sport or combat.

Study question 1: what change would be observed in the position of the scapula at rest, when the serratus anterior is paralysed? (Answer: the medial border of the scapula would project posteriorly away from the thoracic wall.) When the arm is raised, the medial border and inferior angle will move sharply away from the chest wall.

Study question 2: what movements would be lost when the serratus anterior is paralysed? (Answer: lateral rotation of the scapula. Also the patient will not be able to abduct the arm above the horizontal, as this movement is dependent on lateral rotation of the scapula.)

CLINICAL APPLICATION 4.2 Testing cranial nerve XI

Functional assessment of cranial nerves is an essential part of the general physical examination. The distal part of the spinal accessory nerve (cranial nerve XI) is susceptible to injury in the neck due to its superficial position between the muscles. Injury to the spinal accessory nerve can cause diminished or absent function of the upper portion of the trapezius muscle.

Study question 1: using your knowledge of movements of the shoulder girdle, name the movement most severely affected by injury to the spinal accessory nerve. (Answer: elevation of, or shrugging, the shoulder.)

Study question 2: how does the physician test the function of cranial nerve XI? (Answer: the patient is asked to shrug the shoulder with and without resistance. A one-sided weakness of the trapezius indicates injury to the spinal accessory nerve of that side.)

CHAPTER 5
The free upper limb

Introduction

Regions of the free upper limb will be described and dissected in the subsequent chapters. This chapter gives an overview of the free upper limb, with special attention to the superficial veins, nerves, and lymphatics which are best studied in continuity from the shoulder down to the hand.

Surface anatomy

The bones of the upper limb, their main parts, and surface projections, articulations, and movements at the joints are described here. Make use of the dried bones to identify the parts and bony landmarks. The surface anatomy of the upper limb should be appreciated on your own upper limb.

The arm

The **humerus** [Fig. 5.1] is almost entirely covered by the muscles of the arm, so that its outlines can only be felt indistinctly. In the distal part, it expands transversely, and its lateral and medial **margins** (supracondylar ridges) become readily palpable. The lateral and medial margins end inferiorly in the lateral and medial **epicondyles**. The medial epicondyle is more prominent than the lateral epicondyle. In the anatomical position, the epicondyles are in the positions suggested by their names, and the hemispherical head of the humerus faces medially. When the palms of the hands face medially (the arm is semi-pronated), the lateral epicondyle is more anterior, and the head of the humerus is directed posteromedially.

The upper half of the humerus is covered on its anterior, lateral, and posterior surfaces by the deltoid muscle. Inferiorly, the apex of that muscle is attached to the lateral side of the middle of the humerus—the **deltoid tuberosity**. The upper part of the bone consists of the **head**. This is separated by a shallow groove—the **anatomical neck** from the greater (lateral) and lesser (anterior) **tubercles**. Both the head and tubercles are continuous inferiorly with the **body** or **shaft** of the bone through the narrow **surgical neck**. The greater tubercle is the most lateral bony part of the shoulder. The lower half of the bone is covered anteriorly by the biceps and brachialis muscles, and posteriorly by the triceps muscle. The anterior surfaces of the epicondyles and supracondylar ridges give rise to the forearm muscles.

At the midpoint of the anterior surface of the bend of the elbow, find the **tendon of the biceps**. Medial to this, feel the pulsations of the **brachial artery**, and trace it superiorly on the medial side of the arm. The **median nerve** may be palpable, posteromedial to the artery.

The distal end of the humerus articulates with the radius and ulna. There are four named bony prominences at this end. The medial and lateral epicondyles have been described. Immediately lateral to the medial epicondyle is the trochlea. The **trochlea** has a pulley-shaped articular surface for articulation with the ulna. The **capitulum** lies lateral to the trochlea and has a rounded articular surface for the head of the radius. Three bony fossae (depressions) are seen at the lower end of the humerus, immediately above the articular surfaces. On the anterior surface, the **coronoid fossa** lies medially, superior to the trochlea, and the **radial fossa** is

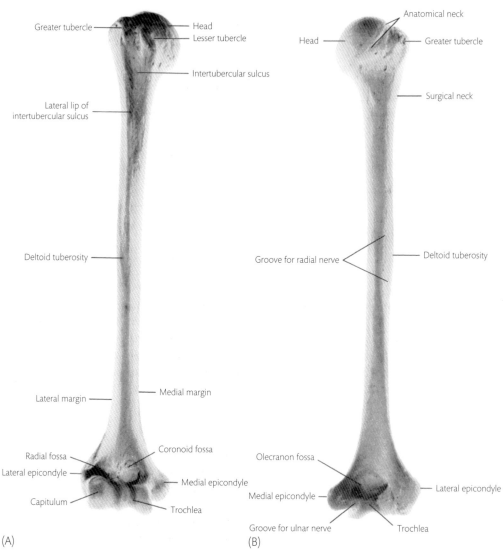

Fig. 5.1 Right humerus. (A) Anterior aspect. (B) Posterior aspect.

lateral, superior to the capitulum. On the posterior aspect, the single **olecranon fossa** lies superior to the trochlea.

The forearm

The two bones of the forearm are the radius (lateral) and the ulna (medial) [Figs. 5.2, 5.3]. Proximally, the trochlear notch of the **ulna** [Fig. 5.2] articulates with the **trochlea of the humerus** [Fig. 5.1]. The ulnar trochlear notch has two processes—the **coronoid process** inferiorly and the **olecranon process** superiorly. The olecranon and coronoid fossa of the humerus are occupied by the olecranon process in full extension of the elbow, and the coronoid process in full flexion.

The proximal part of the ulna (the olecranon) is readily palpable. On its posterior surface is a triangular subcutaneous area which is continuous distally with the **posterior margin** (border) **of the ulna**. The entire length of this posterior margin is palpable. The ulna ends distally in the **styloid process** which projects from the posteromedial aspect of the cylindrical, slightly expanded **head** of the bone [Figs. 5.2, 5.3]. This palpable margin not only allows the entire length of the ulna to be examined for fractures, but also forms the line of separation between the anteromedial flexor group of muscles of the forearm (supplied by the median and ulnar nerves) and the posterolateral extensor group (supplied by the radial nerve) [see Fig. 8.1].

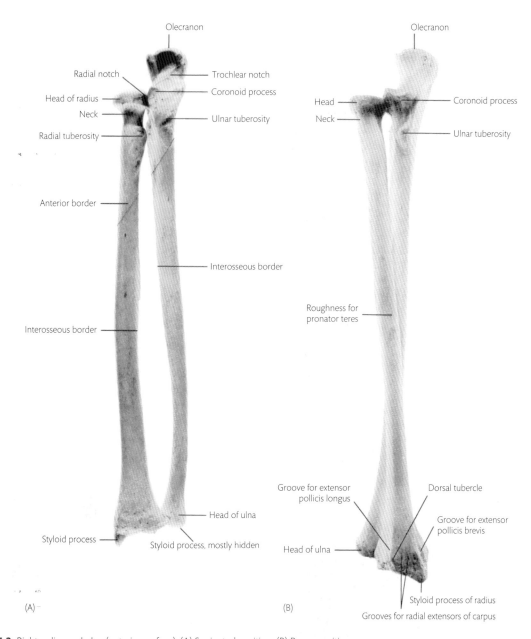

Olecranon

Radial notch

Head of radius

Neck

Radial tuberosity

Trochlear notch

Coronoid process

Ulnar tuberosity

Anterior border

Interosseous border

Interosseous border

Head of ulna

Styloid process

Styloid process, mostly hidden

(A)

Olecranon

Head

Neck

Coronoid process

Ulnar tuberosity

Roughness for
pronator teres

Groove for extensor
pollicis longus

Dorsal tubercle

Groove for extensor
pollicis brevis

Head of ulna

Styloid process of radius

Grooves for radial extensors of carpus

(B)

Fig. 5.2 Right radius and ulna (anterior surface). (A) Supinated position. (B) Prone position.

The proximal end, or **head**, of the **radius** is a short cylinder. Its concave proximal surface articulates with the capitulum of the humerus, and its circumference articulates with the **radial notch of the ulna** and the **annular ligament**. The annular ligament is loop-shaped and attached to the margins of the radial notch on the ulna. It narrows inferiorly to fit the superior part of the **neck of the radius** [Figs. 5.2, 5.3]. This narrowing prevents the head from being pulled out of the ligament when the arm is pulled upon. Palpate the head of the radius just distal to the lateral epicondyle of the

humerus, and feel it rotating within the annular ligament when you pronate and supinate your forearm. The **radial tuberosity** lies on the medial aspect of the radius, distal to the neck. It has the tendon of the biceps brachii attached to its posterior part. Beyond this point, the radius is markedly convex laterally, and only its distal part is readily palpable through the muscles which cover it.

The wrist

At the lower end, the radius expands into a cuboidal mass. The lateral surface of this mass extends

Surface anatomy

55

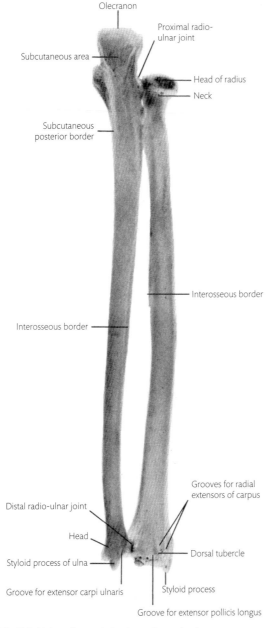

Olecranon

Proximal radio-ulnar joint

Subcutaneous area

Head of radius

Neck

Subcutaneous posterior border

Interosseous border

Interosseous border

Grooves for radial extensors of carpus

Distal radio-ulnar joint

Head

Styloid process of ulna

Dorsal tubercle

Groove for extensor carpi ulnaris

Styloid process

Groove for extensor pollicis longus

Fig. 5.3 Right radius and ulna (posterior surface).

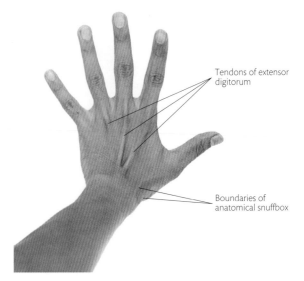

Tendons of extensor digitorum

Boundaries of anatomical snuffbox

Fig. 5.4 Boundaries of the anatomical snuffbox. Copyright Shutterstock.

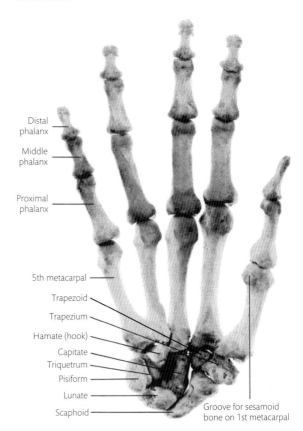

Distal phalanx

Middle phalanx

Proximal phalanx

5th metacarpal

Trapezoid

Trapezium

Hamate (hook)

Capitate

Triquetrum

Pisiform

Lunate

Scaphoid

Groove for sesamoid bone on 1st metacarpal

Fig. 5.5 Palmar aspect of bones of the right hand.

distally to form the blunt **styloid process**. When the thumb is fully extended, i.e. moved laterally, a surface depression—'the **anatomical snuffbox**'—appears on the lateral side of the back of the wrist between the tendons passing to the thumb [Fig. 5.4]. The styloid process of the radius lies in the proximal part of the depression and is covered by tendons of the short extensor and long abductor muscles of the thumb. The bones at the lateral ends of the proximal and distal rows of the carpal bones (**scaphoid** and **trapezium**) and the base of the metacarpal of the thumb [Figs. 5.5, 5.6] can be

felt in the 'snuffbox', distal to the styloid process. Light pressure applied over the trapezium reveals the pulsations of the **radial artery**. The 'radial pulse' is more easily felt where the artery crosses the anterior surface of the distal end of the radius (medial to the styloid process).

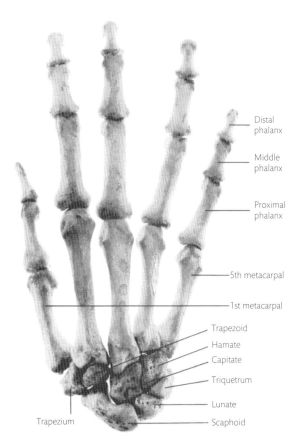

Distal
phalanx

Middle
phalanx

Proximal
phalanx

5th metacarpal

1st metacarpal

Trapezoid

Hamate

Capitate

Triquetrum

Lunate

Scaphoid

Trapezium

Fig. 5.6 Dorsal aspect of bones of the right hand.

Feel your radial and ulnar styloid processes simultaneously. Note that the radial styloid projects further distally than the ulnar styloid—a situation which is altered when the radius is fractured. If the tendon forming the posterior boundary of the 'snuff-box' (extensor pollicis longus) is followed proximally, it curves round the medial surface of the **dorsal tubercle** of the radius which is readily palpable.

The distal end of the radius articulates medially with the ulna (**ulnar notch**) and distally with the lateral two **carpal bones**—the scaphoid and lunate of the proximal row. This forms the only direct articulation of the carpal bones with the bones of the forearm. Forces transmitted from the hand to the forearm pass through the scaphoid and lunate to the radius—a feature which accounts for the fracture of the scaphoid or radius (but not the ulna) from falling on the outstretched hand.

The dorsal surfaces of both rows of carpal bones can be felt through the tendons which cover them, though the individual bones cannot be defined. On the palmar surface of the wrist, only the **pisiform bone** (medially) and the **tubercle of the scaphoid** (laterally) can be felt at the level of

the distal transverse skin crease (junction of the forearm and wrist) when the wrist is fully extended. If the wrist is passively flexed, the pisiform may be gripped between the finger and thumb and moved on the triquetrum bone with which it articulates, and the **tendon of the flexor carpi ulnaris** can be felt passing to its proximal surface [Fig. 5.7]. The **hook of the hamate** can be felt deeply through the proximal parts of the muscles forming the ball of the little finger (**hypothenar eminence**), and the **tubercle of the trapezium** can be felt deeply through the proximal parts of the muscles forming the ball of the thumb (**thenar eminence**). These four palpable bony points lying at the ends of the two rows of the carpal bones—tubercle of the scaphoid, pisiform, tubercle of the trapezium, and hook of the hamate—give attachment to the **flexor retinaculum**. The flexor retinaculum is the deep fascia which connects these bones, maintains the palmar concavity of the carpal bones, and completes the fibro-osseous tunnel through which the flexor tendons and the median nerve pass from the forearm into the hand.

The palm

The skin of the central region of the palm is firmly bound to the thickened underlying deep fascia (**palmar aponeurosis**). The palmar aponeurosis is continuous distally with the deep fascia of the fingers and proximally with the flexor retinaculum and the **tendon of the palmaris longus**. If present, this tendon enters the palm, superficial to the retinaculum, and is the most superficial tendon immediately proximal to the wrist. Contraction of the palmaris longus and extension of the fingers tighten the palmar aponeurosis and stabilize the palmar skin to maintain a firm grip. The distal **skin crease** of the palm lies just proximal to the metacarpophalangeal joints, while that at the roots of the fingers lies approximately 3 cm distal to them [see Fig. 8.10]. The middle skin crease of each finger lies at the level of the proximal interphalangeal joint, and the distal skin crease lies proximal to the distal interphalangeal joint. The **metacarpals** (hand bones) are readily palpated on their dorsal surfaces. When a fist is formed, the **knuckles** are the distal ends of the **heads of the metacarpal bones**, uncovered by the movement of the proximal phalanges on to the palmar surfaces of these heads. The heads of the proximal and middle phalanges of the fingers are similarly exposed.

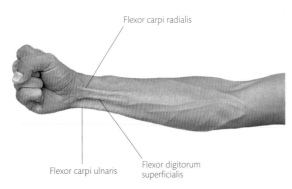

Flexor carpi radialis

Flexor carpi ulnaris

Flexor digitorum superficialis

Fig. 5.7 Flexor tendons at the wrist. Copyright Shutterstock.

The digits

The **thumb** has two phalanges; the other fingers have three. The thumb lies at right angles to the fingers, with its nail facing laterally and not posteriorly. Thus, **flexion** moves the tip of the thumb medially across the palm, while **extension** moves it laterally. **Abduction** swings the tip of the thumb anteriorly; **adduction** moves it to the index finger. The first carpometacarpal joint, between the metacarpal of the thumb and the trapezium, allows for greater freedom of movement, when compared with the carpometacarpal joints of the fingers. To test this, grip the head of each metacarpal in turn, with the thumb and index finger of your other hand on the palmar and dorsal surfaces, and attempt to move it. The metacarpal of the middle finger scarcely moves, while those of the index, ring, and little finger, in that order, have an increasing, but small, range of flexion and extension and slight rotation only in the little finger. None can be abducted or adducted. Next flex your thumb at the metacarpophalangeal joint, and attempt to rotate its metacarpal using the phalanges as a lever. Only a small amount of movement is possible, compared with the free flexion/extension and abduction/adduction at the carpometacarpal joint of the thumb.

Flexion of the **metacarpophalangeal joint** of the thumb is less than 90 degrees. It is 90 degrees in the index and middle fingers and exceeds this in the ring and little fingers. There is some degree of rotation in the ring and little fingers. Check the bones, and note that there is nothing in their contours to prevent rotation. Rotation is limited by ligaments. Also there is very little abduction or adduction at the metacarpophalangeal joint in the thumb, though it is relatively free in the fingers.

The **interphalangeal joint** of the thumb flexes to approximately 90 degrees. The proximal interphalangeal joints of the fingers flex to more than 90 degrees, and the distal interphalangeal joints slightly less than 90 degrees.

The fingers separate on extension and come together in flexion. This is the result of the curve in which the heads of the metacarpals lie and a slight obliquity of the interphalangeal joints. Note also that the tips of all four fingers meet the palm at the same time, despite the differences in their lengths. Check your interphalangeal joints for rotation. This is minimal because of the shape of the articular surfaces of the phalanges.

Cup the palm of your hand by spreading the fingers as though to grasp a large ball. The hollow between the proximal parts of the thenar and hypothenar eminences marks the position of the **flexor retinaculum**. The tightening of the skin on the medial side of the hypothenar eminence is produced by the contraction of the **palmaris brevis** which heaps up the hypothenar skin to form a pad for grasping. Note too that the thumb is slightly flexed at the carpometacarpal joint and rotated medially, so that its palmar surface faces that of the little finger (opposition), which is also rotated laterally. The other three fingers are not parallel to each other but, on flexion, converge to meet the tip of the thumb.

See Dissection 5.1 for instructions on skin reflection of the front of the arm and forearm.

DISSECTION 5.1: Skin reflection of the front of the arm and forearm-1

Objectives

I. To reflect the skin on the front of the arm and forearm.   II. To find the cutaneous vessels and nerves.

Instructions

1. Make incision 5, as shown in Fig. 3.3. Extend the incision along the anterior surfaces of all the fingers, leaving them covered with skin at present to avoid drying of the tissues.

2. Strip the skin and superficial fascia from the deep fascia by blunt dissection.

3. Note and follow the large cutaneous veins and the cutaneous nerves, as they pierce the deep fascia.

Superficial fascia

There are no special features about this fascia in the arm or forearm, but, in the palm, it contains dense bundles of fibrous tissue connecting the skin to the palmar aponeurosis. It is thickened transversely in the webs of the fingers to form the **superficial transverse metacarpal ligament**. On the proximal part of the hypothenar eminence, it contains the **palmaris brevis** which passes from the skin of the medial border of the hand to the palmar aponeurosis.

Superficial veins

The main superficial veins are extremely variable. They begin in the **dorsal venous network** of the hand—an irregular arrangement of veins on the dorsum of the hand, usually with a transverse element 2–3 cm proximal to the heads of the metacarpals. This network receives the dorsal digital veins through the **intercapital veins**, and also communicating veins from the palm which pass through the intermetacarpal spaces. This network drains into a number of veins, of which one or more on the medial side form the **basilic vein** and on the lateral side the **cephalic vein** [Fig. 5.8]. Both the basilic and cephalic veins turn round the corresponding border of the forearm to reach the anterior surface and ascend on the anteromedial and anterolateral surfaces of the forearm [Figs. 5.8, 5.9]. At the elbow, the arrangement of the superficial veins is variable, but they are usually united anterior to the cubital fossa by a **median cubital vein**. Much of the blood in the cephalic vein is transferred to the basilic vein. Another common arrangement is shown in Fig. 5.10. The veins then ascend on the corresponding sides of the biceps muscle. The cephalic vein pierces the deep fascia and runs between the pectoralis major and the deltoid in the deltopectoral groove to the infraclavicular fossa. Here it passes deep to join the axillary vein near the apex of the axilla. The basilic vein pierces the deep fascia at about the middle of the arm. It unites with the brachial veins and runs with the brachial artery to become the axillary vein at the lower border of the axilla [see Fig. 3.12].

Lightly compress your right arm with your left hand, and contract your right forearm muscles by clenching and unclenching your fist. This distends the **superficial veins** and makes them visible. Compare your superficial veins with those of the other students, and note their variability and the presence of a cephalic and a basilic vein in most cases.

Lymph vessels and nodes of the upper limb

It is not possible in an ordinary dissection to display the lymph vessels in any part of the body, and lymph nodes are difficult to find. It is necessary, however, to know the arrangement of the vessels and nodes, because they form a common route for the spread of infection and cancer. The primary source of disease can often be deduced from the nodes which are involved.

In the upper limb, as elsewhere, the lymph vessels and nodes are divided into two groups by the deep fascia—the superficial vessels and nodes, and the deep vessels and nodes.

Deep lymph vessels, which are much less numerous than the superficial vessels, drain structures which are deep to the deep fascia. They accompany the main blood vessels and drain into the axillary lymph nodes. Some of the lymph they contain may have passed through a small number of **deep lymph nodes** which are occasionally found on the arteries of the forearm, in the cubital fossa, and on the brachial artery.

The **superficial lymph nodes** of the upper limb are few in number: (1) one or two lie a little superior to the medial epicondyle near the basilic vein; and (2) a few are scattered along the upper part of the cephalic vein [see Fig. 3.12].

Superficial lymph vessels of the upper limb drain the skin and subcutaneous tissues, and most end in the lateral group of axillary nodes. The larger lymph vessels, unlike the veins, do not unite into larger trunks but run individual courses directly towards the axilla. The general arrangement of superficial lymph vessels is shown in Figs. 3.12 and 5.11. Note the following: (1) the dense palmar plexus drains mainly to the dorsum of the hand to join the posterior vessels of the forearm; (2) the vessels on the posterior surfaces of the forearm and arm spiral upwards round the medial and lateral surfaces to reach the anterior surface and approach the floor of the axilla; most vessels remain superficial, until

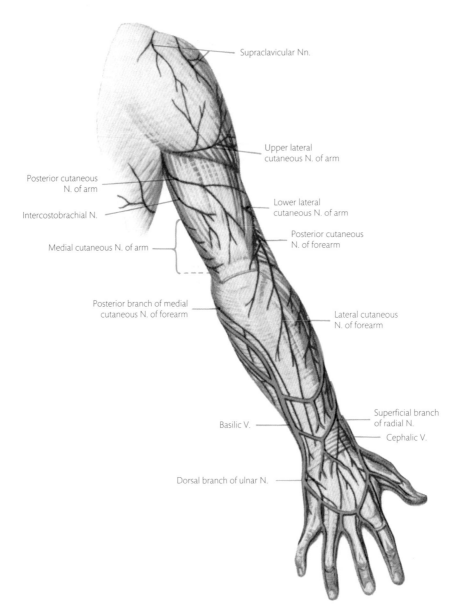

Supraclavicular Nn.

Upper lateral
cutaneous N. of arm

Posterior cutaneous
N. of arm

Lower lateral
cutaneous N. of arm

Intercostobrachial N.

Posterior cutaneous
N. of forearm

Medial cutaneous N. of arm

Posterior branch of medial
cutaneous N. of forearm

Lateral cutaneous
N. of forearm

Superficial branch
of radial N.

Basilic V.

Cephalic V.

Dorsal branch of ulnar N.

Fig. 5.8 Superficial veins and nerves of the back of the upper limb.

they pierce the fascial floor of the axilla; however, some lymphatics on the medial aspect enter the superficial cubital nodes, and efferents from these nodes pass through the deep fascia with the basilic vein; (3) a few vessels from the lateral side of the arm and shoulder run with the cephalic vein into the apical axillary nodes; and (4) vessels from the shoulder and upper parts of the thoracic wall curve round the anterior and posterior axillary folds to enter the pectoral and subscapular groups of **axillary nodes**; those from the walls of the lower parts of the thorax and upper abdomen converge directly on the axilla.

Cutaneous nerves of the upper limb

There are certain general principles about the distribution of nerves to the skin which are of clinical importance.

1. Each nerve which passes to the skin is distributed to a circumscribed area. The area of the upper limb skin supplied by spinal nerves C. 4 to T. 2 is shown in Fig. 5.12.

2. Limb plexuses are formed by the plaiting together of the ventral rami of several spinal nerves. As a result of this: (a) each part of the plexus and each

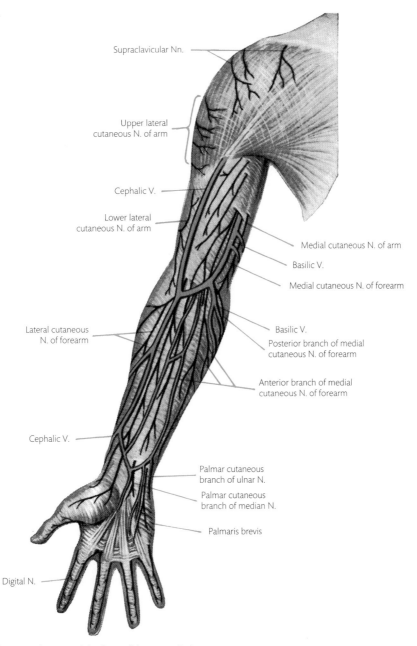

Supraclavicular Nn.

Upper lateral
cutaneous N. of arm

Cephalic V.

Lower lateral
cutaneous N. of arm

Medial cutaneous N. of arm

Basilic V.

Medial cutaneous N. of forearm

Lateral cutaneous
N. of forearm

Basilic V.

Posterior branch of medial
cutaneous N. of forearm

Anterior branch of medial
cutaneous N. of forearm

Cephalic V.

Palmar cutaneous
branch of ulnar N.

Palmar cutaneous
branch of median N.

Palmaris brevis

Digital N.

Fig. 5.9 Superficial veins and nerves of the front of the upper limb.

branch of the brachial plexus contain nerve fibres from more than one ventral ramus—examples: the upper trunk contains fibres from C. 5 and C. 6; the ulnar nerve contains fibres from C. 8 and T. 1; and (b) several of these branches contain some nerve fibres from the same ventral ramus—example: the suprascapular nerve and the axillary nerve contain fibres from C. 5 and C. 6 [see Fig. 3.21]. Thus, the area of distribution of a cutaneous nerve, and consequently the area of sensory loss, when it is destroyed is different from the loss resulting from the destruction of a ventral ramus.

3. Cutaneous nerves supplying adjacent areas of skin overlap with each other to a considerable degree. Thus, the destruction of a single cutaneous nerve leads to a total loss of sensation only in a small area within the area of distribution of that nerve. Surrounding this anaesthetized area, there will be an area of altered sensation due to the presence of nerve fibres from adjacent uninjured nerves.

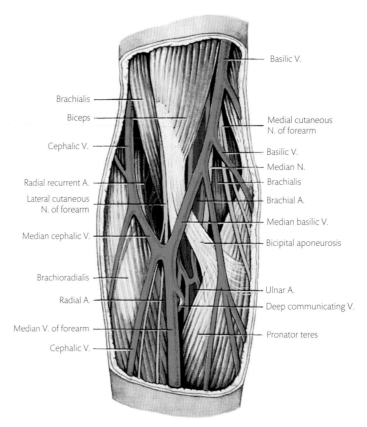

Brachialis

Biceps

Cephalic V.

Radial recurrent A.

Lateral cutaneous
N. of forearm

Median cephalic V.

Brachioradialis

Radial A.

Median V. of forearm

Cephalic V.

Basilic V.

Medial cutaneous
N. of forearm

Basilic V.

Median N.

Brachialis

Brachial A.

Median basilic V.

Bicipital aponeurosis

Ulnar A.

Deep communicating V.

Pronator teres

Fig. 5.10 Commonly seen arrangement of superficial veins at the bend of the elbow.

Each thoracic spinal nerve (except for T. 1 which is involved in the formation of a plexus) supplies a strip of skin (**dermatome**) which overlaps those of adjacent nerves, so that destruction of a single thoracic spinal nerve produces only altered sensation within its dermatome. In the plexus regions, each ventral ramus supplies a circumscribed area of skin in sequence with, and overlapped by, the areas of adjacent ventral rami. The overlap of these dermatomes is accounted for by the presence of nerve fibres from multiple ventral rami in every branch of the plexus.

4. Major branches of the plexus, i.e. the main nerves of a limb, give rise to several cutaneous branches which leave them at different points. Destruction of a nerve before it has given off any branches will produce a different distribution of sensory loss to that which occurs when the nerve is destroyed after giving off one or more branches. It is more important to know the total distribution of these major nerves than that of their individual cutaneous branches. But the ability to

make a detailed diagnosis of the site of an injury depends on knowing the distribution of the individual cutaneous nerves and the approximate site of origin of these nerves from the parent trunk [see Fig. 10.1].

The diagrams of nerve distribution in this book take no account either of the overlap or of the fact that nerve fibres may sometimes pass to their destinations by unusual routes and hence modify the expected clinical effects of destruction of a particular nerve.

5. In both upper and lower limbs, the nerves which pass to the anterior surface supply a greater area of the skin than those which pass to the posterior surface. In the upper limb, this means that a greater part of the skin is supplied by nerves arising from the medial and lateral cords of the brachial plexus which are formed from the anterior divisions of the trunks of the plexus.

Dissection 5.2 continues the study of the cutaneous nerves of the forearm.

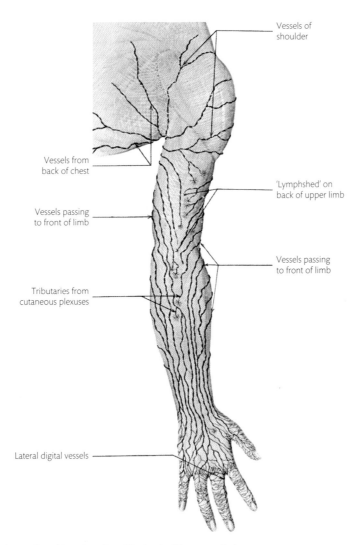

Vessels of shoulder

Vessels from back of chest

Vessels passing to front of limb

'Lymphshed' on back of upper limb

Vessels passing to front of limb

Tributaries from cutaneous plexuses

Lateral digital vessels

Fig. 5.11 Superficial lymph vessels and lymph nodes of the back of the upper limb.

DISSECTION 5.2: Cutaneous nerves of the front of the arm and forearm-2

Objective

I. To continue the study of the cutaneous nerves of the forearm.

Instructions

1. Many of the cutaneous nerves will have been found when the skin and superficial fascia were removed from the upper limb, but their distribution is best determined by reference to Figs. 5.8 and 5.9, since they are very difficult to follow through the superficial fascia.

2. Retain nerves that have been found piercing the deep fascia, so that they can later be traced to their parent nerves.

Cutaneous nerves from the spinal nerves adjacent to the brachial plexus

(a) The **supraclavicular nerves** (C. 3, 4) descend from the neck, cross the superficial surface of the clavicle and acromion, and supply the skin over the upper part of the front of the chest and deltoid muscle to the level of the sternal angle [see Fig. 3.7].

(b) The **intercostobrachial nerve** (T. 2)—this lateral cutaneous branch of the second intercostal nerve enters the axilla from the second intercostal space. It descends obliquely across the axilla, communicates with the medial cutaneous nerve of the arm, and sends branches to the floor of the axilla. It pierces the deep fascia below the axilla to supply the skin on the upper posteromedial part of the arm [Fig. 5.8].

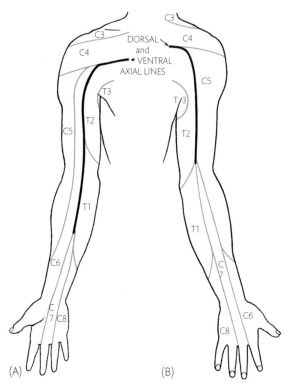

Fig. 5.12 Dermatomes of the upper limb. (A) Front of the upper limb. (B) Back of the upper limb. After Head, 1893, and Foerster, 1933.

Cutaneous nerves from the posterior cord

These supply the posterior surface of the limb. They arise from either the axillary or the radial nerve.

(a) Cutaneous branches of the axillary nerve [Figs. 5.8, 5.9]: the **upper lateral cutaneous nerve of the arm** (C. 5, 6) pierces the deep fascia at a variable point posterior to the lower half of the deltoid muscle. It curves round the posterior border of that muscle and supplies the skin over its lower half.

(b) Cutaneous branches of the radial nerve [Figs. 5.8, 5.9, see also Fig. 10.1]:

(i) The **posterior cutaneous nerve of the arm** (C. 5) arises in the axilla, pierces the deep fascia below the posterior axillary fold, and supplies the skin of the back of the arm from the insertion of the deltoid to the olecranon.

(ii) The **lower lateral cutaneous nerve of the arm** (C. 5, 6) arises posterior to the humerus and pierces the deep fascia below the insertion of the deltoid. It supplies the skin of the lateral side of the arm below that insertion.

(iii) The **posterior cutaneous nerve of the forearm** (C. 6, 7, 8) arises with the lower lateral cutaneous nerve of the arm and pierces the deep fascia below it. It gives some branches to the lateral side of the arm, descends posterior to the lateral epicondyle, and lies in the middle of the back of the forearm. It supplies the skin on the back of the forearm to the level of the wrist or occasionally on to the dorsum of the hand.

(iv) The **superficial branch of the radial nerve** (C. 6, 7, 8) is a terminal branch of the radial nerve. It descends in the forearm between the extensor and flexor muscle groups, passes posteriorly in the distal half of the forearm, and pierces the deep fascia 5 cm superior to the styloid process of the radius. It supplies the lateral two-thirds of the dorsum of the hand, the dorsal surfaces of the thumb, and the lateral two and a half fingers through five **dorsal digital nerves**. These do not supply the terminal parts of the fingers. The area supplied by the nerve varies reciprocally with the other nerves with which it communicates on the dorsum of the hand (ulnar, posterior cutaneous nerve of the forearm, and median).

Cutaneous nerves from the lateral cord

They arise from the musculocutaneous nerve [Figs. 5.8, 5.9, see also Fig. 10.1].

(a) The **lateral cutaneous nerve of the forearm** (C. 5, 6) pierces the deep fascia just lateral to the biceps, 2–3 cm proximal to the bend of the elbow. It divides into anterior and posterior branches which supply the anterolateral and posterolateral surfaces of the forearm, the anterior extending on to the ball of the thumb.

Cutaneous nerves from the medial cord

They arise from either the medial cord or the ulnar nerve.

(a) Cutaneous branches of the medial cord [Figs. 5.8, 5.9, see also Fig. 10.1]:

(i) The **medial cutaneous nerve of the arm** (T. 1, 2) pierces the deep fascia on the medial side of the middle of the arm. It supplies the skin on the medial side of the inferior half of the arm, posterior to the basilic vein.

(ii) The **medial cutaneous nerve of the forearm** (C. 8, T. 1) pierces the deep fascia with the basilic vein. As it descends, it divides into anterior and posterior branches which supply the anteromedial and posteromedial surfaces of the forearm to the wrist. The anterior branch supplies the skin of the distal part of the front of the arm, and together they supply the skin of the medial half of the forearm.

(b) Cutaneous branches of the ulnar nerve (C. 8, T. 1, with fibres of C. 7 received from the median nerve in the axilla) [Figs. 5.8, 5.9, see also Fig. 10.1]: this nerve supplies only skin in the hand and fingers.

(i) The **dorsal branch of the ulnar nerve** (C. 7, 8) arises from the ulnar nerve in the middle of the forearm and descends with it almost to the pisiform bone. It then passes obliquely backwards across the medial surface of the carpus to divide into two **dorsal digital nerves**. These supply the skin of the medial third of the back of the hand and the dorsal surfaces of the little finger and the medial half of the ring finger, except for the terminal part of the fingers which is supplied by the palmar digital branches of the ulnar nerve.

(ii) The **palmar (cutaneous) branch of the ulnar nerve** (C. 7, 8) arises in the distal half of the forearm, pierces the deep fascia anterior to the wrist, and supplies the medial third of the palmar skin.

(iii) Two **palmar digital nerves** (C. 7, 8) arise from the superficial branch of the ulnar nerve, distal to the pisiform bone. The medial nerve is the proper palmar digital nerve to the medial side of the little finger. The lateral nerve is a common palmar digital nerve which divides near the cleft between the little and ring fingers to give a proper palmar digital nerve to the contiguous sides of each. (Palmar and plantar digital nerves and arteries are called '**proper**' when each is distributed only to one finger or toe. The term '**common**' indicates that the nerve or artery is distributed to two adjacent fingers or toes as two proper digital branches.)

Cutaneous nerves from branches of the medial and lateral cords

(a) Cutaneous branches of the median nerve (C. 5, 6, 7 from the lateral cord; C. 8, T. 1 from the medial cord) which supply the skin in the hand [Figs. 5.8, 5.9, see also Fig.10.1]:

(i) The **palmar (cutaneous) branch** (C. 6, 7, 8) arises a little superior to the wrist, pierces the deep fascia just above it, and descends to supply the lateral two-thirds of the palmar skin.

(ii) Five **palmar digital branches** (C. 6, 7, 8) arise in the palm. The medial two are common palmar digital nerves. Each divides near the cleft on the medial and lateral aspects of the middle finger [see Fig. 8.10] to form a proper palmar digital nerve to each side of that cleft. The common palmar digital nerve to the ring and middle fingers communicates with the ulnar nerve. The next palmar digital nerve is the proper palmar digital nerve to the lateral side of the index finger. The lateral two nerves curve round the distal border of the thenar eminence as proper palmar digital nerves to the sides of the thumb. The proper palmar digital nerves not only supply the corresponding parts of the fingers, but also send branches to the dorsal skin on the middle and terminal phalanges.

Dissection 5.3 examines the palmar aponeurosis and the cutaneous nerves of the palm.

65

DISSECTION 5.3: Palmar aponeurosis and cutaneous nerves of the palm

Objectives

I. To examine the palmar aponeurosis. II. To identify and trace the common and proper palmar digital nerves, the dorsal branch of the ulnar nerve, and the superficial branch of the radial nerve.

Instructions

1. Expose the palmar aponeurosis by removing the superficial fascia from the palm. Follow it proximally into continuity with the deep fascia of the forearm and the palmaris longus tendon. Follow it distally to the slip which it sends to the palmar surface of each finger.

2. Look between these slips for the three common palmar digital nerves, and follow them and their branches (proper palmar digital nerves) into the fingers.

3. Identify and follow the proper palmar digital arteries which accompany the nerves.

4. Find the proper palmar digital nerve to the medial side of the little finger on the hypothenar eminence [see Fig. 8.5], and follow it distally.

5. Find the corresponding nerve to the lateral side of the index finger, immediately lateral to the slip of the palmar aponeurosis to that finger.

6. Find the digital nerves of the thumb at the distal margin of the thenar eminence [see Fig. 8.5], and trace them into the thumb.

7. Remove the fat from the medial side of the wrist, distal to the ulnar styloid process, and expose the dorsal branch of the ulnar nerve. Follow it and its dorsal

digital branches, thus confirming the presence of four digital nerves (two palmar and two dorsal) in the little finger, as in each of the digits.

8. Expose the deep fascia on the lateral surface of the lower end of the radius, and find the superficial branch of the radial nerve. Trace its branches to the thumb and fingers, and note its communication with the dorsal branch of the ulnar nerve.

Deep fascia of the upper limb

The following specializations of the deep fascia of the upper limb should be noted. On the dorsal surface of the scapula, a dense layer of fascia extends from the spine of the scapula to the margins of the infraspinous fossa [see Fig. 4.2]. Superolaterally, it splits to enclose the deltoid muscle.

In the arm, the deep fascia is strongest posteriorly where it covers the triceps muscle. Below the insertion of the deltoid, it is thickened on each side and sends strong **medial** and **lateral intermuscular septa** to the corresponding supracondylar lines and epicondyles of the humerus. These septa lie between the triceps muscle posteriorly and the muscles attached to the anterior surface of the distal half of the humerus [see Fig. 6.2].

At the elbow, the deep fascia is thickened by extensions from the triceps and biceps muscles, and by the origin of the forearm muscles from its deep surface. The **bicipital aponeurosis** is a strong slip which extends medially from the tendon of the biceps to the deep fascia and the subcutaneous posterior border of the ulna. The aponeurosis is readily felt by sliding a finger down the medial side of the taut biceps tendon.

The wrist has thickened bands of deep fascia attached to all the subcutaneous bony points (retinacula). The extensor retinaculum binds down the extensor tendons posteriorly and laterally. The flexor retinaculum binds down the flexor tendons and median nerve anteriorly. Both retinacula act as pulleys for the corresponding tendons which slide freely deep to them in synovial sheaths when the wrist is moved.

The **flexor retinaculum** is a strong band (approximately 2 × 2 cm) which is continuous with the deep fascia of the forearm at the distal flexor skin crease of the wrist. Proximally, it is attached to the tuberosity of the scaphoid and the pisiform bone. Distally, it is attached to the tubercle of the trapezium and the hook of the hamate bone, and is continuous with the palmar aponeurosis. It forms the anterior limit of the carpal tunnel. Its superficial surface gives the origin of the thenar and hypothenar muscles.

The **extensor retinaculum** extends from the lateral aspect and the styloid process of the radius to the ulna. Its deep surface is attached to the subcutaneous parts of these bones, and the space deep to it is divided into a number of compartments. The extensor tendons pass through these compartments [see Fig. 1.6]. Distally, the extensor retinaculum is continuous with the thin deep fascia of the dorsum of the hand which fuses, in its turn, with the extensor tendons of the fingers.

In the palm, the deep fascia is thin over the thenar and hypothenar eminences but is thickened between them to form the **palmar aponeurosis**. Distally, the palmar aponeurosis splits into slips passing to each finger. The edges of these slips turn back around the long flexor tendons of the finger, forming a tunnel around them [see Fig. 8.5]. This tunnel is continuous with a dense fibrous tunnel in the finger—the **fibrous flexor sheath**. The posterior margins of the fibrous flexor sheath are attached to the edges of the palmar surfaces of the phalanges. The sheath, along with the bone, produces a fibro-osseous tube, through which the long flexor tendons of the fingers pass to the phalanges. Within the fibrous flexor sheath, the tendons are enclosed in synovial sheaths to facilitate their movement.

See Clinical Applications 5.1 and 5.2 for the practical implications of the anatomy described in this chapter.

CLINICAL APPLICATION 5.1 Intravenous injections

The median cubital vein is most frequently utilized for venepuncture (taking of a blood sample, administering intravenous drugs, transfusing blood), because the vein is large, superficially located, and therefore easily seen and felt.

Study question 1: where is this vein located? (Answer: cubital fossa—superficial fascia.)

Study question 2: which two superficial veins does this vein connect? (Answer: cephalic and basilic.) Distension of these veins is accomplished by applying a tourniquet mid arm and by asking the patient to clench and unclench the fist.

Study question 3: which veins are compressed by the tourniquet at mid arm? (Answer: basilic vein and brachial veins.)

Known complications: thrombosis formation with occlusion of the injected vein is a common consequence of intravenous injection. This obliteration may be asymptomatic or may result in inflammation of the vein—phlebitis. Leakage of the injected drug could lead to injury of the lateral or medial cutaneous nerve of the forearm. Inadvertent puncture of the brachial artery is known to occur.

Study question 4: what firm structure normally separates the median cubital vein from the brachial artery? (Answer: bicipital aponeurosis.)

CLINICAL APPLICATION 5.2 Paraesthesiae over the shoulder

A 10-year-old boy was given an armpit crutch to help him walk after he fractured his right femur. A few days later, he complained of a sensation of numbness and tingling over the outer part of his right shoulder and lateral side of his right upper arm.

Study question 1: what is the sensory innervation to the affected area? (Answer: the upper lateral cutaneous nerve

of the arm, a branch of the axillary nerve.)

Study question 2: what nerve is likely to be compressed? (Answer: axillary nerve.)

Study question 3: what is the probable cause of the injury? (Answer: pressure on the axillary nerve due to improper use of the armpit crutch.)

CHAPTER 6
The shoulder

Surface anatomy

Begin by reviewing the scapula and proximal part of the humerus [see Figs. 4.2, 4.3, 5.1].

Make use of the dried bone to identify the parts of the scapula. The **scapula** is a thin triangular plate of bone which lies at a tangent to the posterolateral surface of the thorax. It has a long, slightly thickened medial border which meets the thin, concave superior border at the **superior angle** and the markedly thickened lateral border (margin) at the **inferior angle**. The lateral angle is the thickest part of the bone. It is truncated (the apex of the angle is cut), so that the end forms the shallow, pear-shaped **glenoid cavity**. The glenoid cavity is continuous with the rest of the scapula through the **neck of the scapula** and faces anterolaterally to articulate with the hemispherical head of the humerus.

The **coracoid** is a thick buttress which extends anterosuperiorly from the neck of the scapula and the upper part of the glenoid cavity to end in the **coracoid process**. The **scapular notch** separates the coracoid laterally from the remainder of the superior border.

The dorsal surface of the scapula is divided into **supraspinous** and **infraspinous fossae** by the **spine of the scapula**. The spine runs from the medial border of the scapula to its neck and increases in height laterally. The posterior surface of the spine (**crest of the spine**) widens laterally to become the flattened **acromion** which projects forwards at the palpable **acromial angle** [see Fig. 4.2]. The acromion and coracoid form two parts of an incomplete bony arch above

the glenoid cavity and the head of the humerus which articulates with it. This **coracoacromial arch** is completed by the **coracoacromial ligament**. Above the coracoacromial ligament, the lateral end of the clavicle articulates with the acromion.

The clavicle is attached to the coracoid process through the powerful **coracoclavicular ligaments**. The acromion and the coracoid process arch forwards, each leaving a space beneath. The subscapularis passes from the subscapular fossa of the scapula beneath the coracoid process. The supraspinatus passes from the supraspinous fossa beneath the acromion. The thick **lateral border of the scapula** gives attachment to the two teres muscles which also pass to the humerus.

The expanded proximal end of the **humerus** consists of the hemispherical articular **head**, which faces medially, upwards, and backwards. The remainder of the expanded end is formed by two **tubercles**—the greater tubercle faces laterally, the lesser tubercle anteriorly. The tubercles are separated from each other by the intertubercular sulcus. This sulcus transmits the tendon of the long head of the biceps muscle which arises from the **supraglenoid tubercle**. The intertubercular sulcus continues inferiorly on the surgical neck and upper part of the body of the humerus as a shallow groove bounded by the **medial** and **lateral lips of the intertubercular sulcus** [see Fig. 5.1]. The lateral lip of the intertubercular sulcus is continuous inferiorly with the anterior limb of the V-shaped **deltoid tuberosity**. The lesser tubercle is the site of insertion of the subscapularis. The greater tubercle has three facets (superior, posterosuperior, and posterior) for the insertion of the supraspinatus, infraspinatus, and teres minor, respectively. The greater and lesser tubercles are separated from the head by a shallow sulcus, the **anatomical neck**. The upper end of the humerus is separated from the body by the **surgical neck**.

Muscles attaching the humerus to the scapula

Muscles attaching the humerus to the scapula are best described in two groups:

(a) Those which have considerable mechanical advantage over the shoulder joint by being attached at some distance from it—deltoid, teres major, coracobrachialis, and biceps brachii (short head).

(b) Those which lie close to the shoulder joint and have a smaller mechanical advantage over it. They help to stabilize the joint in any position and act as the main ligaments of the joint—subscapularis, supraspinatus, infraspinatus, teres minor, and the long heads of the biceps and triceps brachii.

Deltoid

This large muscle forms the bulge of the shoulder. It takes origin from the lateral third of the clavicle, acromion, and spine of the scapula [see Fig. 4.5] and is inserted into the deltoid tuberosity of the humerus [Figs. 6.1, 6.2, 6.3]. **Nerve supply**: axillary nerve. **Actions**: the anterior fibres flex and medially rotate the shoulder; the middle fibres abduct the shoulder, and the posterior fibres extend and laterally rotate the shoulder.

Subscapularis

The subscapularis originates from a wide area on the costal surface of the scapula [see Fig. 4.3]. It is inserted on the lesser tubercle of the humerus [Fig. 6.2]. The fibres fuse with the capsule of the shoulder joint and are separated from it and the lateral part of the costal surface of the scapula by the subscapular bursa [Fig. 6.4]. The subscapular bursa frequently communicates with the cavity of the shoulder joint. **Nerve supply**: upper and lower subscapular nerves. **Actions**: medial rotation

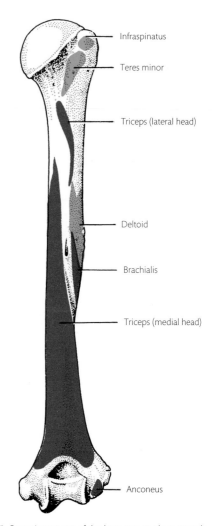

Fig. 6.1 Posterior aspect of the humerus to show muscle attachments.

of the shoulder. Plays an important role in stabilizing the shoulder joint.

Supraspinatus

The supraspinatus arises from the supraspinous fossa of the scapula and is inserted on the superior facet on the greater tubercle of the humerus [see Figs. 4.6, 6.2]. Its fibres pass under the coracoacromial ligament. **Nerve supply**: suprascapular nerve. **Action**: abduction of the shoulder joint.

Infraspinatus

The infraspinatus arises from the infraspinous fossa of the scapula and is inserted on the middle facet on the greater tubercle of the humerus [see Figs. 4.6, 6.1]. **Nerve supply**: suprascapular nerve. **Action**: lateral rotation of the shoulder joint.

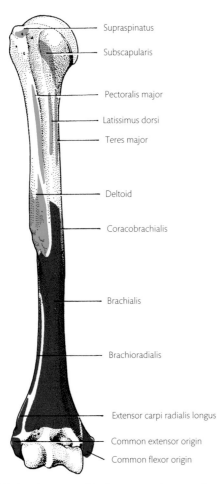

Fig. 6.2 Anterior aspect of the humerus to show muscle attachments.

Supraspinatus
Subscapularis
Pectoralis major
Latissimus dorsi
Teres major
Deltoid
Coracobrachialis
Brachialis
Brachioradialis
Extensor carpi radialis longus
Common extensor origin
Common flexor origin

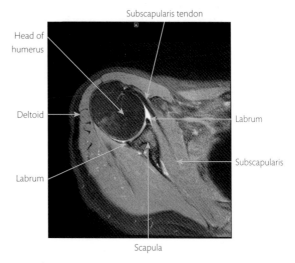

Lateral end of clavicle
Cephalic V.
Deltoid
Cutaneous branches of axillary N.
Upper lateral cutaneous N. of arm
Lateral head of triceps
Brachialis
Lower lateral cutaneous N. of arm
Posterior cutaneous N. of forearm
Brachioradialis
Tendon of triceps
Olecranon
Extensor carpi radialis longus

Fig. 6.3 Deltoid muscle and lateral aspect of the arm.

Teres major

The teres major takes origin from the lateral one-third of the lateral margin of the scapula. Its fibres pass to the anterior surface of the humerus and are inserted into the medial lip of the intertubercular sulcus [see Figs. 4.6, 6.2]. The lower margin is closely related to the latissimus dorsi and forms the posterior axillary fold. **Nerve supply**: lower subscapular nerve. **Actions**: adduction and medial rotation of the shoulder joint.

Teres minor

The teres minor takes origin from the superior two-thirds of the lateral margin of the scapula and is inserted into the posterior facet on the greater tubercle of the humerus [see Figs. 4.6, 6.1]. **Nerve supply**: axillary nerve. **Actions**: lateral rotation and stabilization of the shoulder joint.

Subscapularis tendon
Head of humerus
Deltoid
Labrum
Labrum
Subscapularis
Scapula

Fig. 6.4 MR axial image of the shoulder.

DISSECTION 6.1 Shoulder region-1

Objectives

I. To study the deltoid, infraspinatus, teres minor, and long head of the triceps, and to identify the boundaries of the quadrangular and triangular spaces.   II. To identify and trace the axillary and radial nerves.

Instructions

1. Remove the fascia from the surface of the **deltoid muscle**, and study its attachments. It has a V-shaped origin from the lateral third of the clavicle, the acromion, and the crest of the spine of the scapula. It is inserted into the deltoid tuberosity of the humerus. Note that the long anterior and posterior fibres run parallel to each other on the corresponding surfaces of the shoulder joint. The lateral fibres are short and multipennate to increase the power of this part.

2. Separate the muscle from the spine of the scapula, and turn this part downwards to expose the underlying **infraspinatus muscle**. Remove the dense deep fascia from the surface of the **infraspinatus**. Define its attachments to the infraspinous fossa and the greater tubercle of the humerus.

3. Find the inferior border of the infraspinatus, and separate it from the **teres major** and the **minor muscles** which arise from the lateral margin of the scapula.

4. Turn the detached part of the deltoid forwards; identify the **axillary nerve** (from which the upper lateral cutaneous nerve of the arm arises) and the posterior humeral circumflex vessels supplying its deep surface.

5. Trace these on the surgical neck of the humerus through the **quadrangular space** [Fig. 6.5], inferior to the teres minor and the articular capsule of the shoulder joint.

6. Expose the **long head of the triceps** medial to the quadrangular space. It descends from the **infraglenoid tubercle** of the scapula and passes between the teres minor and the major muscles close to the humerus.

7. Find the branch of the axillary nerve to the **teres minor**, and follow this muscle to its attachments separating it from the teres major.

8. Divide the remainder of the **deltoid** from the acromion and clavicle, and turn it downwards. It lies on the proximal end and surgical neck of the humerus, superficial to the anastomosis of the circumflex humeral vessels [Fig. 6.6].

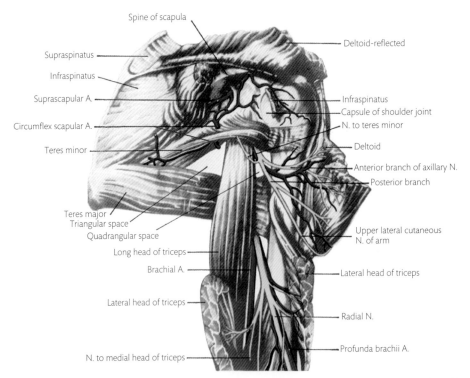

Spine of scapula
Supraspinatus
Infraspinatus
Suprascapular A.
Circumflex scapular A.
Teres minor
Teres major
Triangular space
Quadrangular space
Long head of triceps
Brachial A.
Lateral head of triceps
N. to medial head of triceps
Deltoid-reflected
Infraspinatus
Capsule of shoulder joint
N. to teres minor
Deltoid
Anterior branch of axillary N.
Posterior branch
Upper lateral cutaneous N. of arm
Lateral head of triceps
Radial N.
Profunda brachii A.

Fig. 6.5 Dissection of the scapular region and back of the arm showing the quadrangular and triangular spaces. The lateral head of the triceps has been divided and turned aside to expose the spiral groove on the humerus.

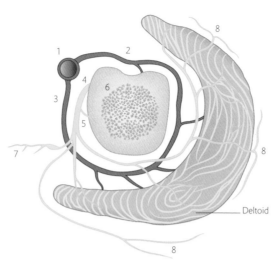

Fig. 6.6 Diagram of the circumflex humeral arteries and axillary nerve. 1. Axillary artery. 2. Anterior circumflex humeral artery. 3. Posterior circumflex humeral artery. 4. Axillary nerve. 5. Articular branch. 6. Humerus. 7. Branch to teres minor. 8. Cutaneous branches.

Dissection 6.1 explores the shoulder region.

Dissection 6.2 continues to explore the shoulder region.

DISSECTION 6.2 Shoulder region-2

Objectives

I. To study the teres major, coracobrachialis, short head of biceps and subscapularis. II. To identify and trace the axillary and radial nerve. III. To explore the subacromial and subscapular bursa.

Instructions

1. On the anterior surface of the scapula, follow the **subscapularis muscle** from the subscapular fossa to the lesser tubercle [Fig. 6.7].

2. Separate it inferiorly from the **teres major**, and trace that muscle to its insertion on the medial lip of the intertubercular crest of the humerus immediately behind the insertion of the **latissimus dorsi**. Both these insertions are lateral to the coracobrachialis and the short head of the biceps which descend in front of them from the coracoid process.

3. Find the **axillary nerve** arising from the posterior cord of the brachial plexus, and follow it to the quadrangular space which, when seen from the front, is between the subscapularis and teres major.

4. Identify the **radial nerve** as it arises from the posterior cord. It descends between the parts of the triceps muscle, after giving branches to the long and medial heads [Fig. 6.5].

5. Remove the fascia covering the **coracobrachialis** and the **short head of the biceps** from the coracoid process to the insertion of the coracobrachialis on the medial aspect of the body of the humerus.

6. Follow the **musculocutaneous nerve** from the lateral cord of the brachial plexus into the medial aspect of the coracobrachialis, and find the branch which it gives to that muscle.

7. Pull these muscles medially, and identify the tendon of the **long head of the biceps**. It lies in the intertubercular sulcus posterolateral to the short head. Follow the long head upwards to the lower border of the lesser tubercle where it disappears deep to the articular capsule of the shoulder joint.

8. Move the fascia covering the superior surface of the greater tubercle of the humerus. It slides easily on the tubercle because of the **subacromial bursa** deep to the fascia.

9. Make a small incision into the bursa, and explore its limits with a blunt seeker. Then open it widely. The bursa separates the superior surface of the humerus and the capsule of the shoulder joint from the acromion and coracoacromial ligament, and makes a secondary synovial socket for the humerus with the coracoacromial arch.

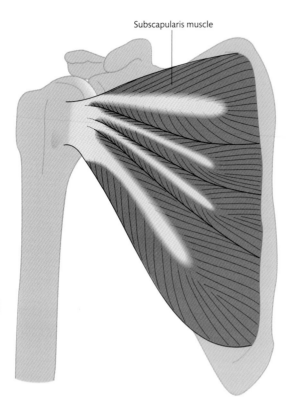

Subscapularis muscle

Fig. 6.7 Diagram showing the attachments of the subscapularis.

Axillary nerve (C. 5, 6)

The axillary nerve is a terminal branch of the posterior cord of the brachial plexus and is formed near the lower border of the subscapularis. It curves back on the lower border of the subscapularis and passes through the quadrangular space with the posterior circumflex humeral artery. It lies medial to the surgical neck of the humerus, immediately inferior to the capsule of the shoulder joint. The nerve gives a branch to the **shoulder joint** and then divides into anterior and posterior branches.

The **posterior branch** supplies the teres minor and the posterior part of the deltoid. It then descends over the posterior border of the deltoid and supplies the skin over the lower half of that muscle as the **upper lateral cutaneous nerve of the arm** [see Fig. 5.8].

The **anterior branch** continues horizontally between the deltoid muscle and the surgical neck of the humerus. It supplies the deltoid and sends a few branches through it to the overlying skin.

➲ The axillary nerve is at risk in downward dislocation of the head of the humerus and in fractures of the surgical neck of the humerus because of its close relation to the joint and the bone [see Fig. 6.11]. When it is damaged, the deltoid and teres minor muscles are paralysed.

Circumflex humeral arteries

The anterior and posterior circumflex humeral arteries are branches of the third part of the axillary artery. Together they form a circular anastomosis at the surgical neck of the humerus [Fig. 6.6]. They supply the surrounding muscles, the shoulder joint, and the upper end of the humerus. They also anastomose with the profunda brachii artery by a descending branch.

Dissection 6.3 continues to explore the shoulder region.

DISSECTION 6.3 Shoulder region-3

Objectives

I. To study the supraspinatus and infraspinatus. II. To identify and trace the suprascapular nerve, suprascapular artery, and circumflex scapular artery. III. To study the coracoacromial ligament, and subacromial and subscapular bursae. IV. To study the acromioclavicular joint.

Instructions

1. Remove the subacromial bursa, and expose the **supraspinatus** passing from the supraspinous fossa, beneath the coracoacromial arch and bursa, to the superior surface of the greater tubercle. The tendon of the supraspinatus is firmly fused to this part of the capsule of the shoulder joint [Fig. 6.8].

2. Cut across the infraspinatus and teres minor muscles at the level of the neck of the scapula. Turn their parts medially and laterally [Fig. 6.9].

3. Find the **suprascapular** and **circumflex scapular arteries** passing deep to the muscles and anastomosing on the posterior surface of the scapula [Fig. 6.9].

4. Find the **suprascapular nerve** as it enters the deep surface of the infraspinatus from the supraspinatus.

The tendons of the teres minor and infraspinatus fuse with the capsule of the shoulder joint as they pass to the greater tubercle of the humerus. There may be a bursa deep to the tendon of the infraspinatus, and this may communicate with the cavity of the shoulder joint [Fig. 6.8].

5. Follow the tendon of the **long head of the triceps** to its attachment on the infraglenoid tubercle, and find the dependent part of the capsule of the shoulder joint lateral to it. The **axillary nerve** passes posteriorly on the surgical neck of the humerus, immediately inferior to this part of the capsule, and sends a branch to it.

6. Cut across the **subscapularis** at the neck of the scapula, and reflect its parts. Laterally, it is fused with the capsule of the shoulder joint. Medially, it is separated from the neck of the scapula and the root of the coracoid process by the **subscapular bursa**. This bursa facilitates movement of the muscle over these bony structures. It communicates with the cavity of the shoulder joint through an aperture in its capsule [Fig. 6.10].

7. Remove the trapezius and the remainder of the deltoid from the capsule of the acromioclavicular joint.

8. Cut away the superior part of the capsule (acromioclavicular ligament) of this joint, and note the articular disc separating the two bones.

9. Identify the **suprascapular artery** and **nerve** crossing the superior margin of the scapula at the scapular notch [Fig. 6.9].

Suprascapular nerve (C. 5, 6)

The suprascapular nerve arises from the upper trunk of the brachial plexus [see Fig. 3.21]. It passes downwards and backwards, superior to the plexus, to join the suprascapular vessels. It enters the supraspinous fossa through the scapular notch. Here it supplies the supraspinatus and gives branches to the acromioclavicular and shoulder joints. The nerve then descends immediately lateral to the root of the spine of the scapula to enter the infraspinous fossa and supply the infraspinatus and shoulder joint.

Suprascapular artery

The suprascapular artery arises from the first branch of the subclavian artery. It enters the supraspinous fossa of the scapula above the scapular ligament,

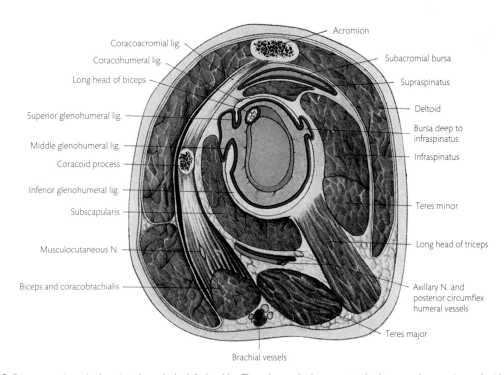

Fig. 6.8 Diagrammatic sagittal section through the left shoulder. The subscapular bursa protrudes between the superior and middle glenohumeral ligaments.

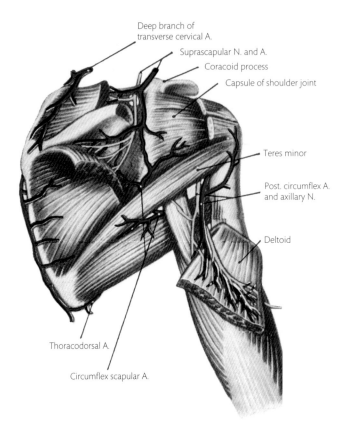

Fig. 6.9 Anastomosing arteries around the scapula. The acromion has been removed to expose the suprascapular artery and nerve.

and runs deep to, and supplies, the supraspinatus. It then passes through the spinoglenoid notch and supplies the infraspinatus. It anastomoses with the circumflex scapular artery and with branches of the transverse cervical artery.

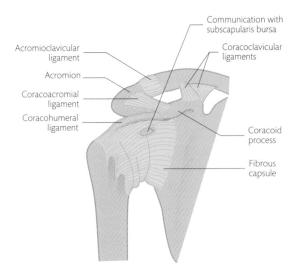

Fig. 6.10 Diagram of the anterior aspect of the right shoulder joint, showing the fibrous capsule, coracoacromial arch, and the coracoclavicular ligaments.

Coracoacromial ligament

The **coracoacromial ligament** is a strong triangular band. Its base is attached to the lateral border of the coracoid process, and its apex to the tip of the acromion. It lies between the subacromial bursa inferiorly and the deltoid muscle superiorly [Fig. 6.10].

Coracoclavicular ligament

The powerful **coracoclavicular ligament** passes between the upper surface of the coracoid process and the clavicle. It has two parts. The posteromedial part is the **conoid ligament**. It is shaped like an inverted cone and is attached above to the **conoid tubercle** of the clavicle [see Figs. 3.4, 6.10]. The anterolateral triangular part is the **trapezoid ligament**. It passes superolaterally to the trapezoid line on the clavicle. The coracoclavicular ligament is the main structure suspending the scapula and hence the upper limb from the clavicle. It supports the acromioclavicular joint and helps to transmit forces from the upper limb to the trunk. ⟳ If the clavicle is broken medial to this ligament, the upper limb sags—a sign characteristic of this fracture.

Shoulder joint

The disproportionately large head of the humerus, the small, shallow glenoid cavity, and the loose articular capsule gives the shoulder joint a wide range of movements but make the joint inherently unstable [see Fig. 6.12]. This instability is overcome by the powerful muscles which closely surround the joint [Figs. 6.4, 6.8]. These muscles support the joint in any position, without restricting movement which ligaments would do. However, there is an increased risk of displacement of the head of the humerus from the glenoid cavity (dislocation) when the joint is suddenly pulled upon. This displacement frequently occurs through the lower part of the joint capsule which is inadequately supported by the long head of the triceps. This inferior

dislocation of the humeral head can result in damage to the adjacent axillary nerve.

Articular capsule

The outer **fibrous membrane** of the articular capsule is a thin, but relatively strong, tubular structure. It is attached to the margin of the glenoid cavity and to the anatomical neck of the humerus, except inferiorly where it extends downwards 1.5–2.0 cm on the surgical neck of the bone [Fig. 6.11]. With the arm by the side, this inferior part of the membrane hangs down in a redundant fold between the teres major and minor muscles. When the arm is abducted to a right angle, this fold is tensed. In the latter position, the lower part of the articular surface of the humeral head lies on this part of the articular capsule, with the long head of the triceps and the teres major muscles supporting it below. Anteriorly, the attachment of the fibrous membrane extends inferiorly (from the anatomical neck) between the tubercles of the humerus bridging over the upper part of the intertubercular sulcus. Deep to it is a synovial-lined tunnel, through which the tendon of the long head of

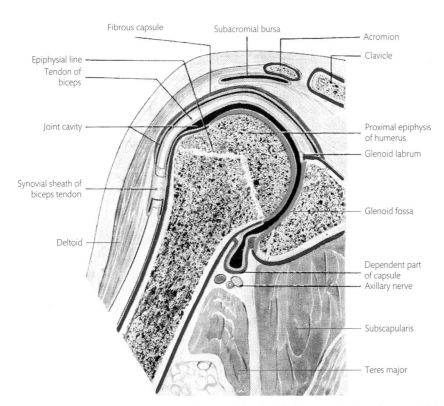

Fig. 6.11 Coronal section through the right shoulder joint. The synovial sheath of the biceps tendon have been partially left in place. Periosteum, red. Articular cartilage, blue.

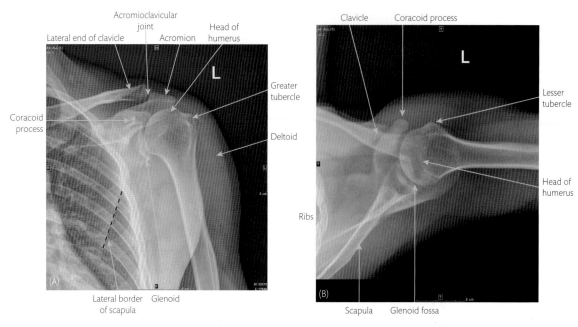

Acromioclavicular joint
Lateral end of clavicle
Acromion
Head of humerus
Coracoid process
Greater tubercle
Deltoid
Lateral border of scapula
Glenoid

L

Clavicle
Coracoid process
Lesser tubercle
Head of humerus
Ribs
Scapula
Glenoid fossa

(A)
(B)

Fig. 6.12 Plain radiographs of the shoulder. (A) Arm is adducted at the shoulder. (B) Superoinferior (axial) view.

the biceps muscle leaves the joint. This is one of three apertures in the fibrous membrane; the other two are extensions of the synovial membrane through the fibrous membrane to form the subscapular and infraspinatus bursae. The **subscapular bursa** is large and more constant. It lies close to the root of the coracoid process and occasionally allows dislocation of the head of the humerus at this point.

There are four slight thickenings of the articular capsule: (1) the **coracohumeral ligament** lies obliquely across the upper surface of the joint from the base of the coracoid process to the superior surface of the greater tubercle of the humerus;

and (2) two or three **glenohumeral ligaments** [see Fig. 6.13] may be visible as thickenings of the anterior part of the membrane, when viewed from the interior of the joint.

The **synovial membrane** lines the fibrous capsule and covers the intracapsular part of the surgical neck of the humerus. The synovial membrane also forms a sheath around the tendon of the long head of the biceps and is continuous with the lining of the bursae which communicate with the joint.

The **nerve supply** of the shoulder joint is by the axillary, suprascapular, and lateral pectoral nerves.

Dissection 6.4 studies the intracapsular parts of the shoulder joint.

DISSECTION 6.4 Shoulder joint

Objective

I. To study the intracapsular parts of the shoulder joint.

Instructions

1. Most of the surface of the thin capsule has already been exposed by the removal of the muscles which closely surround it. These muscles are partly fused to the fibrous membrane, so that they prevent it from passing between the joint surfaces when they contract.

2. Make a vertical incision through the posterior part of the articular capsule of the shoulder joint. Rotate the arm medially, and dislocate the head of the humerus through the cut in the capsule.

3. Identify the **tendon of the long head of the biceps** passing over the superior surface of the head of the humerus within the capsule to reach the supraglenoid tubercle [see Fig. 6.13]. Note that it becomes continuous here with a fibrocartilaginous ring, the **glenoid labrum**. Identify the glenoid labrum which is attached

to the margin of the glenoid cavity and the internal surface of the articular capsule. By surrounding the glenoid cavity, the labrum deepens it.

4. Try to expose the glenohumeral ligaments on the deep surface of the anterior part of the capsule, and note the aperture of the subscapular bursa between them. If necessary, cut through the tendon of the long head of the biceps to increase the mobility of the humerus.

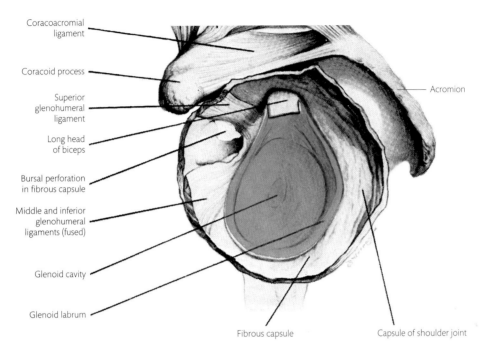

Coracoacromial ligament

Coracoid process

Superior glenohumeral ligament

Long head of biceps

Bursal perforation in fibrous capsule

Middle and inferior glenohumeral ligaments (fused)

Glenoid cavity

Glenoid labrum

Acromion

Fibrous capsule

Capsule of shoulder joint

Fig. 6.13 Left shoulder joint. The articular capsule has been cut across and the humerus removed, together with the surrounding muscles. Articular cartilage and glenoid labrum, blue.

Movements of the limb at the shoulder joint

(Note that movements of the scapula described in Chapter 4 are different from movements of the shoulder joint. The two are associated but should not be confused.)

The wide range of movements which is possible at the shoulder joint is the result of: (1) the nature of the articular surfaces (the large hemispherical head of the humerus fitted to the small, shallow glenoid cavity); (2) a loose-fitting articular capsule; and (3) the replacement of ligaments by a group of muscles. The **glenoid cavity** faces anterolaterally at rest, and its plane is parallel to the axis around which the scapula is rotated in movements of the shoulder girdle. Movement of the shoulder joint can take place independently but is usually accompanied by movements of the shoulder girdle. Even when the scapula is not moved, the muscles would be in tension to maintain a stable scapula on which the limb may be moved.

Flexion

Flexion is carried out by muscles which pass anterior to the shoulder joint (the short head of the biceps, the coracobrachialis, and the clavicular parts of the deltoid and pectoralis major), but the arm can be flexed to the horizontal position only if the inferior angle of the scapula is also pulled forwards on the chest wall (lateral rotation) by the **serratus anterior**, thus turning the glenoid cavity upwards.

Extension

Two sets of muscles extend the shoulder. Extension of the shoulder from the anatomical position is restricted and produced by the posterior fibres of the **deltoid**, assisted initially by the latissimus dorsi. Further extension is completed by elevation of the scapula on the convex thoracic wall by the trapezius and levator scapulae. Extension of the flexed shoulder joint back to the anatomical position against resistance is produced by the latissimus dorsi, the teres major, and the sternocostal part of the pectoralis major, assisted by the rhomboid major and pectoralis minor, both of which rotate the scapula medially.

Abduction

Abduction [Fig. 6.12A] is produced by the middle fibres of the **deltoid** and by the **supraspinatus**, both of which pass superior to the joint. The supraspinatus is responsible for initiating the movement. While the deltoid is contracting, simultaneous contraction of the teres minor and the lower fibres of the subscapularis prevent the humerus from being pulled up against the coracoacromial arch [Fig. 6.13]. The deltoid can abduct the humerus on the scapula to the horizontal, but this movement is associated from the beginning with the **lateral rotation of the scapula** [Fig. 6.14A]. Lateral rotation of the scapula (produced by the serratus anterior and trapezius) permits the humerus to be carried upwards to the vertical position, by turning the glenoid cavity to face superiorly. To confirm this, note the elevation of the shoulder and the lateral projection of the inferior angle of the scapula in full abduction in the living.

Adduction

Adduction against resistance of the arm abducted above the head is first produced by the **latissimus dorsi** and the lowest sternocostal fibres of the **pectoralis major**, and is assisted by the teres major and the medial rotators of the scapula [Fig. 6.14B]. Once the horizontal position has been passed, progressively higher fibres of the pectoralis major are involved. When this movement is not resisted, the muscles which are active in abduction act eccentrically to control the pull of gravity on the limb. This situation is common to every movement where gravity is the driving force. It can be demonstrated in the shoulder by the continuing firmness

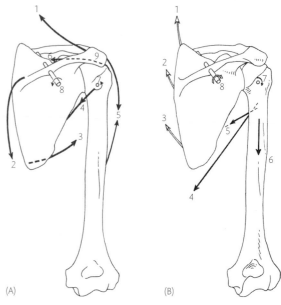

Fig. 6.14 Diagrams to show the direction of pull of muscles producing (A) abduction and (B) adduction of the arm. 7 = axis of abduction of the humerus. 8 = axis of scapular rotation. (A) Abduction of the arm. This action requires two separate movements: (i) lateral rotation of the scapula by the (1) upper and (2) lower fibres of the trapezius, and (3) lower fibres of the serratus anterior; (ii) abduction at the shoulder joint by (5) the deltoid, and (6) the supraspinatus. When the deltoid contracts, it tends to pull the humerus upwards against the acromion (9). This action is counteracted by the teres minor (4). (B) Adduction of the arm. This movement is normally produced by gravity (6). In this case, the arm is lowered to the side by the muscles which produce abduction. When adduction is produced against resistance, two separate movements are involved: (i) medial rotation of the scapula by (1) levator scapulae, (2) rhomboid minor, and (3) rhomboid major; (ii) adduction of the humerus by (5) teres major, (4) latissimus dorsi, and pectoralis major (not shown).

(contraction) of the deltoid as the arm is lowered to the side and its immediate flaccidity when the movement encounters resistance.

Medial and lateral rotation of the humerus

Medial and lateral rotation of the shoulder may occur in any position but are best demonstrated with the arm by the side and the elbow flexed at right angle. The hand can then be swung laterally (lateral rotation of the humerus) or medially (medial rotation of the humerus). In this position, medial rotation is produced by muscles passing to the front of the humerus from the trunk (pectoralis major, latissimus dorsi, subscapularis, teres major, anterior fibres of the deltoid). Lateral rotation results from the contraction of muscles passing to the back of the humerus from the trunk (infraspinatus, teres minor, and posterior fibres of the deltoid).

Muscles, movements, and nerves of the shoulder joint

The action of a muscle crossing the shoulder joint can be predicted not only from its origin and insertion, but also from its relation to the shoulder joint. These details, along with the nerve supply to the muscle, are shown in Table 6.1. In Table 6.2, the muscles are grouped according to their action on the shoulder joint, and the nerve supply of each muscle is repeated. This allows an easy assessment of the degree of paralysis of a particular movement following destruction of a particular nerve. (The tables show only the actions of a particular muscle when it actively shortens.)

→ Axillary nerve injury and the resultant paralysis of the deltoid and teres minor severely affect

Table 6.1 Muscles acting on the shoulder joint

Muscle	Origin	Insertion	Relation to joint	Action	Nerve supply
Pectoralis major	Clavicle, medial two-thirds	Humerus, lateral lip of intertubercular sulcus	Anterior	Flexion and medial rotation	Medial and lateral pectoral nerves
	Sternum Costal cartilages 1–6	Humerus, lateral lip of intertubercular sulcus	Anterior	Adduction and medial rotation	Medial and lateral pectoral nerves
Latissimus dorsi	Lower ribs Thoracolumbar fascia Iliac crest	Humerus, intertubercular sulcus	Inferior	Adduction, medial rotation, extension if flexed	Thoracodorsal nerve
Deltoid	Clavicle, lateral one-third	Humerus, deltoid tuberosity	Anterior	Flexion and medial rotation	Axillary nerve
	Scapula, acromion, spine	Humerus, deltoid tuberosity	Superior Posterior	Abduction, extension, lateral rotation	Axillary nerve
Biceps brachii short head	Scapula, coracoid process	Radius	Anterior	Flexion Stabilization	Musculocutaneous nerve
Biceps brachii, long head	Scapula, supraglenoid tubercle	Radius	Anterior	Flexion Stabilization	Musculocutaneous nerve
Coracobrachialis	Scapula, coracoid process	Humerus, middle of body medially	Anterior	Flexion	Musculocutaneous nerve
Teres major	Scapula, lateral margin inferior one-third	Humerus, medial lip of intertubercular sulcus	Inferior	Adduction, medial rotation	Lower subscapular nerve
Supraspinatus	Scapula, supraspinous fossa	Humerus, greater tubercle superior surface	Superior	Abduction, stabilization	Suprascapular nerve
Infraspinatus	Scapula, infraspinous fossa	Humerus, greater tubercle posterosuperior surface	Posterior	Lateral rotation, stabilization	Suprascapular nerve
Teres minor	Scapula, lateral margin superior two-thirds	Humerus, greater tubercle posterior surface	Posterior	Lateral rotation, stabilization*	Axillary nerve
Subscapularis	Scapula, subscapular fossa	Humerus, lesser tubercle	Anterior	Medial rotation, stabilization*	Upper and lower subscapular nerves
Triceps, long head	Scapula, infraglenoid tubercle	Ulna, olecranon process	Inferior	Stabilization	Radial nerve

* These muscles stabilize the shoulder joint in abduction and prevent the head of the humerus from rising in the glenoid and hitting on the acromion when the deltoid contracts.

Table 6.2 Movements at the shoulder joint

Movement	Muscles	Nerve supply
Flexion	Pectoralis major, clavicular part	Pectoral nerves
	Deltoid, clavicular part	Axillary
	Biceps, short head	Musculocutaneous
	Coracobrachialis	Musculocutaneous
Extension	Deltoid, posterior part	Axillary
	Latissimus dorsi (if shoulder flexed)	Thoracodorsal
	Teres major (if shoulder flexed)	Subscapular
Abduction	Deltoid, acromial part	Axillary
	Supraspinatus	Suprascapular
Adduction	Pectoralis major, sternocostal part	Pectoral
	Latissimus dorsi	Thoracodorsal
	Teres major	Subscapular
Lateral rotation of humerus	Deltoid, posterior part	Axillary
	Infraspinatus	Suprascapular
	Teres minor	Axillary
Medial rotation of humerus	Pectoralis major	Pectoral
	Latissimus dorsi	Thoracodorsal
	Deltoid, clavicular part	Axillary
	Teres major	Subscapular
	Subscapularis	Subscapular
Stabilization*	Subscapularis	Subscapular
	Supraspinatus	Suprascapular
	Infraspinatus	Suprascapular
	Teres minor	Axillary
	Triceps, long head	Radial
	Biceps, long head	Musculocutaneous

The actions of muscles shown in Table 6.2 presuppose a fixed scapula.

* All the muscles of stabilization are attached close to the shoulder joint, have a poor mechanical advantage over it, and are more effective in holding the joint surfaces together than in moving it.

shoulder abduction, extension, and lateral rotation. In such an injury, the arm is held in a position of adduction, medial rotation, and flexion.

See Clinical Applications 6.1 and 6.2 for the practical implications of the anatomy in this chapter.

CLINICAL APPLICATION 6.1 Anastomosis around the scapula

Arteries supplying the muscles on the dorsal surface of the scapula come from two distinct sources. The dorsal scapular artery and the suprascapular artery are branches of the thyrocervical trunk of the subclavian artery. The posterior circumflex humeral artery and the circumflex scapular arteries are branches of the axillary artery. The anastomosis around the scapula [Fig. 6.9] ensures that the mobile scapula is not dependent on only one source.

The anastomosis forms an alternate route through which blood from the first part of the subclavian artery can reach the third part of the axillary artery when the main stem is blocked between these two points. Note that slow occlusion will allow time for collateral circulation to be established. Sudden occlusion is more dangerous, as the collateral circulation may not be ready to take over the increased supply.

CLINICAL APPLICATION 6.2 Rotator cuff injury

A young swimmer came to the doctor with a history of sudden pain in the right shoulder, and inability to sleep on the injured side. After examining the patient, a diagnosis of rotator cuff injury was made.

Study question 1: what are the muscles which form the 'rotator cuff'? (Answer: supraspinatus, infraspinatus, teres minor and subscapularis.)

Study question 2: apart from the movement these muscles bring about at the shoulder, what is the other important function they perform? (Answer: they act as expansile ligaments of the shoulder joint and steady it.) The doctor suspects injury to the supraspinatus.

Study question 3: where is the supraspinatus inserted? What is its action? Under which bony projection does the tendon pass? (Answer: it is inserted into the upper facet on the greater tubercle and produces abduction of shoulder. The tendon passes under the acromion process of the scapula.)

CHAPTER 7
The arm

The deep fascia enclosing the arm sends septa between the groups of muscles to allow them to slide on each other and to give an increased area for origin. Two of these septa—the lateral and medial intermuscular septa—pass to the corresponding supracondylar lines and epicondyles of the humerus, thus dividing the distal part of the arm into anterior and posterior compartments [Fig. 7.1].

Anterior compartment

See Dissection 7.1 for an exploration of the anatomy of the front of the arm.

Biceps brachii and coracobrachialis

The biceps brachii muscle arises from the scapula by two heads—the long and short head. The **short head** arises with the coracobrachialis from the coracoid process. The **long head** of the biceps arises from the supraglenoid tubercle within the shoulder joint. Its tendon runs on the superior surface to the head of the humerus and emerges from the joint through the intertubercular groove. The two heads of the biceps fuse in the distal third of the arm and form a short tendon which passes to the posterior surface of the tuberosity of the radius [see Fig. 7.4]. The biceps tendon also gives off

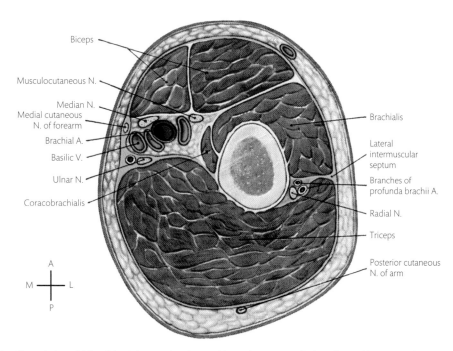

Biceps
Musculocutaneous N.
Median N.
Medial cutaneous N. of forearm
Brachial A.
Basilic V.
Ulnar N.
Coracobrachialis
Brachialis
Lateral intermuscular septum
Branches of profunda brachii A.
Radial N.
Triceps
Posterior cutaneous N. of arm

A
M — L
P

Fig. 7.1 Section through the middle of the right arm showing positions of neurovascular bundles and intermuscular septa. A = anterior; P = posterior; M = medial; L = lateral.

Objectives

I. To study the muscles of the front of the arm.   II. To identify and trace the musculocutaneous, median, and ulnar nerves in the front of the arm.   III. To identify the muscles arising from the lateral supracondylar ridge, the radial nerve, and the profunda brachii artery on the lateral side of the elbow.

Instructions

1. Cut vertically through the deep fascia on the anterior surface of the arm, as far as the elbow. Cut transversely through it at the elbow. Reflect the flaps to uncover the biceps brachii.

2. Lift the biceps brachii, and find the musculocutaneous nerve. Separate the biceps brachii from the brachialis muscle posteriorly. Follow the nerve, and the biceps and coracobrachialis muscles proximally and distally. Neither the tendon of origin of the long head of the biceps nor its tendon of insertion can be followed to the end.

3. Remove the fascia from the brachialis, and define the forearm muscles—the brachioradialis and the extensor carpi radialis longus. They arise from the lateral supracondylar line and the lateral intermuscular septum, and appear to be part of the brachialis but are separated from it by a thin septum which contains the radial nerve and a terminal branch of the profunda brachii artery [Figs. 7.1, 7.2].

4. Find the radial nerve in this situation and its branches to the brachioradialis, extensor carpi radialis longus, and brachialis [Fig. 7.3].

5. Trace the radial nerve proximally to the point where it passes posterior to the humerus. Identify the lower lateral cutaneous nerve of the arm and the posterior cutaneous nerve of the forearm that arise from the radial nerve.

6. Find the principal neurovascular bundle of the arm immediately deep to the deep fascia, medial to the biceps. This bundle includes the median nerve, the ulnar nerve, and the brachial artery and veins. Trace these structures proximally into continuity with the structures in the axilla, and distally to the level of the elbow.

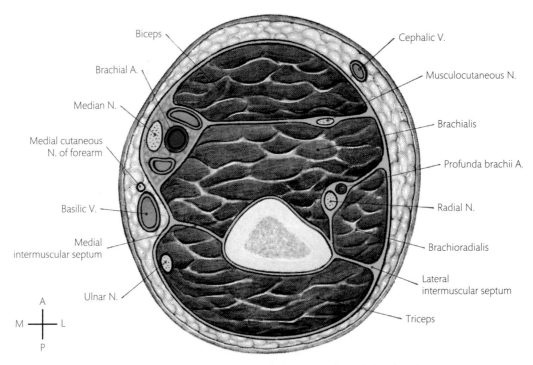

Fig. 7.2 Section through the distal third of the right arm. A = anterior; P = posterior; M = medial; L = lateral.

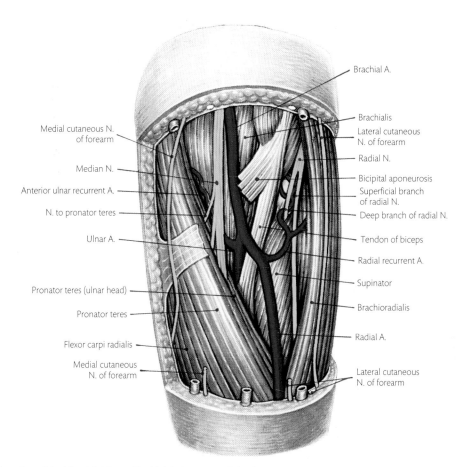

Medial cutaneous N. of forearm

Median N.

Anterior ulnar recurrent A.

N. to pronator teres

Ulnar A.

Pronator teres (ulnar head)

Pronator teres

Flexor carpi radialis

Medial cutaneous N. of forearm

Brachial A.

Brachialis
Lateral cutaneous N. of forearm

Radial N.

Bicipital aponeurosis
Superficial branch of radial N.

Deep branch of radial N.

Tendon of biceps

Radial recurrent A.

Supinator

Brachioradialis

Radial A.

Lateral cutaneous N. of forearm

Fig. 7.3 Dissection of the left cubital fossa. The bicipital aponeurosis has been cut.

the **bicipital aponeurosis**. The bicipital aponeurosis forms a secondary insertion of the biceps to the posterior border of the ulna. The coracobrachialis, which originates from the coracoid process with the short head, is inserted into the middle of the medial surface of the humerus. **Nerve supply**: musculocutaneous nerve. **Actions**: see Action of muscles of the front of the arm below.

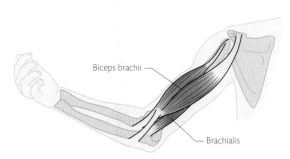

Biceps brachii

Brachialis

Fig. 7.4 Diagram of the biceps brachii showing the two heads of origin and the insertions.

Brachialis

This muscle arises from the anterior surface of the distal half of the humerus [see Fig. 6.2]. It descends across the anterior surface of the elbow joint to be inserted into the coronoid process of the ulna. **Nerve supply**: musculocutaneous nerve, some fibres from the radial nerve. **Actions**: see Action of muscles of the front of the arm below.

Action of muscles of the front of the arm

The short head of the **biceps** and **coracobrachialis** are flexors of the shoulder joint. The long head of the biceps helps to hold the head of the humerus against the glenoid cavity, especially when the arm is abducted. The **brachialis** is a pure flexor of the elbow joint, while the biceps is also a supinator of the forearm because of its attachment to the posterior surface of the radial tuberosity.

The musculocutaneous nerve is the motor supply to all of these muscles. Thus, damage to this nerve interferes with flexion at the shoulder and elbow joints, especially the elbow joint, and weakens supination.

Musculocutaneous nerve (C. 5, 6)

This nerve arises in the axilla from the lateral cord of the brachial plexus. It passes inferolaterally to supply, and then pierce, the coracobrachialis. It then descends between the biceps and brachialis, supplying both muscles, and emerges at the lateral border of the biceps [see Fig. 5.10] as the lateral cutaneous nerve of the forearm.

Principal neurovascular bundle of the arm

Superior to the insertion of the coracobrachialis, this bundle consists of the brachial artery, the basilic and brachial veins, the median, ulnar, and radial nerves, and the medial cutaneous nerve of the forearm. The **radial nerve** is the first to leave the bundle. It passes inferolaterally to the groove for the radial nerve on the posterior surface of the humerus. In the groove, the nerve is accompanied by the **profunda brachii artery** [Fig. 7.5]. Slight traction on that nerve will confirm its continuity with the nerve already exposed on the lateral side of the arm. The **ulnar nerve** is the next to leave the bundle. It passes back through the medial intermuscular septum into the posterior compartment [Fig. 7.6]. Below this level, the **basilic vein** and the **medial cutaneous nerve of the forearm** pierce the deep fascia and enter the superficial fascia. The bundle then contains the **median nerve**, and the **brachial artery** and veins in the lower third of the arm. These structures incline forwards, in front of the brachialis, to lie just medial to the tendon of the biceps at the elbow [Fig. 7.3].

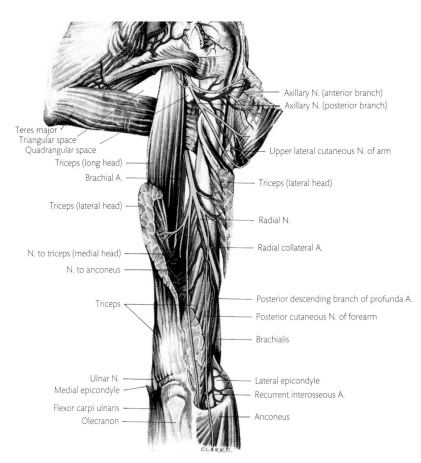

Axillary N. (anterior branch)
Axillary N. (posterior branch)

Teres major
Triangular space
Quadrangular space
Triceps (long head)
Brachial A.

Triceps (lateral head)

N. to triceps (medial head)
N. to anconeus

Triceps

Ulnar N.
Medial epicondyle
Flexor carpi ulnaris
Olecranon

Upper lateral cutaneous N. of arm

Triceps (lateral head)

Radial N.

Radial collateral A.

Posterior descending branch of profunda A.
Posterior cutaneous N. of forearm
Brachialis

Lateral epicondyle
Recurrent interosseous A.

Anconeus

CLARKE.

Fig. 7.5 Dissection of the back of the shoulder and arm. The lateral head of the triceps has been divided and turned aside to expose the radial nerve.

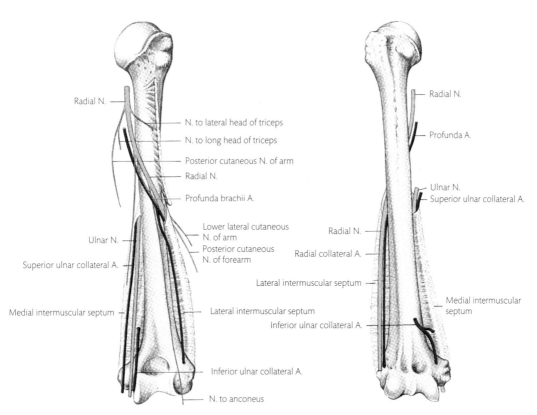

Radial N.

N. to lateral head of triceps

N. to long head of triceps

Posterior cutaneous N. of arm

Radial N.

Profunda brachii A.

Ulnar N.

Superior ulnar collateral A.

Medial intermuscular septum

Lower lateral cutaneous N. of arm

Posterior cutaneous N. of forearm

Lateral intermuscular septum

Inferior ulnar collateral A.

Inferior ulnar collateral A.

N. to anconeus

Radial N.

Profunda A.

Ulnar N.
Superior ulnar collateral A.

Radial N.

Radial collateral A.

Lateral intermuscular septum

Medial intermuscular septum

Fig. 7.6 Diagram to show the relation of the radial and ulnar nerves, and the profunda brachii and ulnar collateral arteries to the humerus. Posterior surface = left; anterior surface = right.

Median nerve (C. 5, 6, 7, 8; T. 1)

This nerve is formed in the axilla by one root each from the medial and lateral cords of the brachial plexus. It descends anterior to the axillary and upper part of the brachial arteries to the medial aspect of the brachial artery in the distal half of the arm. The median nerve does not supply any muscle in the arm but supplies the sympathetic post-ganglionic fibres to the axillary and brachial arteries. It supplies most of the flexor muscles in the anterior aspect of the forearm. In the hand, it supplies the thenar muscles and two lumbricals. It also supplies the skin in the hand and fingers.

Ulnar nerve (C. 8; T. 1)

This nerve is concerned principally with the supply of the small muscles of the hand, some muscles of the forearm, and the skin in the hand and fingers. It does not supply any structures in the axilla or the arm. It arises from the medial cord of the brachial plexus in the axilla and descends posteromedially to the distal part of the axillary artery and the

proximal part of the brachial artery. In the middle of the arm, it pierces the medial intermuscular septum and runs distally in the posterior compartment of the arm. It enters the forearm by passing over the posterior surface of the medial epicondyle [Fig. 7.6].

Brachial artery

The **brachial artery** is the continuation of the axillary artery. It supplies the structures of the arm by branches which accompany the major nerves and by smaller branches which pass directly to the muscles. The **profunda brachii artery** arises from the brachial artery and accompanies the radial nerve. It gives a descending branch on each side of the lateral intermuscular septum [Figs. 7.6, 7.7].

The **superior ulnar collateral branch of the brachial artery** accompanies the ulnar nerve. The **inferior ulnar collateral branch** arises 5 cm above the elbow and sends descending branches on each side of the medial intermuscular septum. These vessels supply adjacent muscles and take part in the anastomosis around the elbow

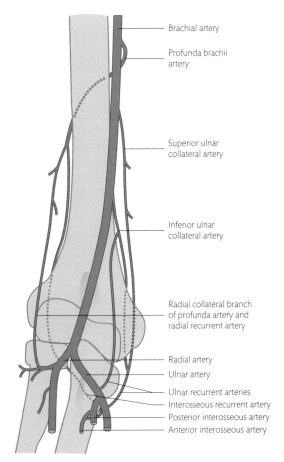

Brachial artery

Profunda brachii artery

Superior ulnar collateral artery

Inferior ulnar collateral artery

Radial collateral branch of profunda artery and radial recurrent artery

Radial artery
Ulnar artery
Ulnar recurrent arteries
Interosseous recurrent artery
Posterior interosseous artery
Anterior interosseous artery

Fig. 7.7 Diagram showing the brachial artery and the anastomosis around the elbow joint.

joint. The **nutrient artery to the humerus** arises from the brachial artery near the middle of the humerus.

Cubital fossa

The cubital fossa is the triangular intermuscular depression at the front of the elbow [Fig. 7.3]. The base of the fossa is an imaginary line drawn between the two epicondyles of the humerus. The medial border is the pronator teres muscle. The lateral border is the brachioradialis muscle, up to a point where it overlaps the pronator teres. The floor is formed by the brachialis and supinator. The median nerve, brachial artery, and tendon of the biceps enter the fossa and are important contents. In the cubital fossa, the brachial artery divides into the radial and ulnar arteries. The radial

artery leaves the fossa at the apex; the ulnar artery leaves by passing deep to the pronator teres. The median nerve supplies muscles medial to it and leaves the fossa through the pronator teres. The tendon of the biceps passes between the forearm bones to reach the radial tuberosity. If the elbow is flexed and the margins pulled apart, the contents of the fossa are seen after the deep fascia covering it has been removed. (The cubital fossa will be dissected with the front of the forearm.)

Posterior compartment

Dissection 7.2 explores the anatomy of the back of the arm.

Triceps brachii

The **long head** of the triceps brachii takes origin from the infraglenoid tubercle of the scapula. The **lateral head** arises from the upper third of the posterior surface of the humerus [see Fig. 6.1]. These two heads descend posterior to the groove for the radial nerve and are joined on their deep surfaces by the **medial head** of the triceps. The medial head arises from the posterior surface of the humerus, distal to the groove for the radial nerve. The three heads form a common tendon which is inserted into the superior surface of the olecranon [see Fig. 8.6] and the surrounding deep fascia. Some of the deep fibres pass to the articular capsule of the elbow joint. These fibres pull up the redundant part of the capsule to avoid it being caught between the olecranon and the humerus in extension of the joint. **Nerve supply**: radial nerve. **Actions**: all three heads of the triceps are extensors of the elbow joint. The long head also acts on the shoulder joint. It is mainly responsible for steadying the humerus in the glenoid cavity, especially when it is stretched across the inferior surface of the joint in abduction of the arm. In abduction of the arm, the long heads of the triceps and biceps lie like supporting cables inferior and superior to the joint, and the long head of the triceps is the main support inferiorly. (For the surface anatomy of the muscles of the arm, see Fig. 7.8.)

Radial nerve

This nerve arises as a branch of the posterior cord of the brachial plexus in the axilla. In the axilla, it gives off the **nerve to the long head of the**

DISSECTION 7.2 Back of the arm

Objectives

I. To study the muscles of the back of the arm.   II. To identify and trace the profunda brachii artery, and the radial nerve and its branches.   III. To follow the ulnar nerve to the back of the medial epicondyle.

Instructions

1. Remove the deep fascia from the back of the arm to expose the triceps muscle which fills the posterior compartment.

2. Superiorly, separate the medially placed long head of the triceps, which arises from the infraglenoid tubercle of the scapula [see Fig. 4.6], from the lateral head, which has a linear origin from the posterior surface of the humerus between the insertions of the teres minor and the deltoid [see Fig. 6.1].

3. Find the radial nerve in the axilla, posterior to the axillary artery. Trace the nerve as far as the triceps, and separate the parts of the triceps by passing a blunt seeker along the nerve in that muscle. Divide and reflect the parts of the lateral head of the triceps where it covers the radial nerve to expose the radial nerve and the profunda brachii artery in the groove on the back of the humerus. The medial head of the triceps takes origin from the humerus, inferior to the groove [Fig. 7.5].

4. Follow the branches of the radial nerve, and check its continuity with the part of the radial nerve already seen between the brachialis and the brachioradialis. Follow this part of the nerve distally. Check its branches to the brachioradialis, extensor carpi radialis longus, and brachialis. Identify its division into superficial and deep branches at the level of the elbow joint [Fig. 7.3].

5. Follow the ulnar nerve into the posterior compartment of the arm with the superior ulnar collateral artery and the branch of the radial nerve to the medial head of the triceps. Trace the ulnar nerve to the back of the medial epicondyle.

6. Remove the connective tissue from the posterior surface of the medial intermuscular septum, and find the posterior branch of the inferior ulnar collateral artery [Figs. 7.5, 7.6].

91

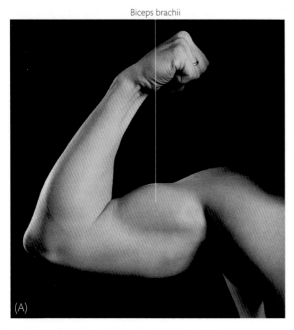
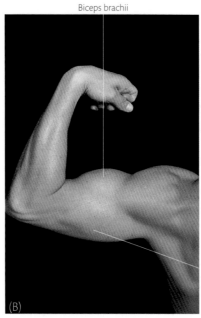

Biceps brachii

Biceps brachii

Triceps brachii

(A)

(B)

Fig. 7.8 Muscles of the arm. (A) Anterior view. (B) Posterior view.

triceps and then passes into the arm, posterior to the brachial artery. Almost immediately, it gives off the **posterior cutaneous nerve of the arm** and a branch to the **medial head of the triceps** (which accompanies the ulnar nerve in the posterior compartment). It then passes inferolaterally into the groove for the radial nerve on the posterior surface of the humerus [see Fig. 5.1B], and winds around this surface of the humerus with the profunda brachii artery. In the groove, the nerve gives off branches to the lateral head of the triceps and a long slender branch which descends through the medial head of the triceps of the anconeus muscle [Fig. 7.5]. Two cutaneous branches—the lower lateral of the arm and the posterior of the forearm—are also given off here.

At the lower end of the arm, the nerve pierces the lateral intermuscular septum and descends in the anterior compartment between the brachialis (medially) and the brachioradialis and the extensor carpi radialis longus (laterally). It divides into superficial and deep branches. The **superficial branch** is a sensory nerve to the back of the fingers and hand [see Fig. 5.8]. The **deep branch** supplies the muscles of the back of the forearm and the joints at the wrist. The radial nerve is sensory to the elbow joint, principally through its branches to the anconeus and the medial head of the triceps, and to the superior and inferior radio-ulnar joints.

See Clinical Applications 7.1 and 7.2 which demonstrate the practical implications of the anatomy explored in this chapter.

CLINICAL APPLICATION 7.1 Fracture of the shaft of the humerus

Mid-shaft fractures of the humerus are common and may damage the radial nerve, as it traverses the groove on the back of the humerus. A knowledge of the muscular and sensory branches given off by the radial nerve, along with the point of origin of these branches, will help you predict what lesions arise from such a fracture.

Study question 1: name the muscles denervated by such an injury. (Answer: triceps, lateral head; anconeus; brachioradialis; extensor carpi radialis longus and brevis. The medial and long heads are supplied before the nerve enters the groove.) Extensor muscles of the forearm and wrist are also paralysed. You will learn about these in Chapter 8.

Study question 2: name the movements likely to be lost or weakened because of this injury. (Answer: loss of

extension of the wrist, hand, and fingers; weakness of supination.)

Study question 3: what sensory nerves will be affected? (Answer: lower lateral cutaneous nerve of the arm, posterior cutaneous nerve of the forearm, superficial branch of the radial nerve.)

Study question 4: what sensory loss will result from this nerve injury? (Answer: loss of sensation over the lateral part of the lower arm, the posterior forearm, the lateral part of the dorsum of the hand, and the dorsal aspect of the lateral three and a half digits, excluding their nail beds.)

Study question 5: name the artery which could be damaged in a fracture of the mid shaft of the humerus. (Answer: profunda brachii artery.)

CLINICAL APPLICATION 7.2 Measurement of blood pressure

Blood pressure is the force exerted by circulating blood upon the walls of blood vessels. It is one of the vital signs of physical well-being. It is measured using a sphygmomanometer, an inflatable rubber cuff connected to a manometer. The cuff is tied around the arm, and the pressure in the cuff inflated till the blood flow through the brachial artery is cut off. The cuff is then deflated slowly, allowing blood flow to resume. A stethoscope placed over the brachial artery at the cubital fossa monitors the start of blood flow in the artery. When the pressure exerted by the cuff is above the systolic pressure, no sounds

are audible, as there is no blood flow. As the cuff pressure falls below the systolic, the sound of spurts of blood flowing past the cuff is heard. When the cuff pressure falls below the diastolic, the blood flow through the brachial artery becomes streamlined (not turbulent any more), and no sound is audible through the stethoscope. The physician measuring the blood pressure makes a note of two pressure readings: (1) when the blood flow first becomes audible with a drop in cuff pressure; and (2) when the blood flow is no longer audible. These two readings give the patient's systolic and diastolic pressures.

CHAPTER 8
The forearm and hand

Introduction

Bones and surface anatomy of the forearm and hand

Begin by revising the palpable parts of the **radius** and **ulna** in your own forearm, and compare these with the bones themselves. Articulate a radius and an ulna parallel to one another, with the head of the radius lying in the radial notch of the ulna and the head of the ulna in the ulnar notch of the radius [see Figs. 5.2, 5.3]. Note the following points.

1. The ulna extends further proximally than the radius. This extension of the ulna is formed by the **trochlear notch** and the **olecranon**.
2. The radius projects further distally than the ulna. The distal end of the radius has markings for the lateral two carpal bones of the proximal row—the **scaphoid** and **lunate**. This is the only articulation between a forearm bone and the carpal bones. Because of this: (a) the bones (and hence the hand) move with the radius in movements of pronation and supination; and (b) forces applied to the hand are transmitted to the radius through these two carpal bones, which are therefore vulnerable to injury.
3. The radius is markedly convex laterally. The radius and ulna are held together by an interosseous membrane attached to the sharp **interosseous borders** on their adjacent surfaces.
4. The anterior surface of the radius is crossed obliquely in its proximal half by its **anterior border**. The distal end of this surface curves forwards to form a flat surface against which the pulsations of the radial artery may be felt (**radial pulse**).
5. Rotate the head of the radius medially in the radial notch of the stationary ulna. When this is done, the distal end of the radius turns around the head

of the ulna and comes to lie medial to the distal end of the ulna. In this position, the posterior surface of the radius is directed anteriorly, and the shaft of the radius crosses the ulna. This movement is **pronation**, and the reverse movement is **supination**. These are the movements at the radio-ulnar joints. Note the following points about pronation and supination: (a) the axis for pronation and supination passes through the centre of the head of the radius proximally and the centre of the head of the ulna distally; (b) any muscle that can rotate the radius medially, e.g. pronator teres, produces pronation, while muscles that rotate it laterally, e.g. biceps brachii, produce supination; (c) in pronation and supination, only the radius moves (there is no rotation of the forearm on the arm); (d) the hand is carried with the radius, and the palm faces posteriorly in pronation (elbow extended); (e) if medial rotation of the humerus is combined with pronation, the palm is brought to face posterolaterally; and (f) testing of the range of pronation is carried out with the elbow flexed.

6. Identify the **subcutaneous posterior border of the ulna**. The flexor muscles are attached to the bones anterior and medial to this and are supplied by the median and ulnar nerves. The extensor muscles are attached lateral to this border and are supplied by the radial nerve [Fig. 8.1]. These two muscle groups abut on each other anteriorly along a line from the lateral side of the tendon of the biceps to the styloid process of the radius.

Superficial structures of the forearm are described in Chapter 5.

Muscles of the forearm

The arrangement of these muscles is complex. In general, both the flexor and extensor groups are arranged in two layers—superficial and deep. In

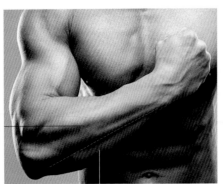

Extensor compartment of forearm

Flexor compartment of forearm

Fig. 8.1 Muscles on the back of the forearm. The subcutaneous posterior border of the ulna (dotted line) separates the flexor muscles medially from the extensor muscles laterally.

Copyright Dean Drobot/Shutterstock.

addition, muscles are grouped together, based on the attachments and actions: (1) muscles that arise from the humerus and pass to the hand (these act on the elbow, the wrist, and, in some instances, the joints of the digits); (2) muscles which arise from the forearm bones and pass to the hand (acting on the wrist and digital joints—but not on the elbow); (3) muscles which arise from both the humerus and the forearm bones and pass to the hand (acting on the elbow, the wrist, and digital joints); (4) muscles which pass from the humerus to the forearm bones (acting on the elbow and the proximal radio-ulnar joint); and (5) muscles which pass between the two forearm bones (acting on radio-ulnar joints).

Front of the forearm and hand

Dissection 8.1 looks at the anatomy of the front of the forearm.

Palmar aponeurosis

This thick, triangular deep fascia lies in the central part of the palm, with its apex at the flexor retinaculum and its base at the level of the heads of the metacarpals. It stabilizes the palmar skin which is firmly

---

DISSECTION 8.1 Front of the forearm

Objectives

I. To study the superficial muscles of the front of the forearm.   II. To identify and trace the brachial, radial, and ulnar arteries, and the median and ulnar nerves.   III. To study the palmaris brevis and palmar aponeurosis.

Instructions

1. Divide the deep fascia of the forearm vertically from the cubital fossa to the proximal margin of the flexor retinaculum. Make a transverse incision just proximal to the retinaculum. Reflect the flaps of the fascia, but avoid cutting the structures deep to it.

2. The muscles uncovered consist of the flexor group medially and the extensor group laterally. Separate the most superficial muscle—the **brachioradialis** [Fig. 8.2]—on the lateral side of the front of the forearm. Follow it to its insertion on the lateral surface of the distal end of the radius.

3. Push aside the tendons of the abductor pollicis longus and extensor pollicis brevis which overlie the insertion of the brachioradialis, as they pass to the base of the thumb [see Fig. 8.21]. Avoid injury to the superficial branch of the radial nerve which crosses their superficial surface.

4. Pull the brachioradialis laterally. This exposes the extensor carpi radialis longus and separates the extensor and flexor groups of muscles.

5. In the groove between the flexors and extensors, identify the **radial artery** and the **superficial branch of the radial nerve**. Follow them distally and proximally [Fig. 8.3]. In this way, find the origin of the artery from the brachial artery in the cubital fossa (occasionally high in the arm) and the branch from the **deep branch of the radial nerve** which supplies the extensor carpi radialis brevis—a muscle deep to the extensor carpi radialis longus.

6. Deep to the extensor carpi radialis brevis is the supinator muscle.

7. Separate the **superficial group of flexor muscles**. These arise from the distal part of the medial supracondylar line and the medial epicondyle of the humerus. Most also have a minor attachment to the coronoid process of the ulna [see Figs. 6.2, 8.4]. These superficial muscles spread out from the medial epicondyle as a narrow fan with a vertical medial edge—the **flexor carpi ulnaris** [Fig. 8.2].

8. The most lateral muscle—the **pronator teres**—arises furthest superiorly and passes obliquely across the

proximal half of the forearm to the point of maximum convexity of the radius [Fig. 8.4]. It passes deep to the radial artery, the superficial branch of the radial nerve, and the extensor muscles overlying the anterolateral surface of the radius [Fig. 8.2].

9. Medial to the pronator teres is the **flexor carpi radialis** (the radial flexor of the wrist), which also takes an oblique course across the forearm. Its tendon disappears deep to the lateral part of the flexor retinaculum, medial to the **radial artery**. Identify this tendon in your own wrist, and feel the pulsation of the radial artery (**radial pulse**) lateral to it on the distal margin of the radius.

10. Medial to the flexor carpi radialis is the **palmaris longus** (if present). Follow its tendon superficial to the flexor retinaculum to join the palmar aponeurosis.

11. Beneath the tendon of the palmaris longus and between it and the flexor carpi radialis, the median nerve becomes superficial, just proximal to the flexor retinaculum [Fig. 8.2].

12. The **flexor carpi ulnaris** is immediately medial to the palmaris longus in the proximal third of the forearm. Further distally, the two muscles separate, and the flexor digitorum superficialis appears between them [Fig. 8.2]. Follow the tendon of the ulnaris to its insertion on the **pisiform** bone.

13. Find the **ulnar artery and nerve** which become superficial between the tendons of the flexor carpi ulnaris and those of the flexor digitorum superficialis, just proximal to the flexor retinaculum. Here the artery and nerve pierce the deep fascia and enter the hand, superficial to the retinaculum, immediately lateral to the insertion of the flexor carpi ulnaris. They then pass deep to the palmaris brevis and divide into their terminal branches [Figs. 8.2, 8.5].

14. The **palmaris brevis** is a thin cutaneous muscle which arises from the palmar aponeurosis and flexor retinaculum. It passes transversely across the proximal 2–3 cm of the hypothenar eminence and is inserted into the skin on the medial side [Fig. 8.5]. It is supplied by the ulnar nerve. ➲ When it contracts, it bunches up the skin over the eminence, thus deepening the concavity of the palm and producing a cushion of skin against which the handle of a tool can be held steadily.

15. Expose the superficial surface of the **flexor carpi ulnaris**. Note its origin from the medial epicondyle, the olecranon, and the proximal two-thirds of the posterior (subcutaneous) border of the ulna [Fig. 8.6].

16. Follow the **ulnar nerve** from the arm, posterior to the medial epicondyle, then between the humeral and ulnar attachments of the flexor carpi ulnaris on its deep surface [see Figs. 7.6, 8.7]. Pull the flexor carpi ulnaris medially, and expose the ulnar nerve on its deep surface lying on the flexor digitorum profundus which covers the ulna. Trace the nerve and the ulnar artery into continuity with the parts exposed at the wrist. Note the branches of the nerve to the flexor carpi ulnaris and flexor digitorum profundus, the **dorsal branch** arising near the middle of the forearm, and the small **palmar branch** [see Fig. 5.9] which arises in the distal half of the forearm. Trace the dorsal branch to the medial side of the forearm.

17. Cut through the middle of the flexor carpi radialis, palmaris longus, and pronator teres muscles, and reflect their parts. Identify the branches of the median nerve entering them proximally [Fig. 8.3].

18. The **flexor digitorum superficialis** is now exposed. Identify the radial head of this muscle attached to the anterior border of the radius, deep to the distal part of the pronator teres [Figs. 8.3, 8.4].

19. Follow the **median nerve** from the cubital fossa between the radial and humero-ulnar heads of the flexor digitorum superficialis. Lift the medial edge of the muscle, and find the nerve on its deep surface. Note its branches to the muscle. A short distance proximal to the wrist, the nerve becomes superficial between the tendons of the flexor carpi radialis and the palmaris longus. It gives off the **palmar branch** of the median nerve which enters the palm, superficial to the flexor retinaculum. The median nerve enters the hand, deep to the flexor retinaculum [Fig. 8.5]. ➲ Identify this position in your own wrist, and note how easily the nerve could be injured by a relatively superficial cut at this point.

20. Turn the tendon of the palmaris longus distally. Note its attachment to the flexor retinaculum and its continuity with the apex of the palmar aponeurosis.

21. Complete the exposure of the superficial surface of the **palmar aponeurosis** and the slips which pass from its distal margin to each of the fingers. Note that the edges of each slip turn posteriorly into the palm, leaving spaces between the slips through which the digital vessels and nerves (and lumbrical muscles) escape from beneath the palmar aponeurosis into the fingers [Fig. 8.5]. Each slip of the aponeurosis is attached: (a) to the phalanges by

fusing with the fibrous flexor sheath (the fibrous tunnel in which the tendons of the long flexors lie); and (b) with the deep transverse metacarpal ligament (described later) [Fig. 8.5]. Confirm this arrangement by pushing a blunt instrument proximally between any two fingers—it passes readily into the palm, deep to the aponeurosis, without having to pierce it.

22. Separate the palmaris longus tendon and the aponeurosis from the surface of the flexor retinaculum. Turn the aponeurosis distally. You will need to separate the edges of the aponeurosis from the thinner deep fascia covering the thenar and hypothenar muscles and divide the septum which passes backwards from each edge. The septa fuse with the fascia anterior to the interosseous muscles and the adductor pollicis [Fig. 8.8]. Avoid injury to the vessels and nerves immediately deep to the aponeurosis.

23. Remove the fat from the interdigital region, and expose the **digital nerves and vessels**, with a **lumbrical muscle** posterior to them [Fig. 8.5].

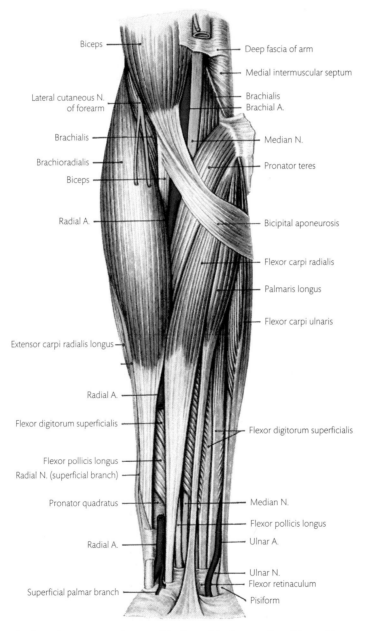

Fig. 8.2 Dissection of superficial muscles, arteries, and nerves of the front of the forearm. Part of the radial artery was removed to show the muscles deep to it.

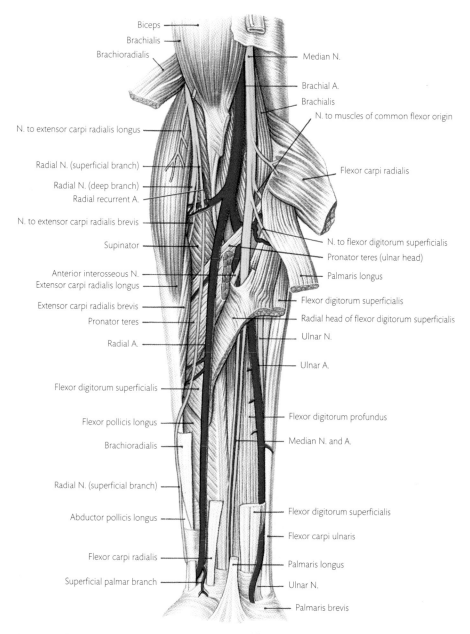

Fig. 8.3 Deep dissection of muscles and nerves of the front of the forearm. The division of the brachial artery is slightly lower than usual.

adherent to it. Medially and laterally, the aponeurosis is continuous posteriorly with the layer of fascia which covers the anterior surfaces of the metacarpals, the interosseous muscles between them, and the adductor pollicis [Fig. 8.8]. Together, these fascial layers surround: (1) the central palmar space; (2) vessels and nerves; (3) long flexor tendons to the fingers; and (4) the lumbrical muscles which arise from the tendons. Distally, at the level of the heads of the metacarpals, the palmar aponeurosis gives off

digital slips to each of the four fingers [Fig. 8.5]. At this point, sheets of fascia pass from the aponeurosis to the metacarpal fascia. Thus, each digital slip forms a tunnel around the flexor tendons. Nerves, vessels, and lumbrical muscles enter the superficial tissues between these slips. ➲ The loose tissue, in which vessels and nerves lie, forms a route for infection to spread from the superficial tissues of the fingers to the central palmar region, from where it can extend behind the flexor retinaculum into the forearm.

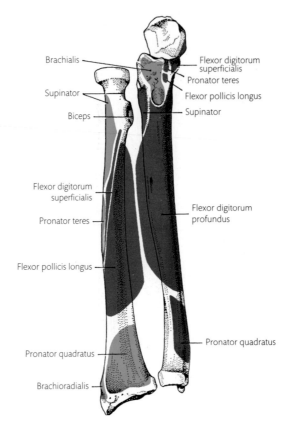

Fig. 8.4 Muscle attachments to the anterior surface of the right radius and ulna.

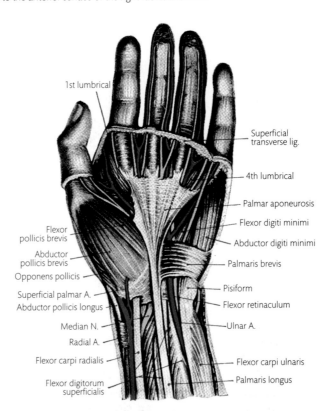

Fig. 8.5 Superficial dissection of the palm to show the palmar aponeurosis. The deep fascia has been removed from the thenar and hypothenar eminences.

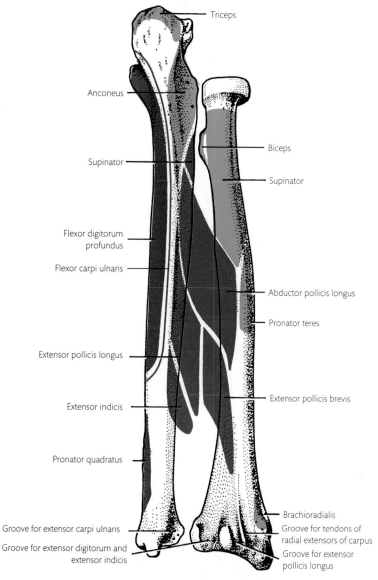

Triceps

Anconeus

Supinator

Flexor digitorum profundus

Flexor carpi ulnaris

Extensor pollicis longus

Extensor indicis

Pronator quadratus

Groove for extensor carpi ulnaris

Groove for extensor digitorum and extensor indicis

Biceps

Supinator

Abductor pollicis longus

Pronator teres

Extensor pollicis brevis

Brachioradialis
Groove for tendons of radial extensors of carpus
Groove for extensor pollicis longus

Fig. 8.6 Muscle attachments to the posterior surface of the right radius and ulna.

Dissection 8.2 begins the dissection of the palm of the hand.

Superficial palmar arch

This arterial arch begins as a terminal branch of the ulnar artery on the flexor retinaculum, distal to the pisiform bone. It runs forwards, medial to the hook of the hamate, and turns laterally, deep to the palmar aponeurosis, to join one of the branches of the radial artery [Fig. 8.10]. The radial branch may form a significant portion of an incomplete arch. The distal point of the arch lies at the same level as

the distal border of the thenar eminence when the thumb is fully extended.

Branches

The principal branches of the superficial palmar arch are the four palmar digital arteries. The most medial is the proper palmar digital artery to the medial side of the little finger. The other three branches are the **common palmar digital arteries** to adjacent sides of two fingers. In the interdigital clefts, the common digital artery receives the corresponding palmar metacarpal artery from the

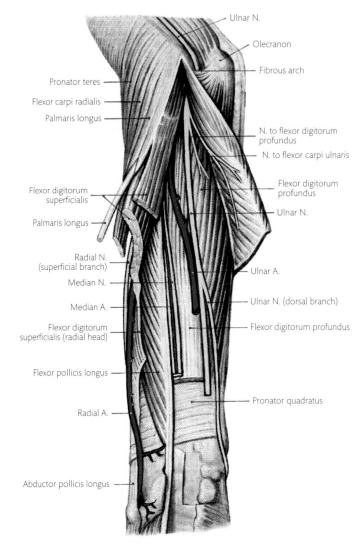

Ulnar N.

Olecranon

Fibrous arch

Pronator teres

Flexor carpi radialis

Palmaris longus

N. to flexor digitorum profundus

N. to flexor carpi ulnaris

Flexor digitorum profundus

Ulnar N.

Flexor digitorum superficialis

Palmaris longus

Radial N. (superficial branch)

Median N.

Ulnar A.

Ulnar N. (dorsal branch)

Median A.

Flexor digitorum superficialis (radial head)

Flexor digitorum profundus

Flexor pollicis longus

Pronator quadratus

Radial A.

Abductor pollicis longus

Fig. 8.7 Deep dissection of the front of the forearm. The elbow is partially flexed, and the forearm semi-pronated. The superficial muscles are cut and reflected. The flexor digitorum superficialis and flexor carpi ulnaris are separated to display deeper structures.

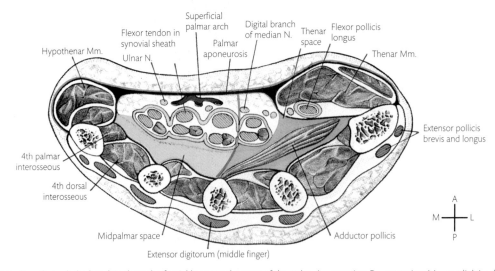

Superficial palmar arch

Flexor tendon in synovial sheath

Digital branch of median N.

Thenar space

Flexor pollicis longus

Hypothenar Mm.

Ulnar N.

Palmar aponeurosis

Thenar Mm.

Extensor pollicis brevis and longus

4th palmar interosseous

4th dorsal interosseous

Midpalmar space

Adductor pollicis

Extensor digitorum (middle finger)

A
M —— L
P

Fig. 8.8 Section through the hand to show the fascial layers and spaces of the palm. A = anterior; P = posterior; M = medial; L = lateral.

DISSECTION 8.2 Palm of the hand-1

Objectives

I. To identify and trace the superficial palmar arch and its branches, the superficial branch of the ulnar nerve, and branches of the median nerve.   **II.** To study the digital fibrous flexor sheath.

Instructions

1. Remove any remnants of the palmaris brevis, and follow the **ulnar nerve** and **artery** distally, superficial to the flexor retinaculum. Note, but do not follow, the deep branch of the nerve (motor) and the deep palmar branch of the artery entering the hypothenar muscles.

2. Follow the superficial palmar arch, which the ulnar artery forms, and trace its branches. Trace the branches of the ulnar nerve (sensory and sympathetic) to the fingers [Fig. 8.9]. The superficial palmar arch is immediately deep to the palmar aponeurosis. Deep to the arch are the branches of the median and ulnar nerves, and further deeper are the long flexor tendons [Fig. 8.8].

3. Pull gently on the **median nerve**, proximal to the flexor retinaculum. This demonstrates its position at the distal edge of the retinaculum. Carefully follow the branches of the median nerve, distal to the retinaculum, but do not disturb the flexor tendons. The nerve gives a short, thick, recurrent (motor) branch into the thenar muscles, close to the distal edge of the retinaculum.

4. The median nerve divides into the **common** and **proper palmar digital nerves** (mainly sensory and sympathetic) to the thumb and lateral two and a half fingers [Fig. 8.10]. The most medial digital branch communicates with the most lateral digital branch of the ulnar nerve.

5. The branch to the lateral side of the index finger supplies the first lumbrical muscle, and the branch to the medial side supplies the second lumbrical.

6. Follow the digital branches at least to the roots of the fingers, and trace them to the tip of one finger. Note the branches which pass dorsally in the distal part of the finger. Through these, the skin on the dorsal surfaces of the distal two phalanges is supplied by the palmar digital nerves.

7. Expose the surface of the **fibrous flexor sheath** in one finger at least, but avoid damage to the tissue surrounding the flexor tendons at its proximal end. Note that the sheath is thick where it lies opposite the bodies of the phalanges but is thinner at the level of the interphalangeal joint.

Front of the forearm and hand

101

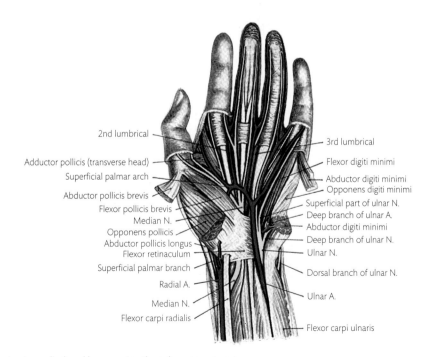

2nd lumbrical
Adductor pollicis (transverse head)
Superficial palmar arch
Abductor pollicis brevis
Flexor pollicis brevis
Median N.
Opponens pollicis
Abductor pollicis longus
Flexor retinaculum
Superficial palmar branch
Radial A.
Median N.
Flexor carpi radialis

3rd lumbrical
Flexor digiti minimi
Abductor digiti minimi
Opponens digiti minimi
Superficial part of ulnar N.
Deep branch of ulnar A.
Abductor digiti minimi
Deep branch of ulnar N.
Ulnar N.
Dorsal branch of ulnar N.
Ulnar A.
Flexor carpi ulnaris

Fig. 8.9 Palmar structures displayed by removing the palmar aponeurosis.

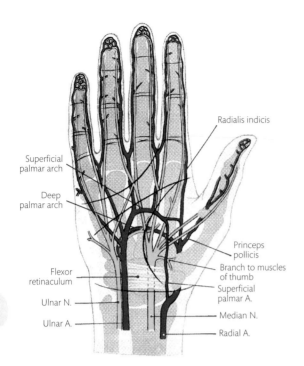

Superficial palmar arch

Deep palmar arch

Flexor retinaculum

Ulnar N.

Ulnar A.

Radialis indicis

Princeps pollicis

Branch to muscles of thumb

Superficial palmar A.

Median N.

Radial A.

Fig. 8.10 Diagram of nerves and vessels of the hand in relation to bones and skin creases.

deep palmar arch. It then divides into two **proper palmar digital arteries** to the adjacent sides of two fingers [Figs. 8.9, 8.10]. The proper palmar digital arteries to each finger form a rich anastomosis in the pulp of the finger and in the nail bed.

Flexor retinaculum

This dense fibrous band unites the ends of the arch of the carpal bones and thus converts the space within the arch into an osteofibrous **carpal tunnel**. The median nerve, the long flexor tendons of the fingers and thumb, and the tendon of the flexor carpi radialis pass through this tunnel. The flexor retinaculum acts as a pulley for these tendons in flexion of the wrist. The retinaculum is continuous with the deep fascia of the forearm and the palmar aponeurosis in the hand.

The flexor retinaculum is attached to the pisiform bone and the hook of the hamate medially and to the tubercle of the scaphoid and the front of the trapezium laterally [see Fig. 5.5]. The attachment to the trapezium is to either side of the groove which lodges the tendon of the flexor carpi radialis, thus forming a separate tunnel for this tendon.

The superficial surface of the retinaculum gives partial origin to the thenar and hypothenar muscles and has the ulnar nerve and vessels, the palmar cutaneous branches of the median and ulnar nerves, and the tendon of the palmaris longus on it.

The space deep to the flexor retinaculum is the 'carpal tunnel'. The tendons of the flexor carpi radialis, flexor pollicis longus, flexor digitorum longus, flexor digitorum superficialis, and the median nerve lie in it [Fig. 8.11A and B].

Fibrous flexor sheaths

Fibrous flexor sheaths are found on the flexor surface of the digits, deep to the superficial fascia. Together with the synovial sheath which lies within them, they form coverings for the long flexor tendons of the fingers [Fig. 8.12]. These thickened sheaths are attached to the sides of the palmar surfaces of the phalanges and of the palmar ligaments of the metacarpophalangeal and interphalangeal joints. It is thick over the surface of the bones, but thinner at the joints to allow flexion. Together with the phalanges, each sheath forms an osteofascial tube and prevents the tendons from springing away from the bone during contraction.

Synovial sheaths of flexor tendons

Synovial sheaths surround tendons wherever they pass through fascial or osteofascial tunnels. In the hand, synovial sheaths are found around tendons, as they pass through the carpal tunnel, and the osteofascial tunnel formed by the phalanges and the fibrous flexor sheaths [Fig. 8.13A]. These sheaths consist of two concentric tubes or layers of smooth synovial membrane joined together at their ends. The layers are separated from each other by a capillary interval (the cavity of the sheath) which contains synovial fluid to lubricate the opposed surfaces as they slide on each other. The inner layer surrounds, and is adherent to, the tendon; the outer layer lines the fibrous or bony canal and is fused with it [Fig. 8.13B]. Tendons may be completely surrounded by the synovial space or suspended in the sheath by a fold of the synovial membrane (**mesotendon**). The mesotendon allows blood vessels to reach the tendon at any point along the sheath (see vincula, Fig. 8.15). ➋ The cavity of a synovial sheath forms a route for rapid spread of infection along its length. When inflamed, the cavity becomes distended with fluid, tense, and painful, and the increased pressure within the sheath may interfere with the blood supply of the tendon.

In the carpal tunnel [Fig. 8.13A], the tendons of the flexor digitorum superficialis and flexor digitorum

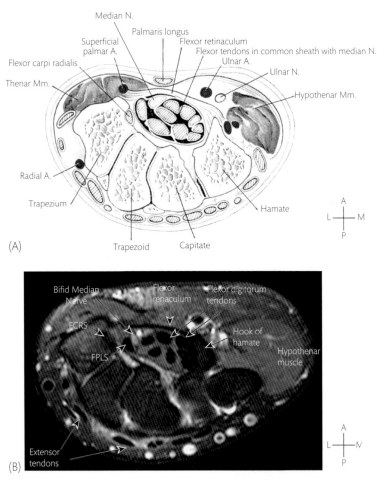

(A)

(B)

Fig. 8.11 (A) Transverse section at the level of the distal row of the carpal bones. The flexor pollicis longus, the median nerve, and the tendons of the two flexors (superficial and deep) of the digits are seen in the carpal tunnel. A = anterior; P = posterior; M = medial; L = lateral. (B) MR image of the hand at the same level. FCRS = flexor carpi radialis; FPLS = flexor pollicis longus.

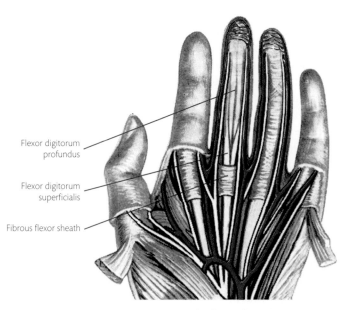

Fig. 8.12 Palmar surface of the middle finger. A window has been cut in the fibrous flexor sheath to show the long flexor tendons.

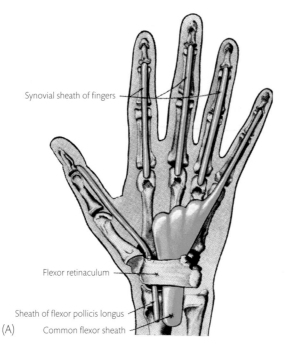

Synovial sheath of fingers

Flexor retinaculum

Sheath of flexor pollicis longus
(A) Common flexor sheath

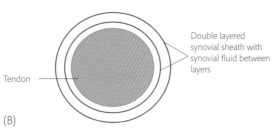

Tendon

Double layered synovial sheath with synovial fluid between layers

(B)

Fig. 8.13 (A) Synovial sheaths of flexor tendons of digits. (B) Schematic drawing to show the relationship of a tendon to the inner and outer layers of the synovial sheath.

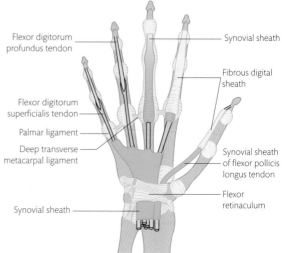

Flexor digitorum profundus tendon

Synovial sheath

Fibrous digital sheath

Flexor digitorum superficialis tendon

Palmar ligament

Deep transverse metacarpal ligament

Synovial sheath of flexor pollicis longus tendon

Flexor retinaculum

Synovial sheath

Fig. 8.14 Relationship between the fibrous flexor sheath, synovial sheath, and long flexor tendons.

profundus are enclosed in a common synovial sheath. More laterally, the tendon of the flexor pollicis longus is enclosed in its own synovial sheath. (The flexor digitorum profundus and flexor pollicis longus will be seen during the deep dissection of the forearm.) These two sheaths may communicate with each other, and both extend 2–3 cm proximally into the forearm, posterior to the tendons. Distally, the sheath for the flexor pollicis longus extends to the terminal phalanx of the thumb. The sheath for the flexor digitorum extends to the middle of the palm for the lateral three digits and to the terminal phalanx of the little finger. The synovial sheaths within the fibrous flexor sheaths of the middle three digits are separate from the common sheath. The synovial sheath of the little finger is incomplete to allow the lumbrical muscles (which are attached to the tendons of the flexor digitorum profundus) to emerge from the sheath. The ten-

don of the flexor carpi radialis has its own synovial sheath. Fig. 8.14 shows the relationship between the fibrous flexor sheath, the synovial sheath, and the long flexor tendons.

Dissection 8.3 continues to study the front of the forearm and the palm of the hand.

Arteries of the flexor compartment of the forearm

The brachial artery divides into the radial and ulnar arteries at the level of the neck of the radius in the cubital fossa. The smaller **radial artery** passes inferolaterally between the brachioradialis and flexor carpi radialis to reach the anterior surface of the distal end of the radius between the tendons of these muscles. Here the artery can be felt readily (radial pulse) against the bone. Except in the initial part of its course, the artery is immediately deep to the deep fascia. It crosses the superficial surface of the pronator teres with the superficial branch of the radial nerve [Fig. 8.3].

The **ulnar artery** passes inferomedially, deep to the median nerve and the muscles arising from the medial epicondyle of the humerus and the coronoid process of the ulna. It lies on the brachialis and flexor digitorum profundus. It meets the ulnar nerve above the middle of the forearm and descends vertically with it to pierce the deep fascia just proximal to the flexor retinaculum, between the tendons of the flexor carpi ulnaris and flexor digitorum superficialis [Fig. 8.3].

DISSECTION 8.3   Front of the forearm and palm of the hand

Objectives

I. To study the long flexor tendons in the hand.   II. To study the deep muscles on the front of the forearm.   III. To identify and trace the branches of the median nerve, ulnar nerve, and anterior interosseous nerve in the forearm.

Instructions

1. Attempt to demonstrate the synovial sheath around the flexor digitorum superficialis tendon. Clean the loose connective tissue (external layer of the sheath) around the tendons, close to the proximal margin of the flexor retinaculum, and note the smooth, slippery internal surface of the sheath and external surface of the tendon. Introduce a blunt probe into the sheath, and try to define its extent. Note that it allows the probe to pass easily into the hand, deep to the flexor retinaculum, but also that the structures here are tightly packed in the carpal tunnel.

2. In one finger, divide the fibrous flexor sheath longitudinally. Note it is thick at the level of the bodies of the phalanges and relatively thin opposite the joints. Examine the extent of the digital synovial sheath.

3. Lift the tendons of the flexor digitorum superficialis and profundus within the digital sheath, and note the vinculae [Fig. 8.15] passing between them and the outer layer of the synovial sheath on the phalanges.

4. Divide the flexor retinaculum by a vertical cut between the thenar and hypothenar muscles. Take care not to damage the median nerve. Establish the continuity of the trunk of the median nerve with the branches found in the hand.

5. Follow the tendons of the flexor digitorum superficialis distally to the fingers. Note how each tendon divides to enclose the corresponding tendon of the flexor digitorum profundus. It is then inserted on the palmar aspect of the middle phalanx, dorsal to the profundus tendon [Fig. 8.15].

6. In the forearm, cut transversely through the humero-ulnar head of the flexor digitorum superficialis. Reflect the distal part of the muscle laterally to uncover the deep muscles of the forearm, the median nerve, and the ulnar artery.

7. Separate the **median nerve** from the deep surface of the flexor digitorum superficialis, and trace it proximally. Find its branches to the muscle and the **anterior interosseous nerve** arising from it in the cubital fossa.

8. Follow the **ulnar artery** to its origin from the brachial artery, and trace its principal branches [see Figs. 7.7, 8.3]. Do not follow the posterior interosseous artery at this stage. Trace the anterior interosseous artery and nerve on the interosseous membrane between the deep flexor muscles of the forearm.

9. Identify the deep muscles of the forearm. These are the **flexor digitorum profundus** medially, the **flexor pollicis longus** laterally, and the **pronator quadratus**. The flexor pollicis longus and flexor digitorum profundus arise from the proximal two-thirds of the ulna and radius [Figs. 8.4, 8.6]. The pronator quadratus is a rectangular muscle which passes transversely between the anterior surfaces of the distal quarters of the radius and ulna.

10. Find the branches of the anterior interosseous artery and nerve to the deep muscles. Note that the artery passes posteriorly through the interosseous membrane at the proximal border of the pronator quadratus.

11. Cut across the flexor digitorum superficialis, distal to the origin of its radial head, and turn its tendons distally. Follow the tendons of the flexor digitorum profundus and flexor pollicis longus through the carpal tunnel into the palm.

12. Note the separation of the tendons of the flexor digitorum profundus in the palm and the four small muscles (**lumbricals**) which arise from them. Follow the lumbrical muscles to their tendons, as they pass with the proper digital vessels and nerves to the lateral side of the base of each finger [Fig. 8.9]. Their tendons will be traced later.

13. Reconfirm the nerve supply to the medial part of the flexor digitorum profundus from the ulnar nerve and the origin of that muscle from the medial and anterior surfaces of the ulna.

14. If possible, follow the anterior interosseous nerve through the pronator quadratus to the anterior surface of the **wrist joint**. It supplies this joint and the **distal radio-ulnar joint**.

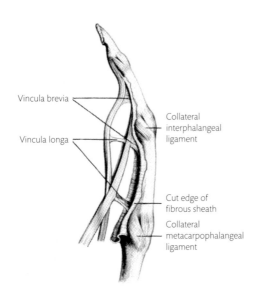

Vincula brevia

Vincula longa

Collateral
interphalangeal
ligament

Cut edge of
fibrous sheath

Collateral
metacarpophalangeal
ligament

Fig. 8.15 Flexor tendons of the finger with the vincula tendinum.

The ulnar artery is the principal source of supply to the forearm; the radial artery is usually the main artery of the hand. Both arteries send **recurrent branches** to anastomose around the elbow joint with branches of the brachial (**ulnar collateral arteries**) and profunda brachii (**radial collateral artery**) arteries [see Fig. 7.7]. Both arteries supply the muscles adjacent to them and give the **palmar** and **dorsal carpal arteries** at the wrist. These arteries anastomose on, and supply, the carpal bones, the surrounding joint tissues, and the adjacent parts of the hand. At the wrist, the radial artery sends a **superficial palmar branch** of variable size into the thenar muscles. It lies superficial to the flexor retinaculum and may anastomose with the superficial palmar arch of the ulnar artery [Fig. 8.9], occasionally forming a large or separate part of it.

The **common interosseous artery** is the principal branch of the ulnar artery in the forearm [see Fig. 7.7]. It passes to the upper border of the interosseous membrane and divides into the anterior and posterior **interosseous arteries**. The posterior interosseous artery passes above the membrane to the back of the forearm. The anterior interosseous artery gives off the long, slender median artery to the median nerve and then descends on the front of the interosseous membrane between the flexor pollicis longus and flexor digitorum profundus to the pronator quadratus [Fig. 8.3]. It supplies these muscles, sends nutrient arteries to the radius and ulna, and pierces the interosseous membrane

at the upper border of the pronator quadratus to enter the back of the forearm.

Nerves of the flexor compartment of the forearm and hand

Median nerve

The median nerve lies medial to the brachial artery at the elbow. It gives branches to the pronator teres, flexor carpi radialis, palmaris longus, flexor digitorum superficialis, and the elbow joint as it lies on the brachialis in the cubital fossa. As it leaves the fossa on the anterior surface of the ulnar artery, it gives off the **anterior interosseous nerve**. This nerve runs with the corresponding artery and supplies the flexor digitorum profundus (lateral half), flexor pollicis longus, and pronator quadratus. It passes posterior to the pronator quadratus to end on the front of the wrist and distal radio-ulnar joints [see Figs. 7.3, 8.3].

The median nerve descends on the deep surface of the flexor digitorum superficialis. Near the wrist, the nerve lies between the tendons of the flexor digitorum superficialis and flexor carpi radialis, deep to the tendon of the palmaris longus. It gives off the palmar cutaneous branch, traverses the carpal tunnel, and divides into six branches near the distal border of the retinaculum. The most lateral branch turns proximally on the retinaculum and enters the thenar muscles to supply the abductor pollicis brevis, flexor pollicis brevis, and opponens pollicis. Medial to this, the mode of division is variable, but commonly three **proper palmar digital nerves** pass, one to each side of the thumb and the radial side of the index finger [Fig. 8.10]. The nerve to the index finger supplies the first lumbrical muscle. A **common palmar digital nerve** passes towards each side of the middle finger. The lateral one supplies the second lumbrical muscle, and the medial one communicates with the common palmar digital nerve from the ulnar nerve. Proximal to the division of the corresponding common palmar digital arteries, each of these nerves divides into two **proper palmar digital nerves**. These nerves pass between the slips of the palmar aponeurosis to enter the subcutaneous tissue of the index, middle, and ring fingers [Fig. 8.9]. They lie anterior to the corresponding arteries.

The proper palmar digital nerves supply the skin on the palmar aspects of the finger and on the dorsal surface of the distal one and a half to two phalanges through the dorsal branches. In the thumb, they frequently supply the skin on the dorsal surface of the terminal phalanx. The areas supplied by the digital nerve overlap to a large extent. ➲ Total destruction of only one of the parent nerves (median, ulnar, or radial) produces an area of complete sensory loss much smaller than the sum of the areas supplied by the individual branches.

Ulnar nerve

The ulnar nerve enters the forearm on the posterior surface of the medial epicondyle of the humerus. It gives a branch to the elbow joint, passes deep to the flexor carpi ulnaris [Fig. 8.7], and gives a branch to it and to the medial half of the flexor digitorum profundus. It descends between these two muscles in the medial part of the front of the forearm and is joined by the ulnar artery. It gives off the **dorsal branch of the ulnar nerve** above the middle of the forearm and becomes superficial on the lateral side of the tendon of the flexor carpi ulnaris, close to the pisiform bone. It pierces the deep fascia with its palmar cutaneous branch and the ulnar artery, passes on to the flexor retinaculum, and divides into deep and superficial branches.

The **superficial branch** supplies the palmaris brevis, passes deep to it, and divides into a **proper palmar digital nerve** to the medial side of the little finger and a **common palmar digital nerve** to the fourth interdigital cleft. The latter communicates with the adjacent common palmar digital nerve from the median nerve and divides into proper palmar digital nerves to the adjacent sides of the ring and little fingers [Fig. 8.10].

The ulnar nerve may transmit nerve fibres from the seventh cervical ventral ramus to the skin of the hand. It receives these C7 fibres either through a communication with the median nerve in the forearm or through a branch from the lateral cord of the brachial plexus in the axilla.

Muscles of the front of the forearm and hand

Extensor muscles

The **brachioradialis** takes origin from high on the lateral supracondylar line of the humerus. It descends in front of the elbow joint, with the extensor carpi radialis longus which arises inferior to it [see Fig. 6.2]. Both flex the elbow joint, though they belong to the extensor group of muscles and

are supplied by the radial nerve. The brachioradialis is inserted into the lateral surface of the distal end of the radius. In addition to flexing the elbow joint, it also partially supinates the fully pronated forearm because of its spiral course through the forearm in this position.

Flexor muscles

The flexor muscles of the forearm are arranged in three groups—superficial, intermediate, and deep groups.

The superficial group consists of the pronator teres, flexor carpi radialis, palmaris longus, and flexor carpi ulnaris. The flexor digitorum superficialis is closely associated with the superficial muscles but forms the intermediate layer. All these muscles take origin from the medial epicondyle of the humerus [see Fig. 6.2], and the fascia between them. Some muscles have a subsidiary attachment to the coronoid process of the ulna [Fig. 8.4]. All these muscles pass anterior to the elbow joint and are weak flexors, though each has other specific actions. All of them are supplied by the median nerve in the cubital fossa, except the flexor carpi ulnaris which is supplied by the ulnar nerve.

The **flexor carpi ulnaris** arises from the olecranon and posterior border of the ulna, in addition to the humeral origin. It passes vertically down and is inserted into the pisiform. It is a flexor of the wrist and an adductor (ulnar deviator) of the hand. The force which it applies to the pisiform is transmitted to the hook of the hamate [Fig. 8.16] by the **pisohamate ligament**, and to the base of the fifth metacarpal by the **pisometacarpal ligament**. Both ligaments are essentially continuations of the tendon.

The **palmaris longus** expands into the palmar aponeurosis and acts to tense it. It stabilizes the palmar skin in grasping an object. It passes anterior to the wrist joint and may assist in its flexion. The muscle is frequently absent.

The **flexor carpi radialis** runs obliquely across the anterior surface of the forearm to the anterolateral surface of the wrist. It passes deep to the lateral end of the flexor retinaculum, grooves the trapezium, and is inserted into the base of the second and third metacarpals (that of the thumb is the first). It is a flexor of the wrist and abductor (radial deviator) of the hand. Acting with the flexor carpi ulnaris, it produces pure flexion of the wrist joint. Because of its

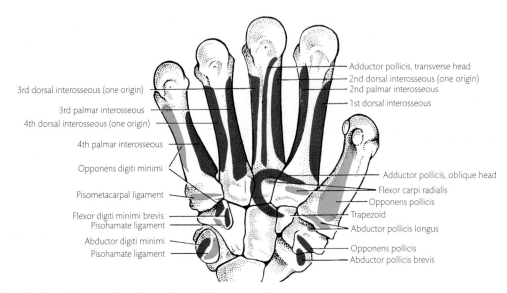

Fig. 8.16 Muscle attachments to the palmar surfaces of the carpus and metacarpus.

oblique course in the forearm, it tends to rotate the hand and radius medially, and so assists pronation.

The **pronator teres** is the most lateral and most oblique of these muscles. It is a pronator (medial rotator of the radius on the ulna) and has increased mechanical advantage by being attached to the most lateral part of the convex radius [Fig. 8.4].

The **flexor digitorum superficialis** lies deep to the other muscles of this group. The humero-ulnar head arises with the other muscles from the medial epicondyle of the humerus and the coronoid process of the ulna. An additional thin **radial head** [Figs. 8.3, 8.4] arises from the anterior border of the radius and straightens the pull of the mus-

cle, so that it passes vertically down the middle of the front of the forearm. Its four tendons enter the palm through the carpal tunnel in the same synovial sheath as those of the flexor digitorum profundus—the common synovial sheath. (The tendons to the middle and ring fingers are anterior to those of the index and little fingers.) One tendon passes into the fibrous flexor sheath of each finger. At the proximal phalanx, each tendon splits into two bands or slips which curve posteriorly on each side of the underlying tendon of the flexor digitorum profundus and are inserted on the palmar surface of the middle phalanx [Fig. 8.17]. The most posterior fibres of each band pass behind the profundus tendon to

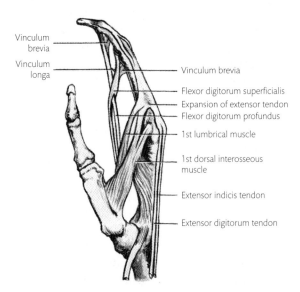

Vinculum brevia

Vinculum longa

Vinculum brevia

Flexor digitorum superficialis
Expansion of extensor tendon
Flexor digitorum profundus

1st lumbrical muscle

1st dorsal interosseous muscle

Extensor indicis tendon

Extensor digitorum tendon

Fig. 8.17 Tendons attached to the index finger.

intermingle with the corresponding fibres of the other band (**chiasma tendinum**) and end in its insertion. Thus, they form an oblique sling around the profundus tendon. The tendons of the flexor digitorum superficialis cross the anterior surfaces of all the joints from the wrist to the proximal interphalangeal joint, and so may flex all of these (the range of movement at the carpometacarpal joints is so small that it may be ignored). Usually they act on the metacarpophalangeal and proximal interphalangeal joints, the wrist being fixed by the extensors. The tendon to the little finger is occasionally missing.

The deep group of flexor muscles arise from the ulna and radius [Fig. 8.4], and consists of the flexor digitorum profundus, flexor pollicis longus, and pronator quadratus.

The **flexor digitorum profundus** arises distal to the coronoid process from the medial and anterior surfaces of the proximal parts of the ulna and the adjacent interosseous membrane. When the fist is clenched, it may be felt contracting through the aponeurotic origin of the flexor carpi ulnaris by placing your fingers medial to the posterior border of the ulna. The four tendons pass through the carpal tunnel and separate in the palm. These tendons give origin to the **lumbrical muscles** from their radial or adjacent sides. Each tendon enters the fibrous flexor sheath of the corresponding finger, deep to the tendon of the flexor digitorum superficialis, traverses the aperture between the slips of the flexor digitorum superficialis tendon, and is inserted into the palmar surface of the base of the distal phalanx [Fig. 8.17]. **Nerve supply**: the lateral half, which passes to the index and middle fingers, is supplied by the anterior interosseous branch of the median nerve; the medial half, which passes to the ring and little fingers, is supplied by the ulnar nerve. **Actions**: this muscle flexes the wrist and fingers, as does the flexor digitorum superficialis. In addition, it also flexes the distal interphalangeal joints and forms the structure from which the lumbricals act. ⊃ When the muscle is paralysed, the obvious effect is the absence of flexion of the terminal phalanges.

The **vincula tendinum** [Fig. 8.17] are thin fibrous slips enclosed in the synovial membrane which transmit blood vessels to the tendons within the digital synovial sheaths. The vincula brevia are triangular and are attached to the tendons immediately proximal to their insertion. The vincula longa are more slender and lie nearer the root of the finger.

The **flexor pollicis longus** arises from the anterior surface of the radius between the attachments of the flexor digitorum superficialis (radial head) and pronator quadratus, and from the interosseous membrane [Fig. 8.4]. The single tendon traverses the lateral part of the carpal tunnel and the palmar surface of the thumb between the muscles of the thenar eminence and adductor pollicis. It enters the fibrous flexor sheath at the base of the proximal phalanx of the thumb and is inserted into the base of the terminal phalanx. **Nerve supply**: the anterior interosseous branch of the median nerve. **Action**: it flexes all the joints of the thumb (including the carpometacarpal joint) and the wrist.

The **pronator quadratus** [Figs. 8.4, 8.7] runs transversely from its origin on the anterior surface of the distal quarter of the ulna to its insertion on the distal quarter of the radius. **Nerve supply**: the anterior interosseous branch of the median nerve. **Action**: pronation.

Dissection 8.4 continues to dissect the palm of the hand.

Fascial compartments of the palm

The deep fascia of the palm covers the muscles in the hand and forms intermuscular septa between them. The fascial compartments of the palm are potential spaces enclosed by septa. Anterior to the central region of the palm is the palmar aponeurosis. Two septa pass posteriorly from the medial and lateral margins of the aponeurosis. On the lateral side, the septum becomes continuous with the fascia covering the palmar aspect of the adductor pollicis. On the medial side, it becomes continuous with the fascia over the medial two interosseous spaces. This central region contains the long flexor tendons of the fingers, the lumbricals, branches of the median and ulnar nerves, and the arteries in the palm. The space is continuous proximally with the carpal tunnel and distally with the superficial tissues of the fingers. It is not directly continuous with the cavities of the fibrous flexor sheaths of the fingers, because these are filled by the digital synovial sheaths. Distal to the common synovial sheath for the flexor tendons, several septa pass between the tendons from the palmar aponeurosis to the fascia covering the metacarpals. Posterior to the structures in the common synovial sheath is a zone of loose connective tissue known as the '**mid-palmar space**' [Fig. 8.8]. ⊃ This space may become distended with fluid in infections of the hand.

DISSECTION 8.4 Palm of the hand-2

Objectives

I. To study the muscles of the thenar eminence, hypothenar eminence, and adductor pollicis.   II. To identify the deep palmar arch and trace its branches.

Instructions

1. Remove the deep fascia from the surface of the thenar and hypothenar eminences. Avoid damage to the branch of the median nerve and the deep branch of the ulnar nerve which supply these muscles.

2. In the **thenar eminence**, the most anterior muscle is the **abductor pollicis brevis**. It covers the **opponens pollicis** completely and the **flexor pollicis brevis** partially [Fig. 8.9]. Pass the handle of a scalpel behind the lateral border of the abductor, and lift it from the underlying muscles. Define its attachments, and cut across it to expose the opponens. Separate the flexor brevis from the opponens; the flexor brevis is inserted, with the abductor brevis, into the anterior aspect of the base of the first phalanx. The opponens pollicis is inserted into the anterior surface of the first metacarpal [Fig. 8.16]. (The use of the terms anterior and posterior in the thumb may be misleading, but necessary because the palmar surface of the thumb faces medially.)

3. All three muscles of the thenar eminence arise from the flexor retinaculum and the tubercle of the trapezium. The flexor has a deep head from the trapezoid and the capitate as well.

4. Cut across the middle of the flexor pollicis brevis, and reflect its parts. This exposes the tendon of the flexor pollicis longus and, behind it, the adductor pollicis passing to the posterior surface of the base of the proximal phalanx.

5. Examine the synovial sheath of the long flexor tendon; then expose and divide the fibrous flexor sheath in the thumb to follow the tendon and its synovial sheath to the terminal phalanx.

6. In the **hypothenar eminence**, separate the **abductor digiti minimi** from the medial side of the **flexor digiti minimi brevis** [Figs. 8.5, 8.9]. Identify and follow the **deep branch of the ulnar nerve** and the deep palmar branch of the ulnar artery between these muscles. Define the attachments of these muscles, and then cut through the middle of the abductor, and reflect its parts to expose the **opponens digiti minimi**. Follow this muscle to its attachments.

7. Cut through the flexor digitorum profundus in the forearm and both ends of the superficial palmar arch in the hand. Turn the distal parts of the flexor digitorum superficialis and profundus towards the fingers. Note the nerves to the lumbricals, as they are reflected with the tendons.

8. Study the remainder of the adductor pollicis, the deep palmar arterial arch, and the deep branch of the ulnar nerve in the palm. Establish the continuity of the last two with the ulnar artery and nerve by tracing them over the medial surface of the hook of the hamate bone. Divide the flexor digiti minimi brevis, if necessary [Fig. 8.9].

9. Follow the artery and nerve laterally on the proximal parts of the bodies of the metacarpals, deep to the long tendons. Find the branches of the nerve which pass to the interosseous muscles between the metacarpals, and trace its branch to the adductor pollicis.

10. Define the attachments of the adductor pollicis [Fig. 8.16]. Cut across the muscle midway between its origins and insertion, and follow the branch of the nerve and the artery between the two parts of the muscle.

11. The deep branch of the ulnar nerve passes to the first dorsal interosseous muscle which is now exposed in the palm.

12. The deep branch of the ulnar artery completes the deep palmar arch by meeting the radial artery entering the palm between the two heads of the first dorsal interosseous muscle. Find the branch of the radial artery which passes to the palmar surface of the thumb (**princeps pollicis**) and the **radialis indicis artery** to the lateral side of the palmar surface of the index finger [Fig. 8.10].

110

➲ Such infections may have tracked to the space from the fingers along the lumbrical muscles or from the digital synovial sheaths.

The adductor pollicis lies in a separate compartment, posterior to the lateral part of the central sheath. ➲ This compartment may also be distended with fluid in infections which involve it, thus forming the '**thenar space**' [Fig. 8.8].

The thenar and hypothenar muscles lie in separate fascial compartments.

➲ Infected puncture wounds of the palm may lead to a collection of fluid between the palmar aponeurosis and the tendons. Fluid in this space cannot escape to the surface, because of the thick aponeurosis, and may involve the tendon sheaths if not drained by surgical incision. Minor injuries of the fingers may also become infected. These lead to considerable effusion of fluid and development of pressure in the dense tissues of the finger. Finger infection may be in the pulp of the finger, distal to the end of the fibrous flexor sheaths or within it in the synovial sheath. If untreated, the pressure may interfere with the blood supply of local tissues and lead to the death of the terminal phalanx if the pulp is involved, or necrosis of the flexor tendons if the flexor sheath is involved. Clearly, if pressure from such infections develops, it must be relieved by opening the sheath and draining the fluid.

Short muscles of the thumb

The **abductor pollicis brevis**, the **flexor pollicis brevis**, and the **opponens pollicis** form the thenar eminence and are innervated by the median nerve. (Occasionally, the flexor and rarely the abductor and opponens are supplied by the ulnar nerve.) All three muscles arise from the lateral part of the flexor retinaculum and from the tubercles of the scaphoid and trapezium [Fig. 8.16].

The opponens pollicis fans out to be inserted on the anterior surface of the first metacarpal. It is covered anteriorly by the abductor pollicis brevis and medially by the flexor pollicis brevis. The abductor pollicis brevis and flexor pollicis brevis are inserted together into the anteromedial surface of the base of the proximal phalanx through a tendon which contains a small sesamoid bone. The abductor pollicis brevis sends part of its tendon into the extensor expansion of the thumb. Through the extensor expansion, it is inserted into the dorsal surface of the base of the distal phalanx and can produce extension of the interphalangeal joint. The flexor pollicis brevis crosses the anteromedial surfaces of the first carpometacarpal and metacarpophalangeal joints and so produces flexion at both joints. The abductor pollicis brevis crosses the anterior surfaces of the same two joints but produces abduction mainly at the carpometacarpal joint. The opponens pollicis acts only on the carpometacarpal joint. It moves the metacarpal towards the centre of the palm and rotates it medially, so that the palmar surface of the thumb is turned to face the palmar surfaces of the fingers.

The **adductor pollicis** is supplied by the deep branch of the ulnar nerve. It lies deep in the palm and takes origin by two heads—the oblique and transverse heads [Fig. 8.16]. The muscles converge on the posteromedial surface of the base of the proximal phalanx of the thumb as a common tendon containing a small sesamoid bone. This muscle draws the thumb posteriorly towards the palm at the carpometacarpal joint, but it may also produce flexion at the metacarpophalangeal joint in the fully opposed thumb.

The **sesamoid bones** of the thumb are small, ovoid bones lying in the tendons and adherent to the capsule of the metacarpophalangeal joint. One flattened surface of each bone is covered with cartilage and slides directly on the cartilage of the palmar surface of the head of the first metacarpal. In a firm grip, sesamoid bones prevent compression of the tendons against the bone and facilitate their movements on the bone.

Movements of the thumb

Movements of the thumb are at right angles to the corresponding movements of the fingers. The **carpometacarpal joint** of the thumb also differs from that of the fingers in possessing a greater degree of mobility. The first carpometacarpal joint is a saddle-shaped joint that permits flexion and extension, and abduction and adduction. (Other carpometacarpal joints allow only a slight degree of gliding movement and no flexion, extension, abduction, or adduction.) The joint surfaces of the first carpometacarpal joint are arranged on a curve, so that flexion is associated with medial rotation of the metacarpal (action of the opponens) and extension with lateral rotation. The range of these movements without rotation is very limited. The metacarpophalangeal and interphalangeal joints of the thumb allow little more than flexion and extension.

Opposition is a complex movement which brings the palmar surface of the distal segment of the thumb into contact with the corresponding surface of a finger. In the thumb, this movement consists of abduction, followed by combined flexion and medial rotation at the carpometacarpal joint, with or without flexion of the other joints of the thumb. Opposition of the thumb must not be confused with simple flexion of all of its joints which can be produced by the flexor pollicis longus acting alone. Simple flexion brings the tip of the thumb into contact with the lateral side of the terminal segment of any flexed finger. It can be carried out by the flexor pollicis longus when true opposition of the thumb is lost due to paralysis of the short muscles of the thumb. This condition is seen when the median nerve is injured, distal to the origin of its anterior interosseous branch supplying the long flexor of the thumb [see Tables 9.9 and 9.10 for muscles and movements of the thumb].

Short muscles of the little finger

The **abductor digiti minimi**, **flexor digiti minimi brevis**, and **opponens digiti minimi** form the hypothenar eminence and are supplied by the deep branch of the ulnar nerve. The **abductor digiti minimi** and **flexor digiti minimi brevis** lie side by side, superficial to the **opponens digiti minimi**. They arise from the flexor retinaculum, the pisiform bone, and the hook of the hamate bone [Fig. 8.16]. The abductor and flexor are inserted together into the anteromedial surface of the base of the proximal phalanx of the little finger. The opponens is inserted along the anteromedial surface of the fifth metacarpal.

The little finger has the most mobile metacarpal of the four fingers, but, even so, lateral rotation of the metacarpal by the opponens is very limited. This movement is supplemented by lateral rotation of the proximal phalanx by the flexor digiti minimi brevis. The flexor digiti minimi brevis also flexes the metacarpophalangeal joint with the flexor digitorum superficialis and profundus.

Deep branch of the ulnar nerve

The deep branch of the ulnar nerve arises from the ulnar nerve on the flexor retinaculum [Fig. 8.9]. It supplies the muscles of the hypothenar eminence and passes deep between the abductor digiti minimi and the flexor digiti minimi brevis with the deep **palmar branch of the ulnar artery**. The nerve and artery turn laterally on the hook of the hamate and cross the palm on the proximal parts of the metacarpal bones, deep to the long flexor tendons. The nerve supplies all interossei muscles, the medial two lumbricals, and the adductor pollicis.

In summary, the deep branch of the ulnar nerve supplies all the muscles in the palm, except the three muscles of the thenar eminence and the lateral two lumbricals. These muscles are supplied by the median nerve. The flexor pollicis brevis frequently receives a branch from the ulnar nerve, in addition to that from the median nerve, and occasionally the ulnar nerve is its only source of supply.

Deep palmar arch

The deep palmar arch is formed by the **radial artery** which enters the palm between the two heads of the first dorsal interosseous muscle. It gives off the **princeps pollicis** and the **radialis indicis arteries** [Fig. 8.10], passes between the heads of the adductor pollicis, runs medially, and unites with the deep palmar branch of the ulnar artery to complete the arch. The deep palmar arch lies a finger's breadth proximal to the superficial palmar arch.

The arch gives a **palmar metacarpal artery** in each of the medial three interosseous spaces. These join the distal ends of the corresponding common palmar digital arteries of the superficial palmar arch and may sometimes replace them.

The **princeps pollicis** passes to the metacarpal of the thumb and divides into the two palmar digital arteries of the thumb, one on each side of the tendon of the flexor pollicis longus.

The **radialis indicis** passes distally between the first dorsal interosseous and the adductor pollicis to become the proper palmar digital artery on the lateral side of the index finger.

Extensor compartment of the forearm and hand

Begin by revising the surface anatomy and cutaneous nerves of the region.

The **posterior cutaneous nerve of the forearm** (a branch of the radial nerve) is the main cutaneous nerve in this region. The **medial** and **lateral cutaneous nerves of the forearm** also spread on to the posterior surface. In the hand, the main supply is from the **superficial branch of the radial nerve** and the **dorsal branch of** the ulnar nerve, often in almost equal proportions. These nerves give rise to the **dorsal digital nerves** to the dorsal aspect of the proximal part of the fingers up to the proximal interphalangeal joints. The cutaneous supply of the dorsal surfaces of the hand and fingers shows considerable variation. Occasionally, the lateral and/or posterior cutaneous nerves of the forearm also supply the dorsum of the hand, and the ulnar nerve regularly supplies a greater area on the dorsum of the hand than on the palmar aspect [see Fig. 5.8].

Dissection 8.5 looks at the back of the forearm.

DISSECTION 8.5 Back of the forearm

Objectives

I. To study the superficial muscles of the back of the forearm.   II. To define the extensor retinaculum.   III. To identify and trace the branches of the posterior interosseous nerve and artery.

Instructions

1. Find the superficial branch of the radial nerve and the dorsal branch of the ulnar nerve on the front of the forearm. Trace both to their distribution on the dorsal surfaces of the hand and fingers.

2. Remove the deep fascia from the back of the forearm, but leave the thickened part at the wrist—the **extensor retinaculum** [Fig. 8.18].

3. As the proximal edge of the retinaculum is defined, try to demonstrate the synovial sheaths of the tendons of the extensor muscles which pass deep to it [Figs. 8.19, 8.20].

4. Separate the superficial muscles from each other, starting with the tendons at the wrist. Because of their limited bony origin, these muscles arise mainly from extensive tendinous sheets between them, so that separation proximally is artificial, but necessary if the deeper structures are to be seen.

5. Completely separate the three anterolateral muscles (brachioradialis, extensor carpi radialis longus, and extensor carpi radialis brevis) from the extensor digitorum [Fig. 8.18], and expose the **supinator** lying deep to them [Fig. 8.21].

6. Expose the **posterior interosseous nerve** emerging from the supinator near its distal border. Follow the branches of this nerve to the extensor digitorum, extensor digiti minimi, extensor carpi ulnaris, and the muscles deep to it. (This nerve is the continuation of the deep branch of the radial nerve.)

7. Pull the brachioradialis and the extensor carpi radialis longus and brevis laterally to expose the radial nerve at the elbow.

8. Complete the exposure of this nerve and its deep branch which gives branches to the supinator and then pierces it. Find the branch to the extensor carpi radialis brevis which arises here. Pull gently on the deep branch to establish its continuity with the posterior interosseous nerve.

9. Find the posterior interosseous artery on the back of the forearm. It emerges between the radius and ulna, immediately distal to the supinator and close to the posterior interosseous nerve. Trace the main branches of the artery.

10. Identify the remaining superficial muscles. The extensor digiti minimi is the separated medial part of the extensor digitorum and leaves it at the extensor retinaculum to pass through a separate compartment, medial to the extensor digitorum. Medial to this is the extensor carpi ulnaris. It is attached to the posterior border of the ulna by the thick deep fascia. Divide the fascia over the extensor carpi ulnaris in the proximal third of the forearm to demonstrate the anconeus [Fig. 8.18].

11. Lift the extensor digitorum, and expose the deep layer of the extensor muscles. Immediately distal to the supinator is the abductor pollicis longus. The other three muscles (extensor pollicis brevis, extensor pollicis longus, and extensor indicis) arise distal to this [Fig. 8.6]. Trace the tendons of these muscles to the extensor retinaculum.

12. Expose the tendons on the back and lateral side of the hand. Note that the thumb, index, and little finger each has two extensor tendons. Identify all these tendons at your own wrist, and note which of them become taut in movements of the wrist and in movements of the fingers and thumb. At the same time, review the position of the flexor tendons on the anterior aspect of the distal part of your forearm.

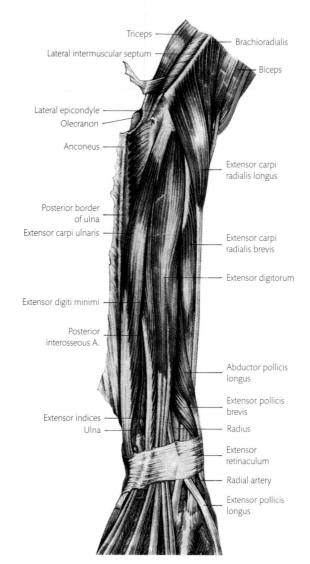

Triceps
Lateral intermuscular septum
Brachioradialis
Biceps
Lateral epicondyle
Olecranon
Anconeus
Extensor carpi radialis longus
Posterior border of ulna
Extensor carpi ulnaris
Extensor carpi radialis brevis
Extensor digitorum
Extensor digiti minimi
Posterior interosseous A.
Abductor pollicis longus
Extensor pollicis brevis
Extensor indices
Ulna
Radius
Extensor retinaculum
Radial artery
Extensor pollicis longus

Fig. 8.18 Superficial dissection of the back of the forearm.

Muscles of the back of the forearm

These may be divided into three groups.

1. The superficial muscles arise from a common origin on the lateral supracondylar line and the lateral epicondyle of the humerus [see Fig. 6.2]. They pass to either: (a) the bones of the forearm [Fig. 8.6]; (b) the bones of the hand [Fig. 8.22]; or (c) the bones of the fingers.
   (i) Centrally placed in the superficial group are the muscles passing to the fingers—the **extensor digitorum** and **extensor digiti minimi**.
   (ii) On either side of the extensor digitorum and extensor digiti minimi are the three extensors of the carpals which are inserted into the metacarpal bones. The **extensor carpi radialis longus** and **brevis** lie laterally, and the **extensor carpi ulnaris** lies medially [Fig. 8.21].
   (iii) Medial and lateral to these, a single muscle from the common origin passes to the radius and ulna. Laterally, the **brachioradialis** passes to the radius; medially, the **anconeus** fans out from the lateral epicondyle to the proximal third of the lateral surface of the ulna [Fig. 8.6].

2. Four deep muscles arise from the forearm bones and the interosseous membrane [Fig. 8.6], and pass to the thumb or index finger. Laterally, the **abductor pollicis longus** and **extensor pollicis brevis** curve over the posterior surface of the radius

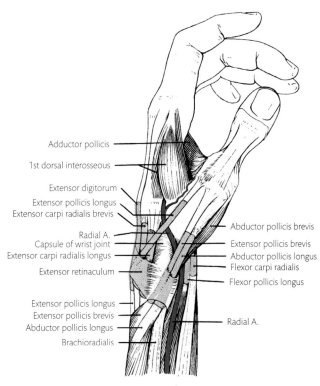

Adductor pollicis

1st dorsal interosseous

Extensor digitorum
Extensor pollicis longus
Extensor carpi radialis brevis

Radial A.
Capsule of wrist joint
Extensor carpi radialis longus

Extensor retinaculum

Extensor pollicis longus
Extensor pollicis brevis
Abductor pollicis longus
Brachioradialis

Abductor pollicis brevis
Extensor pollicis brevis
Abductor pollicis longus
Flexor carpi radialis
Flexor pollicis longus

Radial A.

Fig. 8.19 Dissection of the lateral side of the left wrist and hand, showing the tendons in their synovial sheaths.

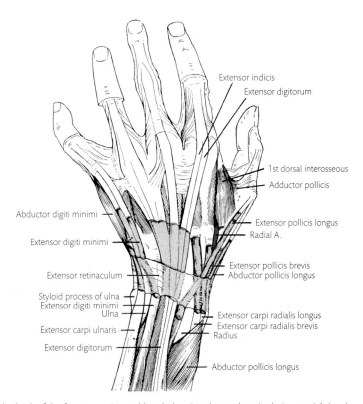

Extensor indicis
Extensor digitorum

1st dorsal interosseous
Adductor pollicis

Abductor digiti minimi

Extensor digiti minimi

Extensor pollicis longus
Radial A.

Extensor retinaculum

Extensor pollicis brevis
Abductor pollicis longus

Styloid process of ulna
Extensor digiti minimi
Ulna

Extensor carpi ulnaris

Extensor digitorum

Extensor carpi radialis longus
Extensor carpi radialis brevis
Radius

Abductor pollicis longus

Fig. 8.20 Dissection of the back of the forearm, wrist, and hand, showing the tendons in their synovial sheaths.

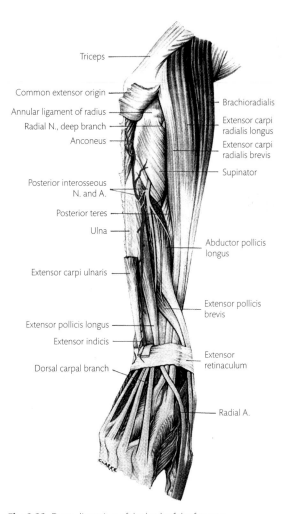

Fig. 8.21 Deep dissection of the back of the forearm.

and the tendons of the lateral three muscles of the superficial group—brachioradialis, and extensor carpi radialis longus and brevis—to the lateral aspect of the base of the first metacarpal. Immediately medial to these is the **extensor pollicis longus**, the tendon of which curves round the medial

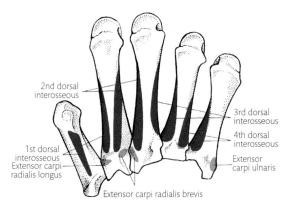

Fig. 8.22 Muscle attachments to the dorsal aspect of the right metacarpus.

side of the **dorsal tubercle of the radius**. More medially, the **extensor indicis** lies medial to the tendons of the extensor digitorum [Fig. 8.21].

3. A single deep muscle—the **supinator**—passes between the two forearm bones. It arises from the lateral surface of the fibrous capsule of the elbow joint and from the upper end of the ulna, distal to the radial notch. It curves round the posterior and lateral surfaces of the radius [Fig. 8.21] and is inserted on the radius between the attachments of the flexor digitorum superficialis [Fig. 8.4] and pronator teres. Figs. 8.23 and 8.24 show the relationship of muscles and tendons to the bones at the upper third of the forearm and wrist.

The **nerve supply** to all these muscles is from the radial nerve and its branches. The brachioradialis, the two extensor carpi radialis, and the supinator are supplied by branches which arise from the radial nerve anteriorly. The remaining muscles, except the anconeus, are supplied by the posterior interosseous nerve which is the continuation of the deep branch of the radial nerve. Thus, injury to the deep branch of the radial nerve in the supinator paralyses only these muscles. (The anconeus is supplied by a branch from the radial nerve to the medial head of the triceps.)

Actions of extensor muscles of the forearm

The actions of the extensor muscles of the fingers and thumb will be dealt with later when the muscles which act with them have been dissected. The action of the brachioradialis has been described earlier.

The **extensor carpi radialis longus** and **brevis** and the **extensor carpi ulnaris** act together to extend the wrist. They also stabilize the wrist in the extended position when the flexor muscles of the fingers act, so that these muscles can apply the full range of their contraction to the fingers. An important point to remember is that, when the wrist is extended, the flexors of the wrist are relaxed. When the wrist is flexed, the fist cannot be closed tightly, because the flexor muscles of the fingers cannot contract sufficiently and the extensor muscles of the fingers cannot stretch adequately to allow this movement. So unless the wrist is extended, a tight fist cannot be formed. Radial extensors of the wrist act with the radial flexor to produce abduction of the wrist. This is an important movement, e.g. in raising a hammer prior to striking with it—which requires the strength of two radial extensors. The **extensor** and **flexor carpi ulnaris** act in a

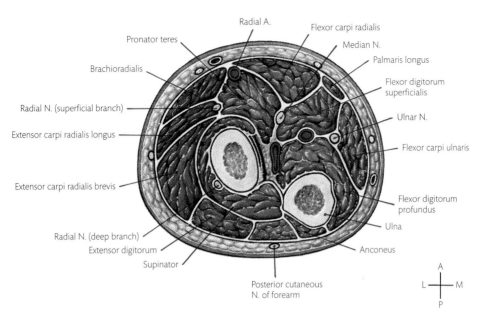

Fig. 8.23 Section through the upper third of the left forearm. A = anterior; P = posterior; M = medial; L = lateral.

similar fashion to produce adduction of the wrist. The flexors and extensors of the wrist act together to fix the wrist, so that fine movements of the fingers can take place on a stable hand.

The **anconeus** holds the ulna firmly against the humerus. It also contracts strongly during pronation, when the distal end of the ulna is displaced laterally by slight medial rotation of the humerus. This occurs in many movements, e.g. in using a screwdriver in the right hand to remove a screw.

The **supinator** supinates the forearm. It is a powerful muscle and acts with the biceps brachii. It may be assisted by the abductor pollicis longus which arises, in part, from the ulna and runs parallel to the supinator.

The **abductor pollicis longus** is inserted into the anterolateral surface of the base of the first metacarpal. It abducts the thumb at the carpometacarpal joint and produces some extension. It also acts with the supinator, as described above.

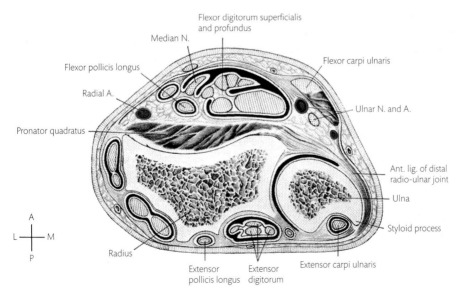

Fig. 8.24 Transverse section through the forearm above the flexor retinaculum, showing the relation of the synovial sheaths to the tendons. A = anterior; P = posterior; M = medial; L = lateral.

Extensor retinaculum and synovial sheaths of extensor tendons

The extensor retinaculum is a thick strip of deep fascia, 2–3 cm wide, which passes across the extensor tendons from the triquetrum and styloid process of the ulna to the sharp anterolateral margin of the distal end of the radius. From the deep surface of the retinaculum, septa extend to the head of the ulna and to each of the bony ridges on the distal end of the radius. The presence of these septa divide the space deep to the retinaculum into a number of tunnels for separate tendons or groups of tendons and their synovial sheaths.

The tendons of the extensor digitorum and extensor indicis lie in a common central synovial sheath. Each of the other tendons usually has its own separate sheath, with the exception of the abductor pollicis longus which lies with the extensor pollicis brevis. The sheaths begin near the proximal edge of the extensor retinaculum and extend for a variable distance on to the corresponding metacarpal. In the case of the extensors of the carpus and the long abductor of the thumb, the sheath ends near the base of the metacarpal to which it is attached. The position of the extensor tendons on the dorsum of the wrist are shown in Table 8.1.

Table 8.1 Position of extensor tendons at the wrist

Tendon palpable	Muscles	Action
Between distal end of radius and bases of second and third metacarpals	Extensor carpi radialis longus and brevis	Extension of wrist
Between distal end of ulna and base of fifth metacarpal	Extensor carpi ulnaris	
Centrally over carpus and bases of third and fourth metacarpals	Extensor digitorum Extensor indicis	Extension of fingers
On fifth metacarpal	Extensor digiti minimi	
From dorsal tubercle of radius along posterior margin of anatomical snuffbox	Extensor pollicis longus	Extension of thumb
From styloid process of radius along anterior margin of snuffbox	Extensor pollicis brevis	
Between styloid process of radius and base of first metacarpal	Abductor pollicis longus	Abduction of thumb

Deep branch of the radial and posterior interosseous nerves

The deep branch of the radial nerve arises at the level of the lateral epicondyle of the humerus. It descends between the brachialis and brachioradialis, and gives branches to the extensor carpi radialis brevis and supinator [see Fig. 7.3]. It enters the supinator, winds obliquely round the lateral and posterior surfaces of the radius within that muscle, and emerges a short distance proximal to the distal border of the supinator, as the posterior interosseous nerve. It gives branches to the surrounding muscles and descends between the extensor digitorum and the abductor pollicis longus on the posterior surface of the interosseous membrane [Fig. 8.21]. In the distal part of the forearm, it accompanies the terminal part of the anterior interosseous artery. It ends on the back of the wrist joint by sending branches to the wrist and the intercarpal joints.

Dissection 8.6 begins the dissection of the back of the hand.

Arteries of the back of the forearm and hand

The **posterior interosseous artery** supplies the muscles on the back of the forearm. It takes part in the anastomosis around the elbow joint and ends in the dorsal carpal rete on the dorsal surface of the wrist. The artery arises from the common interosseous artery in the anterior compartment and passes backwards between the radius and ulna,

---

DISSECTION 8.6 Back of the hand-1

Objective

I. To identify and trace the radial artery on the lateral side and dorsum of the hand.

Instructions

1. Trace the radial artery distally from the anterior surface of the distal end of the radius. It passes through the anatomical snuffbox, deep to the tendons which form the margins, and enters the proximal end of the first intermetacarpal space.

2. Find its dorsal and palmar carpal branches and the dorsal digital arteries which it gives to the thumb and the lateral side of the index finger.

immediately proximal to the interosseous membrane. It appears on the back of the forearm between the supinator and abductor pollicis longus muscles, close to the posterior interosseous nerve. Here it gives muscular branches and sends the interosseous recurrent artery, deep to the anconeus, to the elbow joint anastomosis. The poorly formed remainder of the artery descends between the deep and superficial muscles to the dorsal carpal rete [Fig. 8.21].

The terminal part of the **anterior interosseous artery** pierces the interosseous membrane, 5–6 cm proximal to the distal end of the radius. It descends on the membrane to the dorsal carpal rete with the terminal branch of the posterior interosseous nerve.

The **dorsal carpal rete**—a mesh of anastomosing arteries on the dorsal surfaces of the carpal bones—is formed by the **dorsal carpal branches** of the radial and ulnar arteries and the anterior and posterior interosseous arteries. It supplies the dorsal surfaces of the wrist, the carpal and carpometacarpal joints, and the dorsal surface of the hand and fingers. The rete gives rise to a **dorsal digital artery** to the medial side of the little finger and three **dorsal metacarpal arteries** which lie in the medial three intermetacarpal spaces. Each dorsal metacarpal artery receives **perforating branches** from the deep palmar arch and the corresponding palmar metacarpal artery. It ends by dividing into dorsal digital arteries to each side of adjacent fingers.

The **radial artery** leaves the anterior surface of the radius and passes deep to the tendons of the abductor pollicis longus and extensor pollicis brevis. In the 'anatomical snuffbox', it lies on the scaphoid and trapezium against which it can be palpated. Here it gives off its **palmar** and **dorsal carpal arteries**. The radial artery then passes deep to the tendon of the extensor pollicis longus and gives off **dorsal digital arteries** to both sides of the thumb and the lateral side of the index finger. The artery then turns medially into the palm through the proximal end of the first intermetacarpal space, between the two heads of the first dorsal interosseous muscle [Figs. 8.10, 8.21].

Dissection 8.7 continues the dissection of the back of the hand.

DISSECTION 8.7 Back of the hand-2

Objectives

I. To study the extensor expansion and the insertion of muscles into it.   II. To identify and expose the palmar and dorsal interossei and their tendons.

Instructions

1. Follow the extensor tendons into the fingers and thumb. In each finger, the tendon expands into a sheet as it passes towards the metacarpophalangeal joint and forms a structure known as the **extensor expansion**. Clean the extensor expansion, and note that it is widest at the level of the metacarpophalangeal joint. At this level, the margins of the expansion turn anteriorly on each side of the metacarpal head to be attached to the deep transverse metacarpal ligament.

2. Distal to the metacarpophalangeal joint, the expansion narrows on the dorsal surface of the proximal interphalangeal joint, passing over it to reach the middle and distal phalanges. Over the proximal phalanx, identify the two thickened margins and the central portion of the expansion. Follow the fibre bundles of both parts, as they pass distally.

3. Follow the tendons of the **lumbrical muscles** on the palmar surface of the deep transverse metacarpal ligament into the lateral margins of the expansions.

4. Remove any fat and fascia covering the dorsal surfaces of the intermetacarpal spaces, and expose a **dorsal interosseous muscle** in each space. Trace the muscle distally to its tendon.

5. Divide the dense fibrous tissue which lies between the dorsal parts of the metacarpal heads, and trace part of the tendon into the corresponding margin of the extensor expansion, distal to the metacarpophalangeal joint. (A deeper part of the tendon may be traced into the base of the proximal phalanx.)

6. Identify the deep transverse metacarpal ligament lying between the palmar surfaces of the medial four metacarpal heads.

7. Separate the dorsal interosseous muscle from the two metacarpal bones from which it arises. Turn the muscle distally, and expose the **palmar interosseous muscle** which arises only from the metacarpal of the finger to which it passes. (In the first

intermetacarpal space, the first palmar interosseous muscle is only a slender slip.) Trace the tendon of the palmar interosseous to the extensor expansion and sometimes to the base of the proximal phalanx. The first dorsal interosseous muscle is found on the lateral side of the index finger, and the second on the lateral side of the middle finger. The third and fourth dorsal interossei are found on the medial sides of the middle and ring fingers, respectively. The first and second palmar interosseous muscles are found on the medial side of the thumb and index finger, respectively. The third and fourth palmar interossei are found on the lateral side of the ring and little fingers, respectively. The tendons of the interossei in the medial three spaces lie posterior to the deep transverse metacarpal ligament.

Extensor tendons of the fingers

The four tendons of the **extensor digitorum** pass to the dorsum of the hand. They are linked together by oblique strips of tendinous material—the **intertendinous connections**—proximal to the metacarpophalangeal joints. These connections force the tendons to work together. The index and little fingers each have an additional extensor tendon—**extensor indicis** and **extensor digiti minimi**. These fuse with the corresponding tendon of the extensor digitorum, distal to the connections, and so are able to extend the metacarpophalangeal joints of these fingers alone when the joints of the middle and ring fingers are flexed. The middle and ring fingers cannot be extended individually.

Extensor expansion

The triangular extensor expansion is found on the dorsal aspect of each digit. It forms a hood over the metacarpophalangeal joint and part of the proximal phalanx [Figs. 8.21, 8.25]. Just proximal to the metacarpophalangeal joint, the tendon of the extensor digitorum joins the extensor expansion. The base of the triangle extends anteriorly on each side of the metacarpal head to join the deep transverse metacarpal ligament. Over the proximal phalanx, the lateral margins of the expansion are thickened by the insertion of part of the tendon of the **interossei muscle** and of the tendon of the **lumbricals** (lateral margin only). These thickened margins pass obliquely backwards to the posterior surface of the proximal interphalangeal joint. As they do so, they send tendinous bundles into the tendon of the long extensor in the midline of the extensor expansion [Fig. 8.25]. The main bulk of the extensor digitorum tendon runs through the middle of the extensor expansion and is held in position by strong transverse tendinous bundles at the metacarpophalangeal joint. Distal to the

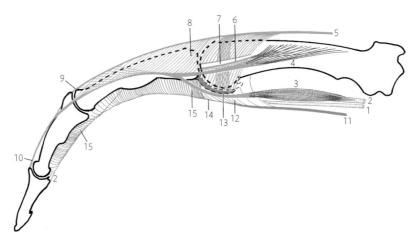

Fig. 8.25 Diagram showing the relationship of the extensor expansion of a finger to the palmar aponeurosis, palmar ligament of the metacarpophalangeal joint, fibrous flexor sheath of the long flexor tendons, and lumbrical and interosseous muscles. 1. Tendon of the flexor digitorum superficialis. 2. Tendon of the flexor digitorum profundus. 3. Lumbrical muscle. 4. Interosseous muscle. 5. Tendon of the extensor digitorum. 6. Deep part of the interosseous tendon passing to the base of the proximal phalanx. 7. Window cut in the extensor expansion. 8. Extensor expansion. 9. Central part of the extensor expansion passing to the base of the middle phalanx. 10. Conjoined lateral and medial parts of the extensor expansion inserting into the terminal phalanx. 11. Palmar aponeurosis with fibres (12) passing to the palmar ligament of (13) the metacarpophalangeal joint, and (14) fibres passing to (15) the fibrous flexor sheath.

metacarpophalangeal joint, the tendon splits into three bundles in the expansion. The central part, joined by bundles from the thick margins of the expansion, crosses the proximal interphalangeal joint and is inserted into the base of the middle phalanx. The other two parts fuse with the margins of the extensor expansion at the level of the proximal phalanx, pass over the posterior surface of the proximal interphalangeal joint, converge and fuse on the dorsal surface of the middle phalanx, cross the posterior surface of the distal interphalangeal joint, and are inserted into the base of the distal phalanx.

At the **metacarpophalangeal** and **interphalangeal joints**, the extensor expansion forms the dorsal part of the **fibrous capsule** of the joint. It is continuous on each side of the joint with the remainder of the fibrous capsule and is held in position by it.

Deep transverse metacarpal ligament and palmar ligaments

The **deep transverse metacarpal ligament** is a strong band which passes between the palmar ligaments of the metacarpophalangeal joints of the medial four digits. These **palmar ligaments** are thick, semi-rigid structures which are firmly attached to the base of the proximal phalanx of each finger. They are only loosely attached to the metacarpal. When the metacarpophalangeal joint is flexed, the palmar ligament slides proximally on the palmar surface of the metacarpal. When the joint is extended, the ligament moves distally on the metacarpal head. Clearly, in each movement, the attachment of the extensor expansion moves with the ligament.

Muscles inserted into the extensor expansion

In addition to the long extensors of the digits, the lumbrical and interosseous muscles are inserted into the extensor expansion.

Lumbrical muscles

The four lumbricals arise from the tendons of the flexor digitorum profundus in the palm of the hand—the first from the lateral side of the tendon to the index finger, the remainder often from the adjacent sides of two tendons. Each passes to the radial side of the corresponding finger, anterior to the metacarpophalangeal joint and the deep transverse metacarpal ligament (except the first), to join the lateral edge of the extensor expansion. **Nerve supply**: the lateral two lumbricals are innervated by the median nerve, and the medial two by the ulnar nerve. **Actions**: these muscles flex the metacarpophalangeal joints of the fingers and extend the interphalangeal joints—the position of the fingers in writing.

Interosseous muscles

These muscles arise from the metacarpal bones [Figs. 8.16, 8.22], the larger dorsal interossei from two adjacent metacarpals and the smaller palmar interossei from the metacarpal of the finger on which they act. They cross the metacarpophalangeal joints, posterior to the deep transverse metacarpal ligament (except for those in the first intermetacarpal space). The **dorsal interossei** pass to the lateral sides of the index and middle fingers and to the medial sides of the middle and ring fingers. Part of the tendon passes deep to the extensor expansion to the base of the proximal phalanx; the remainder joins the corresponding margin of the extensor expansion [Figs. 8.25, 8.26]. **Actions**: dorsal interossei abduct the fingers from the line of the middle finger, extend the interphalangeal joints, and play a part in flexion of the metacarpophalangeal joints (especially the first dorsal interosseous). **Palmar interossei** pass to the medial sides of the thumb and index finger and to the lateral sides of the ring and little fingers. They are inserted into the corresponding margin of the extensor expansion and into the base of the proximal phalanx [Fig. 8.27]. **Actions**: palmar interossei adduct the fingers and the thumb to the line of the middle finger, extend the interphalangeal joints, and play a part in flexion of the metacarpophalangeal joints.

Abduction and adduction at the metacarpophalangeal joints are markedly reduced when these joints are flexed. This is because of tightening of the collateral ligaments and the reduced mechanical advantage of the interossei in the flexed position. **Nerve supply**: all the interossei are supplied by the deep branch of the ulnar nerve [Fig. 8.28].

Movements of the fingers

The fingers are flexed at all joints by the flexor digitorum profundus. They are flexed at the metacarpophalangeal and proximal interphalangeal joints by the flexor digitorum superficialis, and at the metacarpophalangeal joints by the lumbricals and

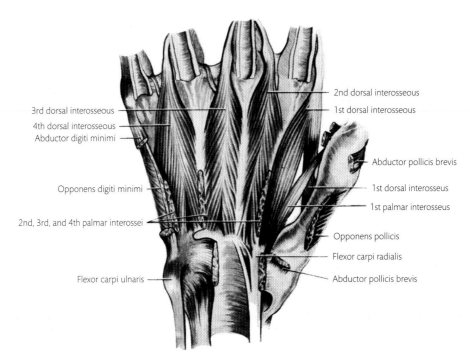

3rd dorsal interosseous
4th dorsal interosseous
Abductor digiti minimi

Opponens digiti minimi

2nd, 3rd, and 4th palmar interossei

Flexor carpi ulnaris

2nd dorsal interosseous
1st dorsal interosseous

Abductor pollicis brevis

1st dorsal interosseus
1st palmar interosseus

Opponens pollicis
Flexor carpi radialis
Abductor pollicis brevis

Fig. 8.26 Dorsal interosseous muscles of the right hand (seen from the palmar aspect).

interossei. ➲ Inability to flex the distal interphalangeal joints occurs in paralysis of the flexor digitorum profundus—a condition which is evident in the ring and little fingers in damage to the ulnar nerve above the elbow.

The fingers are extended together at all joints by the extensor digitorum. The index and little fingers are extended independently at all joints by the extensor indicis and extensor digiti minimi. Extension of the interphalangeal joints is assisted by the lumbricals and interossei. When the metacarpophalangeal joints are fully extended, the deep transverse metacarpal ligament is pulled distally on the metacarpal head, making the attachment to the ligament the only effective insertion of the long extensor tendons. The distal parts of the extensor digitorum and extensor indicis in the extensor expansion are slackened and unable to extend the interphalangeal joints. In this situation (when the metacarpophalangeal joints are fully extended), the interphalangeal joints can only be extended by the **lumbricals** and **interossei**.

➲ Flexion of one finger at the metacarpophalangeal and proximal interphalangeal joints, when the other fingers are extended, leaves the distal phalanx of that finger quite lax—it cannot be either extended or flexed. The distal phalanx cannot be flexed because the flexor digitorum profundus cannot act on a single finger (insufficient separation of the parts of the muscle), and it cannot be extended because the extensor expansion can only extend the distal interphalangeal joint when the proximal interphalangeal joint is extended.

Abduction and adduction of the fingers (but not the thumb) occurs at the metacarpophalangeal

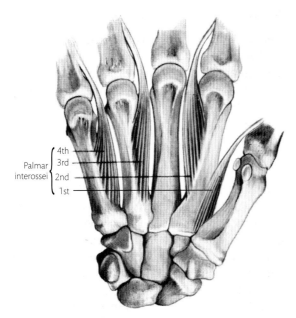

Palmar interossei
4th
3rd
2nd
1st

Fig. 8.27 Palmar interosseous muscles of the right hand.

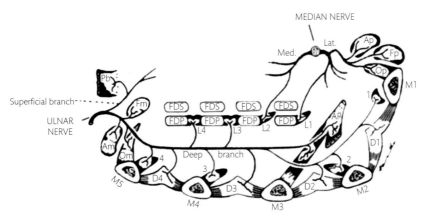

Fig. 8.28 Schematic transverse section through the hand to show the motor distribution of the median and ulnar nerves. 1–4 = palmar interossei 1–4; Am = abductor digiti minimi; Ap = abductor pollicis brevis; AP = adductor pollucis; D1–4 = dorsal interossei 1–4; FDS = flexor digitorum superficialis; FDP = flexor digitorum profundus; Fm = flexor digiti minimi brevis; Fp = flexor pollicis brevis; L1–4 = lumbricals 1–4; M1–5 = metacarpals 1–5; Om = opponens digiti minimi; Op = opponens pollicis; Pb = palmaris brevis.
Reproduced with kind permission of CMC Vellore and Mrs Harsha.

joints. The interossei and abductor digiti minimi produce these movements which have a considerable range when the joints are extended but are limited when they are flexed (see Movements at metacarpophalangeal joints, p. 138). Adduction also occurs in flexion of the fingers and abduction in extension. This is because the axes of the interphalangeal joints do not lie in a straight line, but on an arc of a circle which is concave towards the palm. Confirm this movement in your own hand.

The little finger has the most mobile metacarpal of all the fingers. It can be rotated laterally to a small degree by the opponens digiti minimi, assisted by the short flexor and the abductor. This brings the pulp of the little finger into direct opposition with that of the thumb. Compare this with opposition of the thumb and index finger in your own hand.

Extensors of the thumb

The **extensor pollicis longus** takes origin from the middle third of the posterior surface of the ulna and adjacent interosseous membrane [Fig. 8.6]. Its tendon passes deep to the extensor retinaculum and bends laterally around the dorsal tubercle of the radius. It crosses the tendons of the extensor carpi radialis longus and brevis and runs along the dorsum of the first metacarpal. At the first metacarpophalangeal joint, it is joined by the first palmar interosseous muscle and an extension from the abductor pollicis brevis to form a limited **extensor expansion**.

The **extensor pollicis brevis** and **abductor pollicis longus** arise together—the abductor from the posterior surfaces of the ulna, radius, and interosseous membrane, distal to the supinator, and the extensor brevis from the posterior surfaces of the radius and interosseous membrane, immediately distal to the abductor [Fig. 8.6]. The tendons of both muscles cross the tendons of the brachioradialis and extensor carpi radialis longus and brevis [Fig. 8.21], and pass to the dorsum of the first metacarpal where they form the anterior margin of the 'anatomical snuffbox'. The abductor pollicis longus is inserted to the base of the first metacarpal, and the extensor pollicis brevis continues to the base of the proximal phalanx of the thumb.

These three muscles of the thumb are supplied by the posterior interosseous nerve.

Movements of the thumb

Functionally, the thumb is one half of the hand, for it acts in the opposite direction to the fingers in grasping any object.

The principal movements of the thumb take place at the **carpometacarpal joint**. The movements possible at this joint are flexion, extension, abduction, adduction, and medial and lateral rotation. However, the range of each of these movements varies greatly. The curved saddle shape of the joint freely allows abduction and adduction. Flexion and extension are very slight, unless accompanied by medial rotation in flexion and lateral rotation in extension. These rotatory movements are possible only in abduction, due to the shape of the saddle joint. As such, flexion and extension only occur freely when the thumb is abducted.

Flexion with medial rotation of the abducted thumb is known as **opposition**, because it brings the palmar surface of the thumb to oppose that of one of the fingers.

Movements at the **metacarpophalangeal joint** of the thumb are mainly flexion and extension. A small amount of abduction (produced by the abductor pollicis brevis) and adduction by the adductor pollicis and the first palmar interossei are possible.

Only flexion and extension occur at the **interphalangeal joint**—brought about mainly by the flexor pollicis longus and extensor pollicis longus respectively.

Opposition is produced by the combined action of the abductor pollicis longus and brevis, followed by the action of the opponens pollicis (medial rotation) synchronously with the flexor pollicis brevis. Opposition of the thumb is usually (but not necessarily) accompanied by flexion at the metacarpophalangeal and interphalangeal joints of the thumb.

The flexor pollicis longus is used principally when the tip of the thumb is opposed to the tip of a finger or when power is required. The flexor pollicis brevis is used when the main flexion is at the carpometacarpal and metacarpophalangeal joints. The abductor pollicis brevis is used principally when the thumb is opposed to the little finger; the abductor longus is continuously active during opposition and the reverse movement. In this reverse movement of straightening of the opposed thumb, extension is first produced by the extensor pollicis brevis, which helps to maintain abduction at the carpometacarpal joint. The extensor pollicis longus comes more and more into play, as the movement progresses, helping to produce lateral rotation of the thumb. The extensor pollicis longus may also act as an adductor of the fully abducted thumb, thus assisting the adductor pollicis or mimicking its activity when paralysed.

Confirm these movements in your own hand, and check the contraction of the muscles by noting, as far as possible, their tendons or the hardening of the muscles themselves.

Clinical Applications 8.1, 8.2, and 8.3 explore how the anatomy of the forearm and hand applies to clinical practice.

CLINICAL APPLICATION 8.1 Carpal tunnel syndrome

A 52-year-old domestic worker developed tingling and burning pain over the palmar aspect of the thumb, index, and middle finger. On inspection, the doctor noticed that there was flattening of the thenar eminence.

Study question 1: what forms the thenar eminence? (Answer: muscles of the thenar eminence, the abductor pollicis brevis, the flexor pollicis brevis, and the opponens pollicis.) On examination, it was found that she was not able to abduct or oppose her thumb effectively. She also had decreased sensation over the palmar aspect of the thumb, index finger, middle finger, and lateral part of the ring finger.

Study question 2: if this were due to a nerve lesion, which nerve is affected? (Answer: the median nerve.)

Study question 3: how does the affected nerve enter the hand? Name other structures that lie in the same space at the wrist. (Answer: the median nerve passes deep to the flexor retinaculum (in the carpal tunnel) to enter the hand. Other structures in the carpal tunnel are the tendons of the flexor pollicis longus and flexor digitorum superficialis and profundus.) Death of the tendons due to interference with their blood supply can occur in extreme cases.

CLINICAL APPLICATION 8.2 Tenosynovitis

A 12-year-old schoolgirl pricked her thumb with a needle, just proximal to the interphalangeal joint on the palmar aspect. Over the next few days, she developed pain and swelling over the site of injury which soon spread to the lateral side of the hand and palm up to the wrist. Her parents treated her with painkillers and made her rest. The swelling continued to spread and extended to the lower part of the wrist. Movements of the thumb and wrist became excruciatingly painful, and she developed a fever on the tenth day. She was taken to a hospital. On examination, her entire thumb, lateral side of the hand, and lower part of the forearm were swollen and tender. Movements of the thumb were restricted due to the swelling and painful. There was no lymphadenopathy.

Study question 1: from your knowledge of anatomy of this region, which structure, when infected, is most likely to present with these signs and symptoms? (Answer: synovial sheath of the thumb.)

Study question 2: name the tendon which lies in this sheath. What is the proximal and distal extent of this sheath? (Answer: the tendon of the flexor pollicis longus. The sheath starts from a few centimetres proximal to the flexor retinaculum and ends on the distal phalanx.)

Study question 3: do you think it is possible for the infection to spread outside the sheath? (Answer: Yes.) The radial synovial sheath may communicate with the ulnar (common) synovial sheath for the long flexors, and infection can spread through this communication. The sheath could rupture because of distension, and infection could spread to the surrounding tissue.

CLINICAL APPLICATION 8.3 Dupuytren's contracture

Progressive shortening of the palmar aponeurosis results in a condition known as Dupuytren's contracture. The patient's fingers are flexed, because the aponeurosis is attached to the proximal phalanges through the deep transverse metacarpal ligament. The shortening usually affects the medial part of the aponeurosis, and hence the little and ring fingers. Surgical division of the aponeurosis is required to straighten the fingers.

CHAPTER 9
The joints of the upper limb

Elbow joint

This chapter begins with Dissection 9.1.

The elbow joint is formed by the articulation of the **trochlea** of the humerus with the **trochlear notch** of the ulna, and the **capitulum** of the humerus with the proximal surface of the **head of the radius** [see Figs. 6.2, 8.4]. Its fibrous capsule and joint cavity are continuous with those of the proximal radio-ulnar joint. The elbow joint is essentially a hinge joint with strong radial and ulnar collateral ligaments. The anterior and posterior parts of the fibrous capsule are weak and contain oblique fibres which permit the full range of movements [Fig. 9.1].

Proximally, the anterior part of the fibrous capsule is attached to the medial and lateral epicondyles and the upper margins of the radial and coronoid fossae of the humerus. Distally, it is attached to the coronoid process of the ulna and the annular ligament of the radius.

The posterior part of the capsule is weak. It stretches from a line joining the epicondyles across the floor of the olecranon fossa to the articular margin of the olecranon.

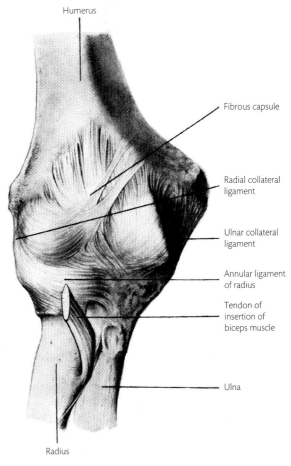

Fig. 9.1 Front of the elbow joint.

Labels: Humerus; Fibrous capsule; Radial collateral ligament; Ulnar collateral ligament; Annular ligament of radius; Tendon of insertion of biceps muscle; Ulna; Radius

DISSECTION 9.1 Elbow joint

Objective

I. To study the fibrous capsule of the elbow joint.

Instructions

1. Separate the muscles from the epicondyles, and reflect them distally. Divide the biceps, brachialis, and triceps, a short distance proximal to the elbow, and turn all three distally.

2. Separate all the muscles from the fibrous capsule of the elbow joint, and remove the loose connective tissue from its external surface, so as to define its parts. Retain the median, ulnar, and radial nerves and the brachial artery.

The **radial collateral ligament** is strong. It passes from the distal surface of the lateral epicondyle to the lateral and posterior parts of the annular ligament of the radius [Fig. 9.1].

The **ulnar collateral ligament** radiates from the medial epicondyle of the humerus to the coronoid process and olecranon of the ulna. The edges of the ligament are thick. The thinner central part is attached to a transverse band that bridges across the interval between these edges [Fig. 9.2]. The ulnar nerve and posterior ulnar recurrent artery lie on the posterior and middle parts of the ligament.

Dissection 9.2 dissects the interior of the elbow joint.

Synovial membrane

As in all synovial joints, the synovial membrane lines the deep surface of the fibrous capsule and the intracapsular non-articular parts of the bones. On the bony fossae—olecranon, coronoid, and radial—the synovial membrane is separated from the fibrous capsule by pads of fat which slide into the fossae when the bony processes are withdrawn during flexion and extension [Fig. 9.3]. The synovial membrane of the elbow joint is continuous with that of the proximal radio-ulnar joint on the lateral side.

The **nerve supply** of the joint is from all the adjacent nerves—median, ulnar, radial, posterior interosseous, and musculocutaneous.

Movements at the elbow joint

The elbow joint is essentially a hinge joint, the main movements of which are flexion and extension. (The movements at the elbow joint are distinct from those which take place at the proximal radio-ulnar joint.) In full flexion, the forearm bones lie parallel to the humerus. In full extension, the ulna is angled laterally, so that the supinated forearm bones make an angle ('**the carrying angle**') of approximately 165 degrees laterally with the humerus. This angulation of the ulna is obscured in pronation when the arm and forearm lie in the same straight line and the radius and ulna cross each other. In addition to being a hinge joint, the humero-ulnar part of the elbow joint is a modified saddle joint which allows some slight abduction and adduction of the ulna. Tables 9.1 and 9.2 summarize the muscles and movements of the elbow joint.

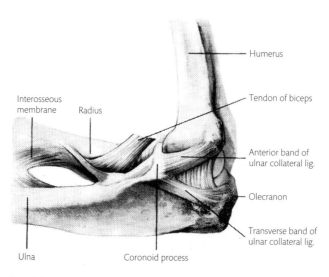

Fig. 9.2 Medial aspect of the elbow joint.

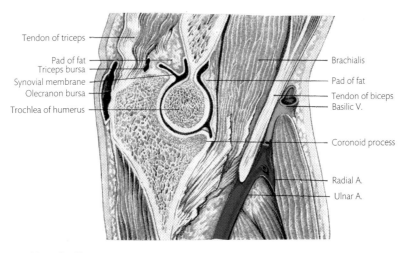

Fig. 9.3 Sagittal section of the right elbow.

Table 9.1 Muscles acting on the elbow joint

Muscle	Origin	Insertion	Action at elbow	Nerve supply
Brachialis	Humerus, anterior surface, distal half	Ulna, coronoid process	Flexion	Musculocutaneous
Biceps brachii	Scapula, coracoid process, supraglenoid tubercle	Radius, tuberosity	Flexion	Musculocutaneous
Brachioradialis	Humerus, lateral supracondylar line	Radius, base of styloid process	Flexion	Radial
Extensor carpi radialis longus	Humerus, lateral supracondylar line	Second metacarpal	Flexion	Radial
Triceps	Scapula, infraglenoid tubercle long head. Humerus, posterior surface. Above groove for radial nerve lateral head, below groove medial head	Ulna, olecranon	Extension	Radial
Anconeus	Humerus, lateral epicondyle	Ulna, lateral surface, proximal one-third	Holds ulna to humerus Abduction of ulna	Radial
Pronator teres	Humerus, medial supracondylar line and medial epicondyle	Radius, lateral surface	Flexion—minor role	Median
Flexor carpi radialis	Humerus, medial epicondyle	First metacarpal	Flexion—minor role	Median

Table 9.2 Movements at the elbow joint

Movement	Muscles	Nerve supply
Flexion	Biceps brachii	Musculocutaneous
	Brachialis	Musculocutaneous
	Brachioradialis	Radial
	Extensor carpi radialis longus	Radial
	Flexor carpi radialis	Median
	Pronator teres	Median
Extension	Triceps	Radial
Ulna, abduction	Anconeus	Radial

Wrist joint

Dissection 9.3 begins the dissection of the wrist.

The **radiocarpal** or **wrist joint** consists of the articulation between the convex surface of the scaphoid, lunate, and triquetrum, with the concave distal surfaces of the radius and the triangular articular disc. The triangular **articular disc** joins the medial edge of the articular surface of the radius to the styloid process of the ulna [Fig. 9.4]. It separates the ulna from the joint. In the resting position of the hand, only the scaphoid and lateral part of the lunate articulate with the two shallow fossae on the distal surface of the radius. The remainder of the lunate is in contact with the articular disc [Fig. 9.4]. The direction of the radiocarpal joint is oblique—the lateral and dorsal margins of the radius extend further distally than the other margins. This reduces the likelihood of posterior dislocation of any of the carpal bones.

Fibrous capsule of the wrist joint

The fibrous capsule passes from the margins of the distal ends of the radius and ulna and the margins of the articular disc to the scaphoid, lunate, and triquetrum. Medially and laterally,

Objective

I. To study the fibrous capsule of the wrist joint.

Instructions

1. Remove the remains of the thenar and hypothenar muscles from their proximal attachments, and separate the flexor and extensor retinacula from the bones.

2. Reflect the flexor and extensor tendons distally.

slightly thickened portions of the fibrous capsule pass from the styloid processes of the radius and ulna to the scaphoid and triquetrum. These are the **radial** and **ulnar collateral ligaments**. The anterior and posterior parts of the fibrous capsule contain fibres which pass obliquely downwards and medially. The synovial membrane, which lines the fibrous capsule and covers the interosseous ligaments of the carpals, may be continuous with that of the distal radio-ulnar joint through a defect in the triangular disc. The nerve supply is through the anterior and posterior interosseous nerves and the dorsal branch of the ulnar nerve.

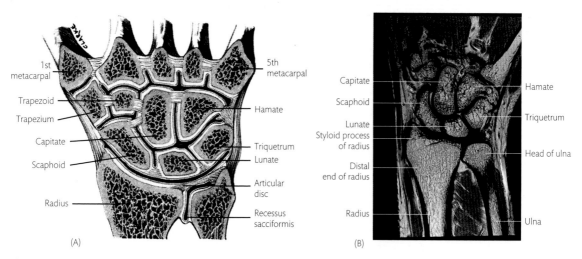

Fig. 9.4 Coronal section through the radiocarpal, intercarpal, carpometacarpal, and intermetacarpal joints to show joint cavities and interosseous ligaments. (A) Schematic drawing. (B) MRI.

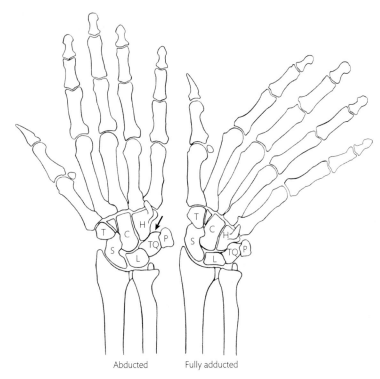

Abducted Fully adducted

Fig. 9.5 Bones of the hand in partially abducted (left) and fully adducted (right) positions of the wrist. In the partially abducted position, the scaphoid articulates with the radius, and the lunate with the articular disc on the ulna. In adduction, the carpal bones slide laterally; the lunate comes into contact with the radius, and the triquetrum with the articular disc. The distal row of carpal bones slides in the concavity of the proximal row. C = capitate; H = hamate; L = lunate; P = pisiform; S = scaphoid; T = trapezium; TQ = triquetrum.

Movements at the wrist joint

The ellipsoid wrist joint has a long radius of curvature transversely which permits abduction and adduction, and a short radius of curvature anteroposteriorly which permits flexion and extension. All these movements are supplemented by similar movements at the **intercarpal joints** [Fig. 9.5]. In adduction, the carpal bones slide laterally, the lunate passing further on to the radius, while the triquetrum comes into contact with the triangular disc.

Because of the two different curvatures of the joint, rotation is not possible. The carpal bones move with the radius in pronation and supination. Thus, the movement of adduction when the hand is pronated deviates the hand laterally, but still towards the ulna which is now lateral to the radius in the distal forearm. For this reason, adduction is commonly called 'ulnar deviation', and abduction 'radial deviation'.

DISSECTION 9.4 Wrist joint-2

Objective

I. To study the interior of the wrist joint.

Instructions

1. Divide the anterior, medial, and lateral ligaments by a transverse incision across the front of the joint.

2. Bend the hand backwards, and expose the articular surfaces.

Dissection 9.4 continues the dissection of the wrist.

Tables 9.3 and 9.4 summarize the muscles and movements of the wrist joint.

Table 9.3 Muscles acting on the wrist joint

Muscle	Origin	Insertion	Action at wrist	Nerve supply
Flexor carpi radialis	Humerus, medial epicondyle	Second and third metacarpal bases	Flexion, abduction	Median
Flexor carpi ulnaris	Humerus, medial epicondyle Ulna, subcutaneous border	Pisiform (hamate and fifth metacarpal)	Flexion, adduction	Ulnar
Extensor carpi radialis longus	Humerus, lateral supracondylar line	Second metacarpal base	Extension, abduction	Radial
Extensor carpi radialis brevis	Humerus, lateral epicondyle	Second and third metacarpal bases	Extension, abduction	Radial*
Extensor carpi ulnaris	Humerus, lateral epicondyle Ulna, posterior border	Fifth metacarpal base	Extension, adduction	Radial*
Extensor digitorum	Humerus, lateral epicondyle	Extensor expansions of fingers	Extension, prevented by radial and ulnar flexors of carpus	Radial*
Extensor digiti minimi	Humerus, lateral epicondyle	Extensor expansion fifth digit		Radial*
Extensor pollicis longus	Ulna, middle third dorsal surface	Thumb distal phalanx		Radial*
Extensor indicis	Ulna, distal to extensor pollicis longus	Second digit extensor expansion		Radial*
Flexor digitorum profundus	Ulna, proximal three-fourths, anterior and medial surfaces	Fingers terminal phalanges	Flexion, prevented by radial and ulnar extensors of carpus	Median** and ulnar
Flexor digitorum superficialis	Humerus, medial epicondyle Ulna, coronoid process Radius anterior border	Fingers middle phalanges		Median
Flexor pollicis longus	Radius, anterior surface middle two-quarters	Thumb distal phalanx		Median**

* Posterior interosseous branch. **Anterior interosseous branch.

Note: Long flexors and extensors of the digits do not bring about flexion or extension of the wrist. This is because flexion is prevented by radial and ulnar extensors of the wrist; and extension is prevented by radial and ulnar flexors of the wrist.

Table 9.4 Movements at the wrist joint

Movement	Muscles	Nerve supply
Flexion	Flexor carpi ulnaris	Ulnar
	Flexor carpi radialis	Median
	Flexor digitorum profundus	Median* and ulnar
	Flexor digitorum superficialis	Median
	Flexor pollicis longus	Median*
	Palmaris longus	Median
Extension	Extensor carpi ulnaris	Radial*
	Extensor carpi radialis longus and brevis	Radial
	Extensor digitorum	Radial*
	Extensor digiti minimi	Radial*
	Extensor pollicis longus	Radial*
	Extensor indicis	Radial*
Abduction	Extensor carpi radialis longus and brevis	Radial
	Flexor carpi radialis	Median
	Abductor pollicis longus	Radial*
Adduction	Flexor carpi ulnaris	Ulnar
	Extensor carpi ulnaris	Radial*

* Anterior or posterior interosseous branch.

Radio-ulnar joints

Proximal radio-ulnar joint

This joint is between the side of the cylindrical head of the radius and the radial notch of the ulna. It is strengthened by the annular and quadrate ligaments.

Annular ligament of the radius

The **annular ligament** is a strong, fibrous collar which encircles the head of the radius and retains it in contact with the radial notch on the ulna [Fig. 9.6]. It is attached to the anterior and posterior margins of the radial notch. It is slightly conical and is loosely attached to the neck of the radius. Thus, the head of the radius is free to turn within the ligament but cannot be pulled down out of it. Proximally, the annular ligament is continuous with, and strengthened by, the lateral and anterior ligaments of the elbow joint [Fig. 9.1]. The weak **quadrate ligament** passes between the neck of the radius and the lower margin of the radial notch of the ulna.

Synovial membrane

The synovial membrane of the proximal radio-ulnar joint is continuous with that of the elbow joint. It lines the deep surface of the annular ligament and is reflected upwards from its distal margin to surround the intracapsular part of the neck of the radius.

Distal radio-ulnar joint

At the distal radio-ulnar joint, the head of the ulna articulates with the ulnar notch of the radius. The bones are held together by the articular disc of the wrist joint, the interosseous membrane, and a weak fibrous capsule.

Articular disc

The triangular, fibrocartilaginous articular disc is the main structure holding the distal ends of the radius and ulna together [Fig. 9.4]. The base of the triangular disc is attached to the distal margin of the ulnar notch of the radius. The apex is attached to a depression at the root of the ulnar styloid process. The disc covers the distal end of the ulna and separates it from the carpal bones. It also separates the distal radio-ulnar joint from the wrist joint. Occasionally, the disc is perforated, and the cavities of the two joints are continuous.

Fibrous capsule of the distal radio-ulnar joint

The fibrous capsule of the distal radio-ulnar joint consists of lax fibres passing between the anterior and posterior borders of the disc and the adjacent surfaces of the radius and ulna. Between these bones, the capsule extends proximally to the distal border of the interosseous membrane enclosing a prolongation of the joint cavity.

Synovial membrane of the distal radio-ulnar joint

The synovial membrane of the distal radio-ulnar joint lines the fibrous capsule and the proximal surface of the articular disc.

Dissection 9.5 describes the dissection of the interosseous membrane.

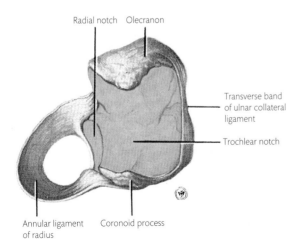

Fig. 9.6 Annular ligament of the radius and proximal articular surfaces of the ulna.

Labels: Radial notch, Olecranon, Transverse band of ulnar collateral ligament, Trochlear notch, Annular ligament of radius, Coronoid process

---

DISSECTION 9.5 Interosseous membrane

Objective

I. To study the interosseous membrane.

Instructions

1. Expose the interosseous membrane by removing the muscles from the back or front of the forearm.

Interosseous membrane of the forearm

This fibrous sheet stretches between the interosseous borders of the radius and ulna and holds these bones together, while allowing movements to take place between them. It begins 2–3 cm distal to the tuberosity of the radius and blends distally with the capsule of the distal radioulnar joint. The fibres run downwards and medially from the radius to the ulna. Forces applied to the radius from the hand (as in a fall on the outstretched arm) are transmitted to the ulna through the interosseous membrane. Such forces are then transferred to the humerus at the elbow joint.

The posterior interosseous vessels pass back between the radius and ulna, proximal to the interosseous membrane. The anterior interosseous vessels pierce the membrane, 5 cm from its distal end. The membrane increases the area of origin for the deep flexor and extensor muscles of the forearm.

Dissection 9.6 explores the superior and inferior radio-ulnar joints.

Movements at the radio-ulnar joints

The movements taking place at the radio-ulnar joints are **supination** and **pronation** [Fig. 9.7]. When the limb is supine, the thumb is directed laterally, and the radius and ulna lie parallel to each other. When the limb is prone, the thumb and styloid process of the radius lie on the medial side; the posterior surfaces of the radius and hand face anteriorly, and the body of the radius lies obliquely

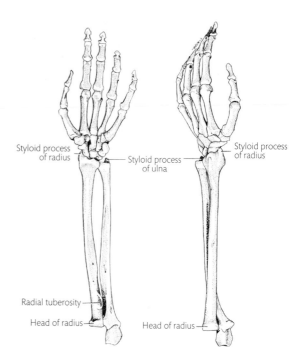

Fig. 9.7 Left forearm and hand bones in the supine (left) and semi-prone (right) positions. Note that the ulna remains stationary and the distal end of the radius rotates around it, carrying the hand with it.

across the anterior surface of the ulna. In pronation, the radius rotates around an axis that passes through the centre of the head of the radius and the head of the ulna. The head of the radius rotates in the annular ligament, while the distal end turns around the stationary ulna, carrying the hand and articular disc with it. As described above, the ulna remains stationary, and the little finger rotates around its own axis. However, pronation and supination can be carried out around the axis of any one of the fingers.

Pronation

Pronation is produced by muscles on the anterior surface of the forearm which run from medial to lateral—pronator teres, pronator quadratus, and flexor carpi radialis. The pronator teres has the maximum mechanical advantage, because it is inserted into the point of maximum lateral convexity of the radius.

Supination

The biceps brachii is a powerful supinator. Its tendon turns round the medial side of the radius into

---

DISSECTION 9.6 Superior and inferior radio-ulnar joints

Objective

I. To study the interior of the superior and inferior radio-ulnar joints.

Instructions

1. Cut through the annular ligament, and divide the interosseous membrane from above downwards.

2. Open the capsule of the distal radio-ulnar joint, and draw the radius laterally to expose the connections of the articular capsule and disc.

Table 9.5 Muscles acting on the radio-ulnar joint

Muscle	Origin	Insertion	Action on radio-ulnar joint	Nerve supply
Pronator teres	Humerus, medial epicondyle and medial supracondylar line	Radius, lateral surface, middle of body	Pronation	Median
Pronator quadratus	Ulna, anterior surface, distal one-fourth	Radius, anterior surface, distal one-fourth	Pronation. Holds radius to ulna	Median*
Flexor carpi radialis	Humerus, medial epicondyle	Second and third metacarpal bases	Pronation	Median
Supinator	Humerus, lateral epicondyle. Ulna, supinator crest	Radius, posterior lateral and anterior surfaces of proximal third	Supination	Radial
Biceps brachii	Scapula, coracoid process. Scapula, supraglenoid tubercle	Radius, tuberosity	Supination (with elbow flexion)	Musculocutaneous
Brachioradialis	Humerus, lateral supracondylar line	Radius, distal end, lateral surface	Supination from pronation to mid position	Radial

* Anterior interosseous branch.

135

the posterior aspect of the radial tuberosity. Thus, it rotates the radius laterally on contraction. Muscles which pass from medial to lateral on the posterior aspect of the forearm also produce supination—supinator and abductor pollicis longus. The brachioradialis can help to start supination of the fully pronated forearm.

With the elbow extended, the range of pronation and supination is apparently increased by the added rotation of the humerus. For this reason, clinical tests for the range of movements at the radio-ulnar joints are always carried out with the elbow flexed at right angles—the position in which the biceps has its maximum supinating power. Tables 9.5 and 9.6 summarize the muscles and movements of the radio-ulnar joint.

Table 9.6 Movements at the radio-ulnar joint

Movement	Muscles	Nerve supply
Pronation	Pronator teres	Median
	Pronator quadratus	Median*
	Flexor carpi radialis	Median
Supination	Supinator	Radial
	Biceps brachii	Musculocutaneous
	Brachioradialis	Radial

* Anterior interosseous branch.

Intercarpal, carpometacarpal, and intermetacarpal joints

There are three separate joint cavities within this complex of articulations between the carpals and metacarpals: (1) the main joint complex; (2) the pisiform (intercarpal) joint; and (3) the carpometacarpal joint of the thumb.

The main joint complex

This is a large single complex joint in which the cavity and synovial membrane are common to the articulations of the carpal bones with each other (intercarpal joints), with the medial four metacarpal bones (carpometacarpal joint), and the bases of these metacarpals with each other (intermetacarpal joints) [Fig. 9.4]. The common fibrous capsule unites the exposed surfaces of all these bones. This intercarpal joint capsule is continuous proximally with the capsule of the wrist joint (though their cavities are separate) and forms three strong intermetacarpal ligaments which limit the cavity distally.

In addition to the intermetacarpal ligaments, **interosseous ligaments** unite each row of carpal bones. The ligaments between the proximal parts of the scaphoid, lunate, and triquetrum bones complete the distal articular surface of the wrist joint and separate its cavity from that of the intercarpal joints. Less regular ligaments unite the distal row of carpal bones and allow continuity of the intercarpal and carpometacarpal joint cavities around them.

Articular surfaces and movements

In each row, the carpal bones articulate with each other by flat surfaces which allow little movement but give some resilience. The joint between the proximal and distal rows is deeply concavo-convex. The capitate and hamate fit into the concavity of the proximal row, and the concave surfaces of the trapezium and trapezoid fit the convex distal surface of the scaphoid [Figs. 9.4, 9.8A and B].

Intercarpal joints

The main movements possible at the intercarpal joints are flexion and extension. The distal row also moves on the proximal row around an anteroposterior axis through the centre of the capitate, producing some abduction and adduction [Fig. 9.5]. Thus, the transverse intercarpal joint increases the range of movements at the wrist and the resilience of the region.

Pisiform joint

This is a small, flat area where the pisiform articulates with the palmar surface of the triquetrum.

The pisiform is held in position against the pull of the flexor carpi ulnaris by the **pisohamate** and **pisometacarpal ligaments**. The joint allows the pisiform to maintain correct alignment during adduction and abduction of the hand.

Medial four carpometacarpal joints

The metacarpal bone of the index articulates with the trapezoid, and that of the middle finger with the capitate [Fig. 9.4]. Both metacarpals have very limited movements. Confirm this on your own hand. The fourth and fifth metacarpals articulate with the hamate. Note that the metacarpal of the ring finger has considerable movement, while that of the little finger is the most mobile. The carpometacarpal joints of the ring and little fingers are flexed when the fist is clenched or the palm 'cupped', and the fifth has slight lateral rotation produced by the opponens digiti minimi.

Carpometacarpal joint of the thumb

The first metacarpophalangeal joint is separate from the rest. This is a saddle-shaped joint with a loose capsule which permits the wide range of movements of the first metacarpal on the trapezium. The thumb lies anterior to the other digits and is rotated, so that its nail faces laterally. Movements

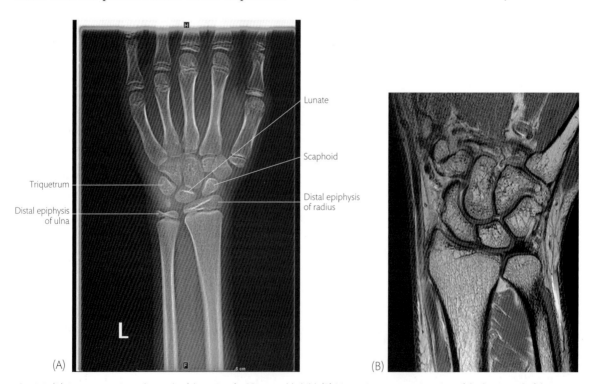

Triquetrum

Distal epiphysis of ulna

Lunate

Scaphoid

Distal epiphysis of radius

(A)   (B)

Fig. 9.8 (A) Anteroposterior radiograph of the wrist of a 12-year-old child. (B) Magnetic resonance imaging of the lower end of the forearm and wrist. See Fig. 9.4B for labels.

of the thumb are thus at right angles to those of the fingers and occur principally at this joint. The first metacarpal may be moved laterally (extension) or medially (flexion) or anteriorly (abduction) or posteriorly (adduction). When the thumb is adducted, the range of flexion and extension is small; when abducted, the range is greatly increased. The metacarpal then moves on an arc of a circle, so that it is medially rotated in flexion and laterally rotated in extension. This movement of flexion with medial rotation of the abducted metacarpal of the thumb is known as **opposition**, for it opposes the palmar surface of the thumb to those of the fingers. It is essential in holding or grasping objects and makes the thumb functionally one-half of the hand.

Intermetacarpal joints

These permit slight movement between the bases of the metacarpals.

Nerve supply

The nerve supply of these joints is from the anterior and posterior interosseous nerves, the dorsal and deep branches of the ulnar nerve, and the superficial branch of the radial nerve.

The wrist, intercarpal, and intermetacarpal joints are visualized in the living by X-rays and magnetic resonance imaging. Study Figs. 9.8A and B, and compare them with Fig. 9.4.

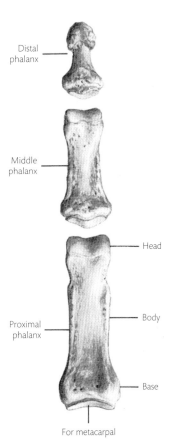

Distal phalanx

Middle phalanx

Proximal phalanx

Head

Body

Base

For metacarpal

Fig. 9.9 Phalanges of a finger, palmar view. By comparison, in the foot, the base of the proximal phalanx is large, and the bodies are much thinner.

Metacarpophalangeal joints

These are condyloid joints in which the convex head of the metacarpal fits into the shallow fossa on the base of the proximal phalanx [Fig. 9.9]. In the thumb, the metacarpal surface is flatter and less extensive than in the other metacarpals, for the range of movements is smaller in the thumb.

Fibrous capsules of metacarpophalangeal joints

The fibrous capsule is thickened anteriorly to form the palmar ligament, and on each side to form a collateral ligament. On the dorsal surface, it is replaced by the extensor expansion, a mechanism which allows for full range of flexion with continuous support for the dorsal surfaces of the joints.

The **collateral ligaments** are strong, oblique bands which extend from the dorsal surface of the metacarpal heads to the sides of the base of the proximal phalanx anteriorly [see Fig. 8.15].

The **palmar ligament** is a thick, fibrous plate attached firmly to the base of the proximal phalanx, but loosely to the neck of the metacarpal. Its position varies with movements of the metacarpophalangeal joint. In full flexion, the plate lies on the palmar surface of the body of the metacarpus. It moves on to the palmar surface of the head when the joint is straightened and on to its distal surface in full extension. In the medial four digits, the margins of the palmar plate give attachment to the: (1) **deep transverse metacarpal ligaments**; (2) **fibrous flexor sheath**; (3) slips of the **palmar aponeurosis**; (4) **collateral ligaments**; and (5) transverse fibres of the **extensor expansion**. Thus, the palmar aponeurosis and the transverse fibres of the extensor expansion are tightened when the plate is drawn on to the distal aspect of the metacarpal head in full extension. This holds the extensor digitorum tendon in place and prevents it from extending the interphalangeal joints when the metacarpophalangeal joint is extended. When the metacarpophalangeal joints are straight or flexed, the extensor digitorum can extend the interphalangeal joints.

Sesamoid bones

A small, oval sesamoid bone is buried on each side of the palmar ligament of the metacarpophalangeal joint of the thumb, where the tendons of the adductor pollicis and flexor pollicis brevis fuse with the ligament. Each bone articulates with the corresponding surface of the head of the metacarpal. The tendon of the flexor pollicis longus lies in the groove between them. Smaller sesamoid bones may be found in the palmar ligaments of the other joints, particularly in the index and little fingers.

Movements at metacarpophalangeal joints

Based on the shape of the joint surfaces, flexion, extension, abduction, and adduction take place at the metacarpophalangeal joint. (Some amount of passive rotation is possible, but no voluntary rotation.) Abduction and adduction movements of the fingers are possible when the joint is extended and the collateral ligaments are relaxed. These movements are severely restricted in flexion because of the tightening of the collateral ligaments. Because the metacarpals are arranged in an arc convex dorsally, the fingers converge on flexion and diverge on extension.

In **precision movements**, flexion of the metacarpophalangeal joints of the medial four digits is produced mainly by the interossei and lumbricals. Extension of these joints is produced by the extensor digitorum and by the extensor indicis and extensor digiti minimi in the index and little fingers. The extensors of the index and little fingers permit isolated extension of the index and little fingers when the middle and ring fingers are flexed at the metacarpophalangeal joints.

In the **metacarpophalangeal joint of the thumb**, the range of movements is much less in all directions. (A wide range of movements occurs at the carpometacarpal joint of the thumb.) Flexion is produced by the flexor pollicis brevis and longus, abduction and adduction by the short

abductor, adductor, and first palmar interossei, and extension by the long and short extensor muscles.

Interphalangeal joints

The interphalangeal joints have the same arrangement as the metacarpophalangeal joints, except that the articular surfaces only permit a hinge-like movement of flexion and extension (no abduction and adduction) [Fig. 9.9].

The flexor digitorum profundus flexes all the joints of the fingers. The flexor digitorum superficialis acts only on the proximal interphalangeal and meta-carpophalangeal joints. Extension at the interphalangeal joints is produced by the long extensors of the digits and also by the interosseous and lumbrical muscles acting through the extensor expansion. When the metacarpophalangeal joints of the fingers are fully extended, the long extensors are unable to act on the interphalangeal joints (see above) which can then only be extended by the lumbricals and interossei. The **lumbricals** and **interossei** also flex the metacarpophalangeal joints. ➔ When the lumbricals and interossei are paralysed, the long extensor muscles produce full extension of the metacarpophalangeal joint, and the long flexor muscles of the fingers act unopposed to flex the interphalangeal joints and produce the '**claw hand**' which is characteristic of this paralysis.

In the thumb, the single interphalangeal joint is acted upon by the flexor and extensor pollicis longus, and sometimes by the extensor pollicis brevis. The abductor pollicis brevis (supplied by the median nerve) may be partly inserted into the extensor expansion and able to produce extension. ➔ Thus, some extension of the interphalangeal joint of the thumb may still be possible when all the extensor muscles of the thumb are paralysed by damage to the radial nerve.

The muscles acting on, and the movements of, the fingers and thumb are summarized in Tables 9.7, 9.8, 9.9, and 9.10. In these tables, the following abbreviations are used: CM = carpometacarpal joint; DIP = distal interphalangeal joint; IP = interphalangeal joint; MP = metacarpophalangeal joint; PIP = proximal interphalangeal joint.

See Clinical Application 9.1 for a discussion of the condition known as claw hand.

Table 9.7 Muscles acting on the fingers

Muscle	Origin	Insertion	Action on fingers	Nerve supply
Flexor digitorum superficialis	Humerus, medial epicondyle. Radius anterior border	Middle phalanges	Flexion, MP, and PIP	Median
Flexor digitorum profundus	Ulna, proximal two-thirds, anterior and medial surfaces	Distal phalanges	Flexion, all joints	Median* and ulnar
Lumbricals	Tendons of flexor digitorum profundus	Middle and distal phalanges via extensor expansion	Flexion MP, extension IP	Median and ulnar
Extensor digitorum	Humerus, lateral epicondyle	Extensor expansion	Extends all joints all fingers. If MP fully extended, IP not extended	Radial*
Dorsal interossei	Adjacent sides, metacarpals 1–5	Corresponding proximal phalanx, base through extensor expansion	Abduction of MP of index, middle, and ring fingers. Extension IP	Ulnar
Palmar interossei	Metacarpals, medial side 1 and 2, lateral side 4 and 5	Corresponding proximal phalanx, base through extensor expansion	Adduction of MP of thumb, index, ring, and little fingers. Extension IP	Ulnar
Abductor digiti minimi	Pisiform. Flexor retinaculum	Proximal phalanx, base medial side	Abduction MP (and CM) little finger	Ulnar
Flexor digiti minimi	Hamate, hook. Flexor retinaculum	Proximal phalanx, base medial side	Flexion CM and MP	Ulnar
Opponens digiti minimi	Hamate, hook	Fifth metacarpal, medial side	Lateral rotation of metacarpal. Flexion CM	Ulnar
Extensor indicis	Ulna, posterior surface	Extensor expansion	Extension all joints index finger	Radial*
Extensor digiti minimi	Humerus, lateral epicondyle	Extensor expansion	Extension all joints little finger. Abduction MP	Radial*

* Anterior or posterior interosseous branch.

Table 9.8 Movements of fingers

Movement	Muscles	Nerve supply
Flexion		
All fingers All joints: MP, PIP, DIP	Flexor digitorum profundus	Median* (index and middle) Ulnar (ring and little)
MP and PIP	Flexor digitorum superficialis	Median
MP only	Lumbricals	Median (index and middle)
	Lumbricals	Ulnar (ring and little)
	Interossei	Ulnar
CM and MP, little finger	Flexor digiti minimi	Ulnar
CM only, little finger	Opponens digiti minimi	Ulnar
Extension		
All fingers All joints: MP, PIP, DIP	Extensor digitorum	Radial*
Index: MP, PIP, DIP	Extensor indicis	Radial*
Little finger: MP, PIP, DIP	Extensor digiti minimi	Radial*
IP only when MP fully extended	Lumbricals	Median (index and middle) Ulnar (ring and little)
	Interossei	Ulnar
Abduction at MP		

(Continued)

Table 9.8 Movements of fingers (*Continued*)

Movement	Muscles	Nerve supply
All fingers, except little finger	Dorsal interossei	Ulnar
Little finger	Abductor digiti minimi	Ulnar
Adduction at MP		
All fingers, except middle	Palmar interossei	Ulnar
Opposition at CM of little finger	Opponens digiti minimi	Ulnar

* Anterior or posterior interosseous branch.

Table 9.9 Muscles acting on the thumb

Muscle	Origin	Insertion	Action on thumb	Nerve supply
Flexor pollicis longus	Radius, anterior surface middle two-quarters	Distal phalanx, base	Flexion all joints	Median*
Flexor pollicis brevis	Trapezium, tubercle. Flexor retinaculum	Proximal phalanx, base	Flexion CM and MP	Median
Abductor pollicis brevis	Scaphoid, tubercle. Flexor retinaculum	Proximal phalanx, anterior aspect	Abduction CM and MP	Median
Opponens pollicis	Trapezium, tubercle. Flexor retinaculum	Metacarpal, anterior surface	Medial rotation and flexion of CM	Median
Abductor pollicis longus	Radius and ulna, dorsal surfaces distal to supinator	Metacarpal base, anterior aspect	Abduction of CM, some extension	Radial*
First palmar interosseous	First metacarpal, base	Proximal phalanx base	Adduction of MP	Ulnar
Adductor pollicis	Metacarpal, base of 2 and 3, body of 3	Proximal phalanx base posterior aspect	Adduction CM and MP	Ulnar
Extensor pollicis longus	Ulna, posterior surface middle third	Distal phalanx	Extension all joints, especially with CM laterally rotated	Radial*
Extensor pollicis brevis	Radius, posterior surface	Proximal (and distal) phalanx base	Extension of CM, MP (and IP), especially when thumb opposed	Radial*

* Anterior or posterior interosseous branch.

Table 9.10 Movements of the thumb

Movement	Muscles	Nerve supply
Flexion		
All joints	Flexor pollicis longus	Median*
CM and MP	Flexor pollicis brevis	Median
CM only	Opponens pollicis	Median
Extension		
All joints	Extensor pollicis longus	Radial*
CM and MP (IP)	Extensor pollicis brevis	Radial*
CM only	Abductor pollicis longus	Radial*
IP only	Abductor pollicis brevis	Median
Abduction		
CM only	Abductor pollicis longus	Radial*
CM and MP	Abductor pollicis brevis	Median

Table 9.10 Movements of the thumb (*Continued*)

Movement	Muscles	Nerve supply
Adduction		
CM and MP	Adductor pollicis	Ulnar
MP only	First palmar interosseous	Ulnar
Opposition		
Medial rotation, CM	Opponens pollicis	Median

* Anterior or posterior interosseous branch.

CLINICAL APPLICATION 9.1 Ulnar claw

Claw hand is an abnormal hand position that develops due to damage of the ulnar and/or median nerves. The affected fingers are hyperextended at the metacarpophalangeal joints, and flexed at the distal and proximal interphalangeal joints. The primary cause of this deformity is the paralysis of the lumbricals and interossei which normally flex the metacarpophalangeal joint and extend the interphalangeal joints. When they are paralysed, the extensor action of the long extensors on the metacarpophalangeal joint and the flexor action of the long flexors on the interphalangeal joint are unopposed. Patients with a claw hand will be unable to abduct and adduct their fingers (due to paralysis of the interossei).

An ulnar claw results from a lesion in the ulnar nerve in the hand. The third and fourth lumbricals are paralysed, resulting in clawing of the fourth and fifth fingers. As the ulnar nerve also supplies the interossei, they too are paralysed. The lumbricals of the index and middle fingers are not affected, and clawing of these fingers is not seen (even though the interossei are paralysed).

A paradoxical condition is seen when the ulnar nerve is damaged at the elbow. The effects of the lumbrical paralysis are unchanged. But because, in this condition, the medial half of the flexor digitorum profundus is also denervated, flexion of the interphalangeal joints of the ring and little fingers is weak. The claw-like appearance of the hand is reduced (and not worsened, as one would expect from a higher-level injury). As reinnervation and healing occur along the ulnar nerve after a high lesion, the claw hand deformity will get worse as the patient recovers. Claw hand can be demonstrated in yourself. Fully extend your fingers at all joints, and note the taut extensor tendons on the back of your hand. Keeping the metacarpophalangeal joints fully extended, flex your interphalangeal joints, and note that this can be done without any movement of the extensor tendons.

CHAPTER 10
The nerves of the upper limb

Introduction

An **upper limb neurological examination** is part of general neurological examination and is used to assess the integrity of motor and sensory nerves which supply the upper limb.

Sensory distribution

Fig. 10.1 shows the cutaneous distribution of the main nerves of the upper limb. Clinical Applications 10.1 and 10.2 at the end of this chapter will explore the practical application of this knowledge.

Motor distribution

Injury to a motor nerve will result in paralysis of the muscles supplied by it and an inability to move the joint on which the paralysed muscles act. For example, injury to the musculocutaneous nerve will paralyse the biceps brachii and brachialis, and make flexion of the elbow difficult or impossible. Clearly, if only the biceps and brachialis are paralysed, some flexion of the elbow will be possible by other muscles such as the brachioradialis and pronator teres. If the only muscle moving a joint in a certain direction is paralysed, the loss of that movement will be total. For example, paralysis of the flexor digitorum profundus will result in total inability to flex the distal interphalangeal joint of the fingers. Where a nerve innervates muscles in more than one segment of the limb (shoulder, arm, forearm, hand), the effects of injury to the nerve depend on the level of injury. For example, when the median nerve is damaged at the wrist, muscles supplied by it in the forearm are not paralysed—only those in the hand are.

Fingers of the hand are simply indicated by their name, e.g. 'index' for 'index finger'. CM = carpometacarpal. DIP = distal interphalangeal. IP = interphalangeal. MP = metacarpophalangeal. PIP = proximal interphalangeal.

Median nerve

Table 10.1 shows the effects of injury to the median nerve. (See Fig. 10.2 for an overview of the median nerve.)

Ulnar nerve

Table 10.2 shows the effects of injury to the ulnar nerve. (See Fig. 10.3 for an overview of the ulnar nerve.)

Musculocutaneous nerve

Table 10.3 shows the effects of injury to the musculocutaneous nerve. (See Fig. 10.4 for an overview of the musculocutaneous nerve.)

Axillary nerve

Table 10.4 shows the effects of injury to the axillary nerve. (See Fig. 10.5 for an overview of the axillary nerve.)

Subscapular nerve

Table 10.5 shows the effects of injury to the subscapular nerve.

Thoracodorsal nerve

Table 10.6 shows the effects of injury to the thoracodorsal nerve.

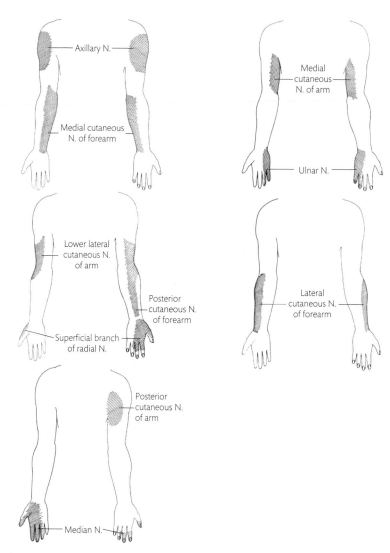

Fig. 10.1 Cutaneous distribution of nerves in the upper limb.

Table 10.1 Effects of injury to the median nerve

Joint involved	Movement affected/deformity produced	Explanation for loss/weakness of movement
Effect on shoulder joint	None	None of the muscles that move the shoulder joint are supplied by median nerve
Effect on elbow joint	Flexion, minimal weakness	Pronator teres and flexor carpi radialis are paralysed (important flexors—the biceps and brachialis are not supplied by the median nerve)
Effect on radio-ulnar joints	Pronation lost	Pronator teres and pronator quadratus are paralysed
Effect on wrist joint	Flexion weakened	Flexor carpi radialis, palmaris longus, flexor digitorum superficialis, flexor pollicis longus, and part of flexor digitorum profundus are paralysed
	Ulnar deviation	Unopposed action of flexor carpi ulnaris (as flexor carpi radialis is paralysed)

Table 10.1 Effects of injury to the median nerve (*Continued*)

Joint involved	Movement affected /deformity produced	Explanation for loss/weakness of movement
Effect on thumb movements	Flexion of IP joint lost	Flexor pollicis longus (only flexor) is paralysed
	Flexion of CM and MP joints weakened	Flexor pollicis longus is paralysed. Weak movement brought about by adductor pollicis
	Abduction of CM joint weakened	Abductor pollicis brevis is paralysed. Weak movement brought about by abductor pollicis longus
	Opposition lost	Opponens pollicis is paralysed
Effect on MP joints of fingers	Flexion weakened	Flexor digitorum superficialis and flexor digitorum profundus in lateral two fingers are paralysed. Weak flexion brought about by interossei (all fingers), medial two lumbricals (medial two fingers), and flexor digiti minimi (little finger)
Effect on PIP joints of lateral two fingers	Flexion lost	Flexor digitorum superficialis and profundus are paralysed
	Extension weakened	Lumbricals are paralysed. Weak extension brought about by extensor digitorum and interossei
Effect on PIP joints of medial two fingers	Flexion weakened	Flexor digitorum superficialis is paralysed. Weak flexion is brought about by flexor digitorum profundus
Effect on DIP joints of lateral two fingers	Flexion lost	Flexor digitorum profundus is paralysed
Effect on DIP joints of medial two fingers	None	Flexor digitorum profundus is uninvolved

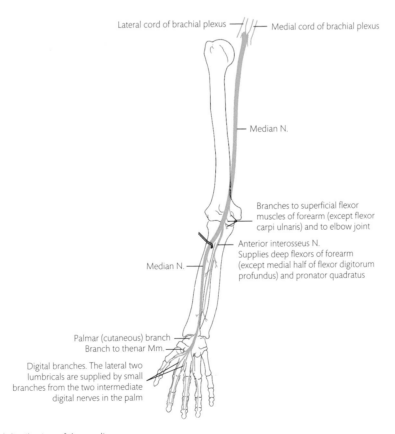

Lateral cord of brachial plexus — Medial cord of brachial plexus

Median N.

Branches to superficial flexor muscles of forearm (except flexor carpi ulnaris) and to elbow joint

Anterior interosseus N. Supplies deep flexors of forearm (except medial half of flexor digitorum profundus) and pronator quadratus

Median N.

Palmar (cutaneous) branch
Branch to thenar Mm.

Digital branches. The lateral two lumbricals are supplied by small branches from the two intermediate digital nerves in the palm

Fig. 10.2 Course and distribution of the median nerve.

Table 10.2 Effects of injury to the ulnar nerve

Joint involved	Movement affected/deformity produced	Explanation for loss/weakness of movement
Effect on shoulder joint	None	None of the muscles that move the shoulder joint are supplied by ulnar nerve
Effect on elbow joint	None	None of the muscles that move the elbow joint are supplied by ulnar nerve
Effect on wrist joint	Weakened wrist flexion	Flexor carpi ulnaris and part of flexor digitorum profundus are paralysed
	Radial deviation	Unopposed action of flexor carpi radialis
Effect on radio-ulnar joints	None	None of the muscles that move the radio-ulnar joints are supplied by ulnar nerve
Effect on thumb movement	None	Although adductor pollicis is paralysed, long flexor and extensor of the thumb together mimic the action of the adductor
Effect on CM joints of little finger	Opposition is lost	Opponens digiti minimi is paralysed
Effect on MP joints of all fingers (medial four digits)	Abduction and adduction lost	All interossei and abductor digiti minimi are paralysed
Effect on MP joints of medial two fingers	Flexion weakened	Flexor digitorum profundus, lumbricals, and flexor digiti minimi are paralysed. Weak flexion is brought about by flexor digitorum superficialis
Effect on PIP joints of medial two fingers	Flexion weakened	Flexor digitorum profundus is paralysed. Weak flexion is brought about by flexor digitorum superficialis
Effect on PIP joints of all fingers	Extension weakened in all fingers	Interossei are paralysed. Lumbricals of medial two fingers are paralysed
	No IP joint extension of medial two fingers if MP joint is fully extended	Extension possible only when extensor digitorum, extensor indicis, and extensor digiti minimi are not extending MP joint
Effect on DIP joints of medial two fingers	Flexion lost	Flexor digitorum profundus is paralysed

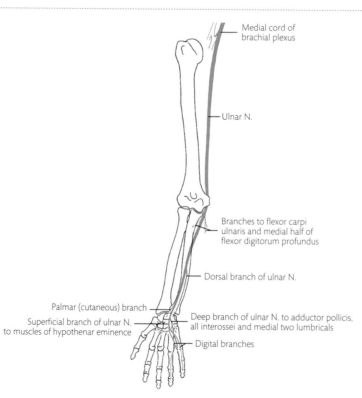

Fig. 10.3 Course and distribution of the ulnar nerve.

Table 10.3 Effects of injury to the musculocutaneous nerve

Joint involved	Movement affected	Explanation for loss/weakness of movement
Effect on shoulder joint	Flexion weakened	Coracobrachialis and short head of biceps are paralysed. Weak flexion brought about by deltoid and pectoralis major
	Stability in abduction lost	Long head of biceps is paralysed. Some stability maintained by deltoid, supraspinatus, and subscapularis
Effect on elbow joint	Flexion severely weakened	Biceps brachii and brachialis are paralysed. Some weak flexion is brought about by brachioradialis, extensor carpi radialis longus, pronator teres, and flexor carpi radialis
Effect on radio-ulnar joints	Supination weakened	Biceps brachii paralysed. Weak supination is brought about by supinator and brachioradialis

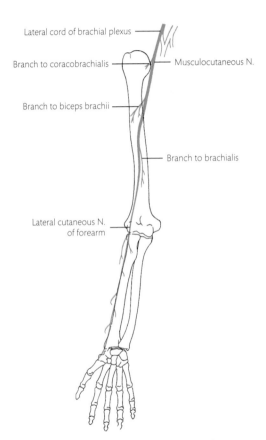

Fig. 10.4 Course and distribution of the musculocutaneous nerve.

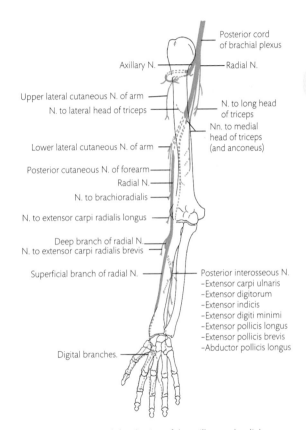

Fig. 10.5 Course and distribution of the axillary and radial nerves.

Table 10.4 Effects of injury to the axillary nerve

Joint involved	Movement affected	Explanation for loss/weakness of movement
Effect on shoulder joint	Abduction severely weakened	Teres minor and deltoid are paralysed. Weak abduction is brought about by supraspinatus
	Extension severely weakened	Deltoid and teres minor are paralysed . Weak extension is brought about by latissimus dorsi
	Lateral rotation of humerus weakened	Teres minor is paralysed. Weak lateral rotation is brought about by infraspinatus

Table 10.5 Effects of injury to the subscapular nerve

Joint involved	Movement affected	Explanation for loss/weakness of movement
Effect on shoulder joint	Instability and tendency for anterior dislocation	Subscapularis is paralysed
	Medial rotation of humerus weakened	Teres major is paralysed. Weak medial rotation is brought about by pectoralis major and deltoid

Table 10.6 Effects of injury to the thoracodorsal nerve

Joint involved	Movement affected	Explanation for loss/weakness of movement
Effect on shoulder joint	Medial rotation of humerus is weakened	Latissimus dorsi is paralysed
	Inability to pull the body upwards with the upper limb	Latissimus dorsi is paralysed

Radial nerve

Table 10.7 shows the effects of injury to the radial nerve. (See Fig. 10.5 for an overview of the radial nerve.)

Suprascapular nerve

Table 10.8 shows the effects of injury to the suprascapular nerve.

Table 10.7 Effects of injury to the radial nerve

Joint involved	Movement affected	Explanation for loss/weakness of movement
Effect on shoulder joint	Minor instability of shoulder in abduction, with tendency for downward dislocation in this position	Long head of triceps brachii is paralysed
Effect on elbow joint	Extension lost	Triceps is paralysed
Effect on radio-ulnar joint	Supination weakened	Supinator is paralysed. Weak supination is brought about by biceps brachii
	Elbow flexion in mid-prone position weakened	Brachioradialis, extensor carpi radialis longus and brevis are paralysed. Weak movement is brought about by brachialis, biceps brachii, and pronator teres
Effect on wrist joint	Markedly weakened radial deviation	Extensor carpi radialis longus and brevis are paralysed. Weak radial deviation brought about by flexor carpi radialis
	Wrist extension is lost—'wrist drop'	Extensor carpi ulnaris* and extensor digitorum* are paralysed
	Weakened ulnar deviation of wrist	Extensor carpi ulnaris* is paralysed. Weak ulnar deviation is brought about by flexor carpi ulnaris
Effect on MP and IP joints	Extension lost at MP joints Extension weakened at IP joints	Extensor pollicis longus*, extensor pollicis brevis*, and abductor pollicis longus* are paralysed. Weak extension of IP joints brought about by interossei and lumbricals
Effect on MP joints—index	Independent extension lost	Extensor indicis* is paralysed
Effect on MP joints—little	Independent extension lost	Extensor digiti minimi* is paralysed
Effect on CM, MP, and IP joints of thumb	Extension is lost—thumb	Extensor pollicis longus* and extensor pollicis brevis* are paralysed. Some extension is brought about by abductor pollicis brevis
	Thumb abduction is weakened	Abductor pollicis longus* is paralysed. Weak abduction is brought about by abductor pollicis brevis

* Posterior interosseous branch.

Table 10.8 Effects of injury to the suprascapular nerve

Joint involved	Movement affected	Explanation for loss/weakness of movement
Effect on shoulder joint	Difficulty with initiating abduction	Supraspinatus is paralysed. Abduction brought about by deltoid (teres minor and subscapularis assist deltoid by holding down humeral head)
	Lateral rotation of humerus weakened	Infraspinatus is paralysed. Some lateral rotation is brought about by posterior fibres of deltoid and teres minor

Long thoracic nerve

Table 10.9 shows the effects of injury to the long thoracic nerve.

Table 10.9 Effects of injury to the long thoracic nerve

Joint involved	Movement affected/deformity produced	Explanation for loss/weakness of movement
Effect on shoulder girdle	Protraction of scapula weakened	Serratus anterior is paralysed. Some protraction is brought about by pectoralis major and minor
	Lateral rotation of scapula weakened	Serratus anterior is paralysed. Some lateral rotation is brought about by trapezius
	Scapula not held against ribs–'winged scapula'	

CLINICAL APPLICATION 10.1 Cervical rib syndrome

The costal element of the seventh cervical vertebra is normally incorporated into its transverse process soon after birth. Rarely, it may persist and give rise to a condition known as 'cervical rib'. The presence of a cervical rib can cause thoracic outlet syndrome due to compression of the lower trunk of the brachial plexus. Study question 1: which part/parts of the plexus supplying the upper limb is most likely to be affected in this condition? (Answer: brachial plexus—T. 1 root, and lower trunk.)

A patient with a symptomatic cervical rib could experience a dull, aching pain radiating down the medial side of the arm, forearm, and hand, with numbness in the little and ring fingers. Study question 2: name the nerves supplying the skin of these regions. What are they branches of? (Answer: (i) medial cutaneous nerve of the arm—medial cord of the brachial plexus; (ii) medial cutaneous nerve of the forearm—medial cord of the brachial plexus; (iii) and (iv) superficial branch of the ulnar nerve and dorsal branch of the ulnar nerve—ulnar nerve.)

On examination of the patient, there was wasting of all the intrinsic muscles of the hand, except the abductor and flexor pollucis brevis. Study question 3: what is the innervation of these muscles of the hand? (Answer: ulnar nerve.)

Study question 4: would any forearm muscles be affected? If so, which ones? (Answer: yes—medial half of the flexor digitorum profundus and flexor carpi ulnaris.)

CLINICAL APPLICATION 10.2 Motor assessment of upper limb musculature

Motor examination of the upper limb in a patient with spinal cord injury provides a reliable and quick way to localize the level of the lesion. Five muscles of the upper limb, one primarily supplied by each of the five segmental nerves C. 5 to T. 1, are tested. The integrity of each spinal segment is evaluated by the ability of a muscle supplied by it to bring about a particular movement of a joint [Table 10.10]. (The strength of the muscle is scored on a 5-point scale not included here.)

Table 10.10 Motor assessment of upper limb musculature

Spinal segment (myotome)	Primary movement	Prime muscle causing movement
C. 5	Elbow flexion	Biceps brachii
C. 6	Wrist extension	Extensor carpi radialis longus
C. 7	Elbow extension	Triceps
C. 8	Finger flexion*	Flexor digitorum profundus
T. 1	Finger abductors (little finger)	Abductor digiti minimi

* Distal interphalangeal joint of the middle finger.

Reference: *Standard neurological classification of spinal cord injury* by American Spinal Injury Association (ASIA).

CHAPTER 11
MCQs for part 2: The upper limb

The following questions have four options. You are required to choose the most correct answer.

1. **The supraclavicular nerves supply the skin down to a horizontal line at the level of**
   A. clavicle
   B. first costal cartilage
   C. second costal cartilage
   D. third costal cartilage

2. **The anterior axillary wall consists of the following muscles, EXCEPT**
   A. pectoralis major
   B. pectoralis minor
   C. subclavius
   D. subscapularis

3. **The intercostobrachial nerve communicates with the**
   A. medial cutaneous nerve of the arm
   B. medial cutaneous nerve of the forearm
   C. median nerve
   D. musculocutaneous nerve

4. **The inferior angle of the scapula corresponds approximately to the level of the**
   A. sixth thoracic spine
   B. seventh thoracic spine
   C. eighth thoracic spine
   D. ninth thoracic spine

5. **Retraction of the scapula is caused by the following muscles, EXCEPT**
   A. rhomboid major
   B. rhomboid minor
   C. upper fibres of the trapezius
   D. middle fibres of the trapezius

6. **The nerve supply of the latissimus dorsi is by the**

   A. long thoracic nerve

   B. dorsal scapular nerve

   C. suprascapular nerve

   D. thoracodorsal nerve

7. **The bones felt in the anatomical snuffbox are all, EXCEPT**

   A. styloid process of the radius

   B. scaphoid

   C. lunate

   D. trapezium

8. **The upper lateral cutaneous nerve of the arm arises from the**

   A. musculocutaneous nerve

   B. axillary nerve

   C. radial nerve

   D. median nerve

9. **The following arteries are involved in the anastomosis around the scapula, EXCEPT**

   A. suprascapular artery

   B. subscapular artery

   C. transverse cervical artery

   D. internal thoracic artery

10. **The axis of movement of supination and pronation passes through the centre of the head of the radius proximally and the**

    A. centre of the head of the ulna distally

    B. styloid process of the radius distally

    C. centre of the pisiform distally

    D. hook of the hamate distally

11. **The structures that pass in the carpal tunnel are all, EXCEPT**

    A. flexor carpi ulnaris

    B. flexor digitorum superficialis

    C. flexor digitorum profundus

    D. flexor pollicis longus

12. **The anterior interosseous nerve is a branch of the**

    A. ulnar nerve

    B. median nerve

    C. radial nerve

    D. musculocutaneous nerve

13. Carpal tunnel syndrome is caused due to compression of the

A. ulnar nerve
B. median nerve
C. anterior cutaneous nerve
D. posterior cutaneous nerve

14. The muscle producing adduction of the wrist is

A. flexor carpi ulnaris
B. flexor carpi radialis
C. extensor carpi radialis longus
D. extensor carpi radialis brevis

15. The action of lumbricals is

A. flexion of the metacarpophalangeal joint and extension of the interphalangeal joint
B. flexion of the metacarpophalangeal joint and flexion of the interphalangeal joint
C. extension of the metacarpophalangeal joint and flexion of the interphalangeal joint
D. extension of the metacarpophalangeal joint and extension of the interphalangeal joint

Please go to the back of the book for the answers.

PART 3
The lower limb

155

CHAPTER 12
Introduction to the lower limb

Introduction

The parts of the lower limb are the hip and buttock, the thigh, the leg, and the foot.

The hip and buttock together make up what is called the **gluteal region**. This overlies the side and back of the pelvis, from the waist down to the groove (**gluteal fold**). It extends from the waist to the buttock inferiorly, and to the depression on the lateral side of the hip. The hip and buttock are not clearly distinguished from each other. The **hip** (*coxa*) is the upper part of the region in a lateral view; the **buttock** (*natis*) is the rounded bulge behind. The **natal cleft** is the groove between the buttocks. The lower part of the sacrum and coccyx (the end of the backbone) can be felt in the natal cleft. The perineum lies in front of the buttocks and continues forwards between the thighs.

The skeleton of the hip and buttock is the **hip bone**. It consists of three parts—the **ilium, ischium**, and **pubis**. These three bones fuse together at the **acetabulum** [Fig. 12.1] where the head of the femur articulates with the hip bone. The **ilium** is the large upper part. It has a crest at its superior margin which can be felt in the lower margin of the waist. The **ischium** is the posteroinferior part on which the body rests when sitting. The **pubis** is the anterior part. It can be felt in the lower part of the anterior abdominal wall. In the midline, it meets its fellow of the opposite side in the **pubic symphysis** (*symphysis* = union)—a joint between the right and left pubic bones.

The right and left hip bones, together with the sacrum and coccyx, make up the skeleton of the pelvis [Fig. 12.1]. The two hip bones together are

sometimes called the **pelvic girdle**. Anteriorly, they articulate with each other at the pubic symphysis. Posteriorly, they articulate with the sides of the sacrum at the two **sacro-iliac joints**.

The **thigh** (*femur*) extends from the hip to the knee. The thigh bone **femur** articulates at its upper end with the hip bone to form the hip joint. At the **knee joint**, the femur articulates with the **tibia** and with the **patella** (kneecap). The proximal extent of the thigh is the gluteal fold posteriorly, the groove of the groin (**inguinal region**) anteriorly, the perineum medially, and the surface depression on the side of the hip laterally. The greater trochanter of the femur can be felt through the skin, immediately anterior to the depression. The ham (*poples*) is the lower part of the back of the thigh and the back of the knee. The depression on the back of the knee is the **popliteal fossa**.

The **leg** (*crus*) extends from the knee joint to the ankle joint. The term 'leg' is never used in anatomical descriptions to refer to the entire lower limb, as it frequently is in colloquial speech. The soft, fleshy part of the back of the leg is the **calf** (*sura*).

The bones of the leg are the **tibia**, or shin bone, and the **fibula**. They lie side by side, with the slender fibula laterally. The tibia and fibula articulate with each other at their upper and lower ends— the superior and inferior tibiofibular joints. Along their length, they are united by the **interosseous membrane**. The lower ends of the tibia and fibula form prominences at the sides of the ankle—the **medial** and **lateral malleoli** which are readily felt. The medial and lateral malleoli hold the first bone of the foot (the **talus**) between them to form the **ankle joint**. At the knee joint, the superior surface of the proximal end of the tibia is flattened

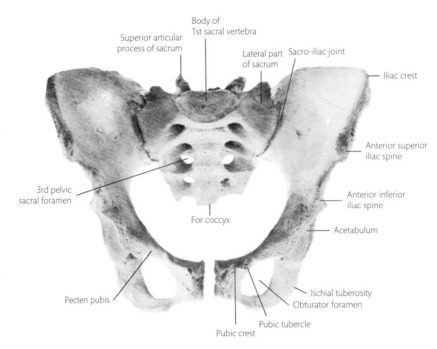

Superior articular
process of sacrum

Body of
1st sacral vertebra

Lateral part
of sacrum

Sacro-iliac joint

Iliac crest

Anterior superior
iliac spine

Anterior inferior
iliac spine

Acetabulum

3rd pelvic
sacral foramen

For coccyx

Pecten pubis

Ischial tuberosity

Obturator foramen

Pubic tubercle

Pubic crest

Fig. 12.1 The bony pelvis seen from the front (without the coccyx).

to form the tibial condyles which articulate with the femur. The proximal end of the fibula (head) does not take part in the knee joint. It reaches up to the inferolateral surface of the lateral tibial condyle. A large part of the tibia is subcutaneous and easily felt.

The fibula is mainly covered by muscles which are attached to it, so that only its head and distal quarter are easily felt.

The **foot** extends from the point of the heel to the tips of the toes. Its superior surface is the **dorsum**; its inferior surface is the **sole** (*planta*). The bones of the foot, from proximal to distal, are the tarsal bones, the metatarsals, and the phalanges. The **tarsal bones** are in two rows. The proximal row consists of two large bones—the **talus** and the **calcaneus**, with the talus resting on the calcaneus. The calcaneus is the largest bone of the tarsus and forms the skeleton of the heel. The talus articulates with: (1) the superior surface of the calcaneus; (2) the tibia and fibula to form the ankle joint; and (3) the **navicular** distally. The navicular lies between the proximal and distal row of the tarsal bones. The navicular articulates proximally with the talus and distally with the three cuneiforms. The distal row of tarsal bones consists of the **cuboid bone** laterally, and the three wedge-shaped **cuneiform bones** (*cuneus* = a wedge)—the **medial**, **intermediate**, and **lateral cuneiforms**—medially. The cuboid articulates

proximally with the calcaneus and distally with the lateral two metatarsals. The cuneiforms articulate with the navicular proximally and with the medial three metatarsals distally. Between the tarsal bones are the intertarsal joints.

The five **metatarsal bones** are set side by side. They are numbered 1 to 5 from the medial side. The proximal ends—the **base of the metatarsals**—articulate with the tarsal bones at the tarsometatarsal joints, and the base of the medial four metatarsals articulate with each other at the intermetatarsal joints. Each metatarsal has a **head** at the distal end which articulates with the base of the proximal phalanx of the corresponding toe at the metatarsophalangeal joint. The **toes** (digits) are numbered from the medial side. The first is the big toe, or **hallux**; the fifth is the little toe, or **digitus minimus**. The bones of the toes are the **phalanges**. The hallux has two phalanges; each of the other toes has three, though the middle and distal phalanges of the little toe may be fused together. The proximal end of the phalanx is its base; the distal end is its head. The phalanges articulate with each other at the **interphalangeal joints**.

There are several **sesamoid bones** in the lower limb. The largest is the patella. The others are small and inconstant, except for two which are always present on the plantar surface of the metatarsophalangeal joint of the big toe.

CHAPTER 13
The front and medial side of the thigh

Introduction

Before starting to dissect, study the surface anatomy of the region on yourself or on another living subject, and relate this to the appropriate dried bones.

Surface anatomy and bones

The **hip bone** [Figs. 13.1, 13.2] is made up of three bones—the **ilium**, **ischium**, and **pubis**.

The ilium is large, flat, slightly curved, and directed upwards. The pubis and ischium lie inferiorly, the pubis more anteromedially, and the ischium more posterolaterally. The **obturator foramen** is a large aperture in the hip bone between the pubis and ischium. The ilium, ischium, and pubis meet at a narrow, thick central part which has the **acetabular fossa** for articulation with the head of the femur. The pubis and ischium are fused together by a bar of bone, inferior to the obturator foramen. This is the **ischiopubic ramus** and

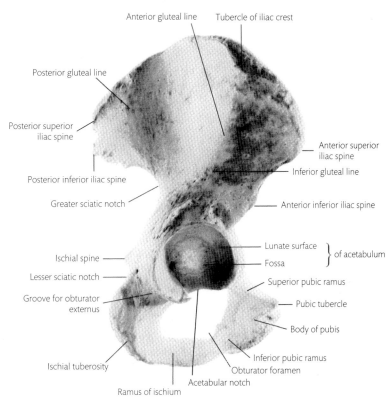

Fig. 13.1 Right hip bone seen from the lateral side.

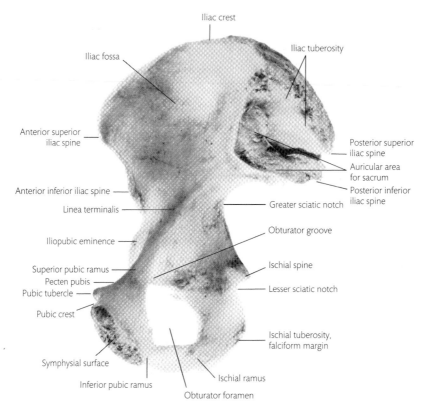

Fig. 13.2 Right hip bone seen from the medial side.

is formed by the union of the **inferior ramus of the pubis** and the **ramus of the ischium**. In the region of the acetabulum, the ilium fuses with the superior ramus of the pubis at the **iliopubic eminence** [Fig. 13.2], and with the ischium at the rough ridge on the posterior surface of the acetabulum.

The **greater sciatic notch** is a deep, curved depression, or notch, on the posterior margin of the ilium, immediately above the acetabulum. The medial aspect of the ischium has a shallow **lesser sciatic notch**, separated from the greater sciatic notch by the **spine of the ischium**. Immediately inferior to the lesser sciatic notch, the ischium expands to form the **ischial tuberosity**.

The **body of the pubis** [Fig. 13.1] articulates with its fellow of the opposite side through a median fibrous joint—the **pubic symphysis**. The pubic symphysis may be felt at the lower end of the abdominal wall. Draw your finger laterally from the pubic symphysis on the anterosuperior surface of the body of the pubis. This surface is the **pubic crest** which ends in a small, blunt prominence—the **pubic tubercle**—laterally. The tubercle is less easily felt in the male, because

it is covered by the spermatic cord. Lateral to the pubic tubercle, a resilient band can be felt in the inguinal groove between the anterior surface of the thigh and the abdomen. This is the **inguinal ligament**. On the bone, note a sharp ridge which curves posterolaterally on the superior ramus of the pubis from the pubic tubercle to the iliopubic eminence. This is the **pecten pubis**. Fibres of the inguinal ligament stretch posteriorly to the pecten and form the **lacunar ligament**. Below and behind the pubic symphysis, the two **inferior pubic rami** diverge to form the **pubic arch**. Each inferior pubic ramus unites with the corresponding **ramus of the ischium** to form the **ischiopubic ramus**. The ischiopubic ramus forms the boundary between the thigh and perineum, and is palpable through its length.

Find the **iliac crest** at the lower margin of the waist. Trace it forwards. It slopes downwards and slightly medially to end in a rounded knob—the **anterior superior iliac spine**. This may be grasped between the finger and thumb in a thin individual. The inguinal ligament stretches from this spine to the pubic tubercle. On the bone, a notch on the anterior margin of the ilium separates the anterior superior iliac spine from the **anterior inferior iliac spine** which lies immediately above the acetabulum. The anterior inferior iliac spine has two parts—the upper for attachment of the tendon of the rectus femoris muscle, and the lower for attachment of the iliofemoral ligament of the hip joint. Trace the outer lip of the iliac crest posteriorly, until you feel a low prominence—the **tubercle of the iliac crest**. This is the widest part of the pelvis. Further posteriorly, the iliac crest turns downwards to end in the **posterior superior iliac spine** at the level of the second sacral vertebra.

The outer **gluteal surface** of the ilium is marked by three ridges, or gluteal lines, which curve upwards and forwards across it. These **gluteal lines** (posterior, anterior, and inferior) are formed by the attachment of the deep fascia between the **gluteal muscles**. The portion between the lines marks the areas of attachment of these muscles to the ilium [Fig. 13.1].

The **greater trochanter of the femur** can be palpated indistinctly, immediately in front of the surface depression on the side of the hip [Fig. 13.3]. The top of the trochanter lies at the level of the pubic crest. The **head of the femur** can be felt indistinctly, even though it is deeply buried in muscles. To do this on yourself, place your finger just below the inguinal groove at the **mid-inguinal point**, i.e. midway between the anterior superior iliac spine and the pubic symphysis. Press firmly, and rotate your limb medially and laterally. The head will be felt moving behind the muscles. With lighter pressure, the **femoral artery** can be felt pulsating at the same spot.

Study the main features of the femur, with reference to Figs. 13.3 and 13.4.

The spherical **head of the femur** fits into the acetabulum where it articulates with the C-shaped **lunate surface**. The lunate surface is a broad strip of articular bone at the periphery of the acetabulum which partially surrounds the central non-articular **acetabular fossa**. This fossa is continuous interiorly with the floor of the **acetabular notch** between the ends of the lunate surface. The acetabular notch is converted into a foramen by the **transverse ligament of the acetabulum** which bridges the notch and completes the acetabular margin. The transverse ligament of the acetabulum and the margin of

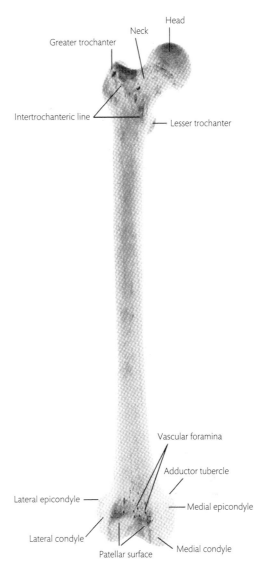

Fig. 13.3 Right femur (anterior aspect).

the acetabular fossa give attachment to the **ligament of the head of the femur**. This ligament contains connective tissue and small blood vessels, is covered by a synovial membrane, and attached on the femur to the non-articular **pit of the head of the femur**. The ligament of the head of the femur may transmit some small blood vessels through foramina in the pit to the head of the femur.

The head of the femur is continuous with the **neck** of the femur which joins it to the shaft. Two bony prominences—the **greater** and **lesser trochanters**—mark the junction of the neck with the shaft. The neck meets the shaft posteriorly at a prominent, rounded ridge (the

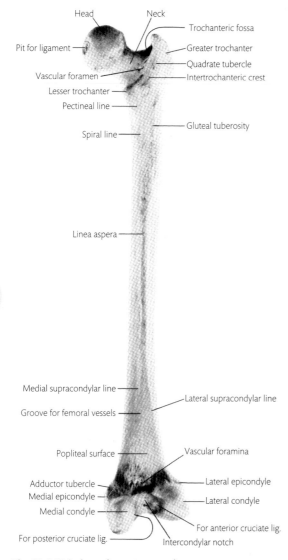

Head   Neck

Trochanteric fossa

Pit for ligament

Greater trochanter

Quadrate tubercle

Vascular foramen

Intertrochanteric crest

Lesser trochanter

Pectineal line

Gluteal tuberosity

Spiral line

Linea aspera

Medial supracondylar line

Lateral supracondylar line

Groove for femoral vessels

Popliteal surface   Vascular foramina

Adductor tubercle   Lateral epicondyle

Medial epicondyle   Lateral condyle

Medial condyle

For anterior cruciate lig.

For posterior cruciate lig.   Intercondylar notch

Fig. 13.4 Right femur (posterior aspect).

intertrochanteric crest) which extends from the **greater trochanter** above to the **lesser trochanter** below. Anteriorly, the neck meets the shaft in a rough **intertrochanteric line** which extends between the two trochanters. This line gives attachment to the powerful **iliofemoral ligament**—a thickening of the fibrous capsule of the hip joint.

The **neck** forms an angle of approximately 125 degrees with the body of the femur. A thick bar of bone in the lower part of the neck transmits compressive forces applied by the weight of the body on the head of the femur. The surface of the neck is ridged longitudinally by bundles of fibres (**retinaculae**) which are continuous with

the fibrous capsule of the hip joint and transmit blood vessels to the neck. Note the foramina on the neck of the femur for these vessels. These vessels form the main blood supply for the head and neck of the femur. The greater trochanter projects upwards and medially over the neck. The bony depression on its medial side is the **trochanteric fossa**.

The **shaft of the femur** is covered by muscles and cannot be felt easily. It is convex anteriorly, particularly in its proximal half. Most of its surface is smooth, except for a linear elevation (the **linea aspera**) posteriorly in its middle two-quarters. Superiorly and inferiorly, the medial and lateral lips of the linea aspera separate. Superiorly, these diverging lines pass on either side of the lesser trochanter and the **pectineal line** which descends from it. The continuation of the medial lip forms the **spiral line** anteriorly, and the continuation of the lateral lip forms the rough **gluteal tuberosity** posteriorly. The spiral line becomes continuous above, with the intertrochanteric line on the anterior surface of the femur. A faint bony ridge along the lower margin of the greater trochanter joins the intertrochanteric line anteriorly, with the gluteal tuberosity posteriorly. Inferiorly, the lips of the linea aspera diverge to form the medial and lateral **supracondylar lines** [Fig. 13.4]. These lines form the boundaries of the flattened **popliteal surface of the femur**. The lateral supracondylar line continues down to the lateral epicondyle. The medial line continues to the **adductor tubercle** on the medial epicondyle of the femur but is interrupted where the femoral artery crosses it to become the popliteal artery.

The distal end of the shaft of the femur widens into the **medial** and **lateral** condyles. Posteriorly, the condyles are separated by a wide **intercondylar fossa**. Anteriorly, the condyles unite in the grooved **patellar surface**. The lateral surface of this groove is wider and projects further forwards than the medial surface. The margin of the lateral surface may be felt, proximal to the patella, when the knee is flexed. The **medial** and **lateral epicondyles** are flattened, conical projections from the surface of each condyle [Figs. 13.3, 13.4]. Each epicondyle shows some additional bony features. The lateral epicondyle gives attachment to the lateral head of the muscle **gastrocnemius**. Below the lateral epicondyle is a fossa with a groove running posteriorly from it. The **tendon** of the **popliteus** is attached to the fossa and lies in the groove when the knee is flexed. The posterior surface of the medial epicondyle is marked by the attachment of the medial head of the gastrocnemius. The adductor tubercle lies superior to the medial epicondyle.

Identify the condyles of the femur and their epicondyles on your own knee. The condyles of the tibia and femur can be differentiated by the movement of the tibia when the knee is flexed and extended. Grasp the **patella**, and try to move it. The patella is mobile when the knee is extended but becomes rigid when the knee is flexed. Feel the strong **patellar tendon (patellar ligament)** which stretches from the patella to the **tibial tuberosity** (a blunt prominence on the front of the upper end of the tibia). This tendon becomes taut when the knee is flexed. During flexion, the patella slides on to the distal end of the femur, and the upper part of the patellar surface is exposed.

With the knee straight, a muscular strip with three tendons posterior to it can be felt on the medial side of the knee, posterior to the medial epicondyle. When the knee is flexed, these tendons project back. The muscles and tendons on the posterior medial side of the knee are the **sartorius**, **gracilis**, and **semitendinosus**. Another tendon, more deeply placed and less readily felt, is that of the **semimembranosus**. On the lateral side, a single stout tendon can be felt, posterior to the lateral epicondyle, when the knee is bent. This is the tendon of the **biceps femoris**. Trace it down to the **head of the fibula**. Anterior to this tendon and separated from it by a depression is a broad, tendon-like structure which is best felt when standing with the knee slightly bent. This is the **iliotibial tract**, a strip of thickened deep fascia of the thigh. Through the iliotibial tract, two muscles—the gluteus maximus and tensor fasciae latae—are inserted into the lateral condyle of the tibia.

Proximal to the medial epicondyle of the femur is a fleshy swelling. This is the lowest part of the **vastus medialis** muscle [Fig. 13.5]. When the knee is bent, a shallow groove appears, posterior to this part of the muscle. Press your finger into the groove, and feel the tendon of the **adductor magnus** muscle. Slide your finger distally on the tendon to the adductor tubercle where the tendon is attached. The fleshy swelling proximal to the lateral epicondyle is the lowest part of the vastus lateralis [Fig. 13.5].

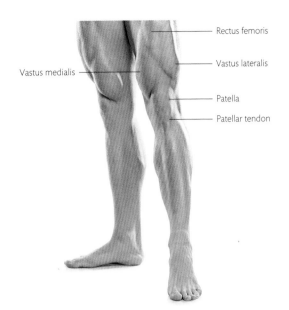

Fig. 13.5 Front of the knee, lower part of the thigh, and upper leg, illustrating the visible bony elevations and muscle masses.

Copyright I T A L O/Shutterstock.

Labels: Rectus femoris; Vastus lateralis; Patella; Patellar tendon; Vastus medialis

Front of the thigh

Dissection 13.1 instructs how to reflect the skin on the front of the thigh.

Superficial fascia

Close to the inguinal ligament, the superficial fascia of the thigh consists of a thick superficial layer and a deeper membranous layer which are continuous with the same two layers in the anterior abdominal wall. The membranous layer of the superficial abdominal fascia (from the abdomen) descends and is attached to the deep fascia of the thigh along a line parallel and approximately

---

DISSECTION 13.1 Skin reflection

Objective

I. To reflect the skin on the front of the thigh.

Instructions

1. Make incisions 9 and 10 [Fig. 13.6] through the skin.

2. Reflect the skin from the superficial fascia, and turn it laterally.

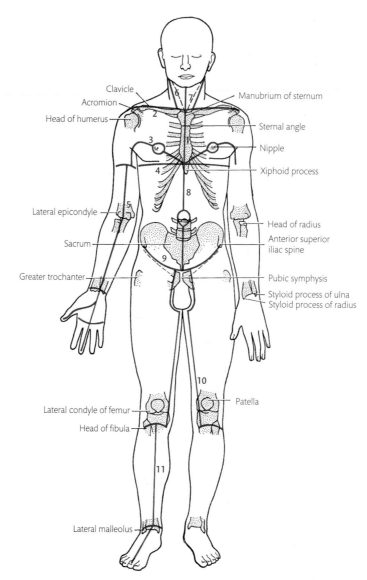

Clavicle
Acromion
Head of humerus
Manubrium of sternum
Sternal angle
Nipple
Xiphoid process
Lateral epicondyle
Head of radius
Anterior superior iliac spine
Sacrum
Greater trochanter
Pubic symphysis
Styloid process of ulna
Styloid process of radius
Patella
Lateral condyle of femur
Head of fibula
Lateral malleolus

Fig. 13.6 Landmarks and incisions.

1 cm inferior to the inguinal ligament [Fig. 13.7]. At the pubic tubercle, the line of fusion extends downwards across the front of the body of the pubis and the margin of the inferior pubic ramus to the ischial tuberosity. This arrangement permits communication between the perineum and the tissue deep to the membranous layer in the anterior abdominal wall. This is the same plane that is invaded by fluid tracking from the perineum into the abdominal wall, e.g. in rupture of the urethra in the male. The fusion of the abdominal fascia to the fascia of the thigh separates the tissue of the anterior abdominal wall and perineum from the thigh [Fig. 13.7].

If the abdomen is being dissected at the same time as the lower limb, Dissection 13.2 should be carried out.

The **femoral sheath** is an extension of the fascia lining the abdominal cavity. It surrounds the upper 4 cm of the femoral artery and vein. The femoral vein lies posterior to the saphenous opening (a defect in the deep fascia) and the femoral artery lies behind its lateral margin. Medial to the vein, and within the sheath, is the tubular **femoral canal**, through which a femoral hernia may occur (see Clinical Application 13.1). A hernia in this position lies posterior to the thin cribriform fascia covering the saphenous opening and can push it

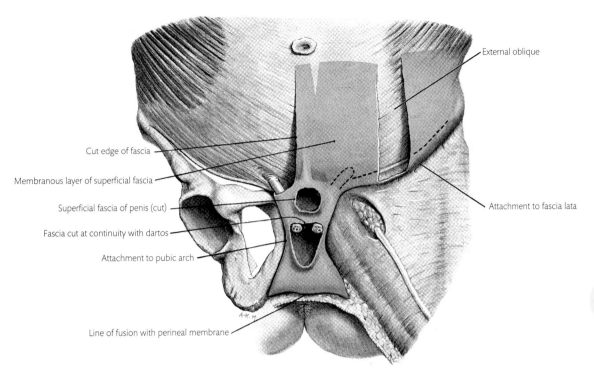

External oblique

Cut edge of fascia

Membranous layer of superficial fascia

Superficial fascia of penis (cut)

Fascia cut at continuity with dartos

Attachment to pubic arch

Attachment to fascia lata

Line of fusion with perineal membrane

Fig. 13.7 Diagram showing continuity of the membranous layer of the superficial fascia of the abdominal wall, perineum, and thigh.

DISSECTION 13.2 Superficial veins

Objectives

I. To explore the continuity of fascial planes and spaces from the abdomen to the perineum and from the abdomen to the lower limb.   II. To expose the upper part of the long saphenous vein and the tributaries in this area.   III. To identify the superficial arteries.   IV. To demonstrate the saphenous opening and cribriform fascia.

Instructions

1. If the abdomen has not been dissected, make a horizontal incision through the entire thickness of the superficial fascia of the anterior abdominal wall from the anterior superior iliac spine to the midline.

2. Raise the superficial fascia inferior to the cut, and pass the fingers downwards between the membranous layer of the fascia and the underlying aponeurosis of the external oblique muscle [Fig. 13.7].

3. Appreciate that little resistance is felt to the passage of the fingers, till the line of fusion of the membranous layer with the deep fascia of the thigh is reached at the fold of the groin.

4. Note that the fingers cannot be carried into the thigh because of this line of fusion.

5. Pass the fingers medially along this line, and find the opening into the perineum, just medial to the pubic tubercle. Note that a finger can easily be passed into the perineum.

6. In the male, the finger passes beside the spermatic cord towards the scrotum; in the female, it passes into the base of the labium majus.

7. Revert back to the dissection of the lower limb. Find the **long saphenous vein** in the superficial fascia of the medial part of the anterior surface of the thigh. Trace the vein downwards to the knee and upwards to the point where it turns sharply backwards through the deep fascia to enter the femoral vein.

8. As the upper part is exposed, note the lower group of **superficial inguinal lymph nodes** scattered along the vein and the delicate, thread-like lymph vessels which enter them.

9. Three small veins enter the long saphenous vein at its upper end. Follow these and the small superficial

inguinal branches of the femoral artery. They pierce the deep fascia and supply the adjacent skin and lymph nodes. The **superficial external pudendal vessels** pass medially to the external genital organs; the **superficial epigastric** runs superiorly to the anterior abdominal wall, and the **superficial circumflex iliac** runs towards the lateral part of the groin [Fig. 13.8]. (When tracing these vessels, note the upper group of superficial inguinal lymph nodes which lie scattered along the lower border of the inguinal ligament. They vary greatly in number and size.)

10. Find the ilio-inguinal nerve just below the pubic tubercle. Trace its branches to the skin of the upper

medial part of the thigh. It also sends branches to the external genital organs.

11. Lift the upper end of the long saphenous vein, and note that it turns backwards over a sharp edge of the deep fascia.

12. Follow this edge round the lateral side of the vein and upwards towards the inguinal ligament. This is the falciform margin of the **saphenous opening** [Fig. 13.8]. From this margin, the thin **cribriform fascia** passes in front of the opening and the femoral vessels in the femoral sheath.

13. Remove the cribriform fascia to expose the femoral sheath. Take care not to damage the structures which pierce the cribriform fascia or lie posterior to it.

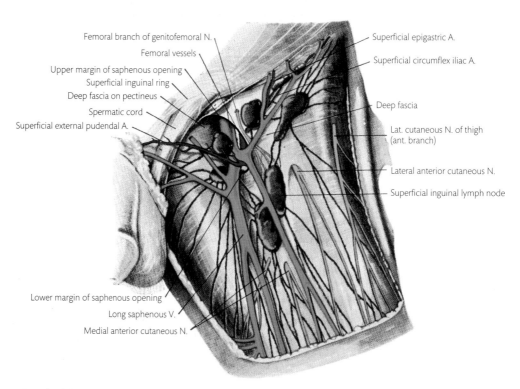

Fig. 13.8 Superficial dissection of the proximal part of the front of the thigh. The saphenous opening and the superficial lymph nodes and lymph vessels of the groin are displayed.

forwards, producing a swelling medial to the upper end of the long saphenous vein. Such a swelling may be mistaken for distension of the vein, especially as both swellings are connected with the abdomen and are made more obvious by raising the intra-abdominal pressure, e.g. by coughing.

Saphenous opening

The saphenous opening overlies the upper part of the femoral vein. The deep fascia over the opening is thin and perforated, and gets the name **cribriform fascia** (*cribrum* = a sieve). The cribriform fascia and saphenous opening transmit the long saphenous vein, one or more of the superficial inguinal arteries, and efferent lymph vessels from the superficial inguinal lymph nodes. The saphenous opening lies approximately 3–4 cm inferolateral to the pubic tubercle and is about 3 cm long and 1.5 cm wide. Except on the medial side, the opening is limited by the sharp **falciform margin** of the thicker deep fascia which surrounds it [Fig. 13.8].

Superficial inguinal lymph nodes

The superficial inguinal lymph nodes lie in the superficial fascia and are arranged in the shape of a T. The upper nodes are below, and roughly parallel to, the inguinal ligament. The lower nodes are placed vertically along the upper part of the long saphenous vein [Fig. 13.8].

The superficial inguinal lymph nodes receive almost all the lymph from the skin and superficial fascia below the level of the umbilicus. This includes: (1) the skin and superficial fascia of the trunk below the level of the umbilicus, including the perineum (anal canal, lower vagina, and urethra—the only parts of the perineum not drained by the superficial inguinal nodes are: (a) the testis which drains to the lumbar lymph nodes and (b) the glans penis or glans clitoris which drain to the deep inguinal lymph nodes); (2) the skin and superficial fascia of the lower limb, except the heel and lateral part of the foot which drain into the deep nodes in the popliteal fossa; (3) in addition, a few lymph vessels from the fundus and body of the uterus also reach the superficial inguinal lymph nodes along the round ligament of the uterus.

The superficial inguinal lymph nodes are connected together by many lymph vessels. The efferents pass through the cribriform fascia to the deep inguinal lymph nodes on the femoral vessels and the external iliac nodes on the external iliac vessels in the abdomen.

Long saphenous vein

This is the longest superficial vein of the lower limb. It begins on the medial side of the dorsum of the foot and runs up to end in the femoral vein by piercing the cribriform fascia. In the leg, it first lies anterior to the medial malleolus, then on the medial surface and medial border of the tibia and the posteromedial surface of the knee. In the thigh, it ascends to enter the femoral vein through the saphenous opening.

The long and short saphenous veins form parallel channels with the deep veins (plantar and tibial veins) of the lower limb. Venous blood in the lower limb has to flow against gravity, and several mechanisms exist in both superficial and deep veins to aid this. Blood in the deep veins is pushed up against gravity by the pumping action produced by contraction of the surrounding muscles. No such mechanism aids blood flow in the superficial veins. However, the saphenous vein has several communications with the deep veins, through veins that pierce the deep fascia. These are the perforators, and they contain valves which direct blood from the superficial to deep. Flow of blood through the valved perforators keeps blood from collecting in the superficial veins.

Another mechanism for combating stagnation of blood in the low-pressure long saphenous vein is the presence of valves. Valves divide the column of blood in the vein into segments. Blood from each segment drains into the deep veins through the perforators. In this way, pressure on the walls of the distal part is kept low.

⊃ The system breaks down when there is no muscular contraction to empty the deep veins, or if the valves in the communicating vessels become incompetent. When valves become incompetent, muscular contraction forces blood into the superficial veins, instead of pushing it up. The pressure in the superficial veins rises, and they will eventually dilate and lead to further incompetence of the valves and worsening of the situation (see Clinical Application 18.1).

Dissection 13.3 traces the cutaneous nerves.

Cutaneous nerves

The front and medial sides of the thigh are supplied by the following cutaneous nerves:

1. Directly from the lumbar plexus: ilio-inguinal nerve, femoral branch of the genitofemoral nerve, lateral cutaneous nerve of the thigh.
2. From the femoral nerve: anterior cutaneous branches to the thigh, saphenous nerve.
3. From the obturator nerve: occasional branch to the medial side of the thigh.

The **ilio-inguinal nerve** (L. 1) emerges just lateral to the pubic tubercle (through the superficial inguinal ring) and is distributed to the scrotum or labium majus and the medial side of the thigh.

DISSECTION 13.3 Cutaneous nerves on front of thigh

Objective

I. To clean and trace the cutaneous nerves on the front of the thigh.

Instructions

1. Strip the superficial fascia down from the front and lateral side of the thigh by blunt dissection. Leave the deep fascia in place.

2. With the assistance of Figs. 13.8 and 13.9, find the cutaneous nerves as they pierce the deep fascia, and follow them distally.

3. Note how most of these nerves terminate in the patellar plexus, anterior to the patella.

4. Check for the presence of a prepatellar bursa between the skin and the lower part of the patella.

The **femoral branch of the genitofemoral nerve** (L. 1, 2) is small and difficult to find. It enters the thigh, posterior to the inguinal ligament, and pierces the deep fascia, lateral to the saphenous opening. This nerve supplies an area of skin immediately below the inguinal ligament.

The **lateral cutaneous nerve of the thigh** (L. 2, 3) enters the thigh, posterior to the lateral part of the inguinal ligament. It gives a posterior branch that pierces the deep fascia and supplies an area of skin over the greater trochanter. The remainder of the nerve pierces the deep fascia lower down. It descends on the lateral side of the thigh to the patella, sending branches to the skin of the lateral and anterior surfaces of the thigh.

Three **anterior cutaneous branches** arise from the femoral nerve (L. 2, 3) in the front of the thigh. They supply the skin of the anterior and medial surfaces of the thigh and the upper part of the medial surface of the leg. The more medial branches pierce the deep fascia more distally [Fig. 13.9].

The **saphenous nerve** (L. 3, 4) arises from the femoral nerve and descends with the femoral artery, deep to the sartorius muscle. It sends an **infrapatellar branch** through that muscle to supply the skin medial to the knee and distal to the patella. The main nerve pierces the deep fascia, posterior to the sartorius, at the knee. It supplies the skin of the medial surface of the leg and the medial surface of the foot

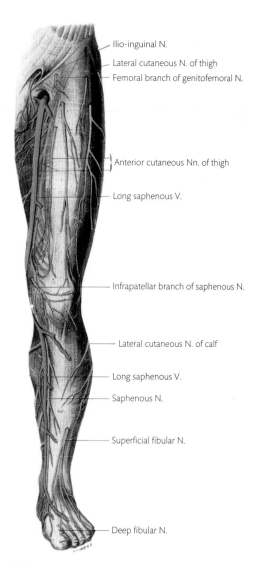

Fig. 13.9 Cutaneous nerves on the front of the lower limb.

up to the proximal end of the big toe. It descends on the leg with the long saphenous vein [Fig. 13.9].

Patellar plexus

The patellar plexus is a cutaneous nerve plexus formed by branches of the lateral cutaneous nerve of the thigh, the lateral and intermediate anterior cutaneous branches of the femoral nerve, and the infrapatellar branch of the saphenous nerve. The plexus supplies the skin over the patella, the patellar ligament, and the proximal part of the tibia anteriorly. The individual nerve fibres entering the plexus do not anastomose but merely run in the same connective tissue sheath.

Dissection 13.4 is the dissection of the deep fascia of the thigh.

DISSECTION 13.4 Deep fascia of the thigh

Objective

I. To expose the deep fascia and establish its attachments.

Instructions

1. Complete the exposure of the deep fascia of the front and lateral side of the thigh. (Do not remove the cutaneous nerves, so that they may be followed to their origins later.)

2. Trace the deep fascia upwards to the iliac crest, inguinal ligament, and the body of the pubis.

Fascia lata

The deep fascia of the thigh is called the **fascia lata**. Like the deep fascia elsewhere in the body, it is continuous with the periosteum of the underlying bones, either directly where the bone is subcutaneous, or indirectly through intermuscular septa. The upper part of the fascia lata is attached around the root of the lower limb to: (a) the iliac crest laterally; (b) the inguinal ligament anteriorly; (c) the body of the pubis, ischiopubic rami, and ischial tuberosity medially; and (d) the sacrotuberous ligament and sacrum posteriorly. Below, at the knee, the fascia lata fuses with the patella, the femoral

and tibial condyles, and the head of the fibula. Posteriorly, it is continuous with the dense fascia covering the popliteal fossa.

The fascia lata is thin medially and where it forms the cribriform fascia over the saphenous opening. Laterally, it forms the **iliotibial tract**, a thickened band stretching from the iliac crest to the lateral tibial condyle. Two muscles—**gluteus maximus** and **tensor fasciae latae**—are inserted into the tract. Through the insertion into the iliotibial tract, they help stabilize the pelvis on the thigh and maintain extension of the knee while standing.

From the deep surface of the fascia lata, three intermuscular septa pass to the linea aspera of the femur. These medial, posterior, and lateral intermuscular septa separate the thigh into three compartments, each of which contains a group of muscles and the vessels and nerves which supply them [Fig. 13.10]: (1) the anterior compartment lies anteriorly and laterally; it contains the extensor muscles and the femoral nerve; (2) the medial compartment contains the adductor muscles and the obturator nerve; and (3) the posterior compartment contains the flexor muscles (hamstrings) and the sciatic nerve. The extensor group consists principally of four large muscles (quadriceps femoris) which are inserted into the patella. Their tendinous fibres continue over the anterior surface of the patella as the patellar tendon which attaches the patella to the tibial tuberosity.

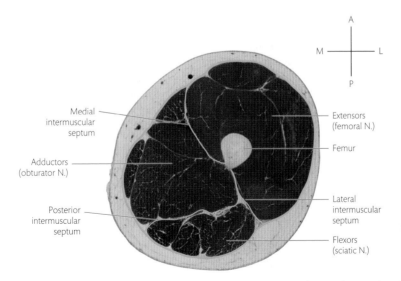

Fig. 13.10 Section of the thigh to show the arrangement of muscles and intermuscular septa forming the osteofascial compartments of the right thigh. A = anterior; P = posterior; M = medial; L = lateral.

Image courtesy of the Visible Human Project of the US National Library of Medicine.

Patellar bursae

A number of fluid-filled bursae are present around the knee joint. These allow free movement of the skin on the underlying tissues, e.g. in kneeling, and movement of the deep tissues on each other. There are two or three subcutaneous bursae between the skin and the front of the patella, the lower part of the patellar ligament, and the tibial tuberosity.

There are two deep bursae: (1) a large **suprapatellar bursa** separates the tendon of the quadriceps femoris from the front of the femur. It extends upto a hand's breadth above the patella and is usually continuous with the cavity of the knee joint; (2) a **deep infrapatellar bursa** lies between the tibial tuberosity and the patellar ligament.

Inguinal ligament

The free lower border of the aponeurosis of the external oblique muscle of the abdomen forms the inguinal ligament. (The external oblique muscle is seen in Fig. 13.7, and the inguinal ligament in Fig. 13.11.) The inguinal ligament extends from the anterior superior iliac spine laterally to the pubic tubercle medially. The free edge of the aponeurosis is curved back on itself to form a groove on the abdominal aspect. The fascia lata is attached to the length of the ligament, exerts traction on it, and makes the inguinal ligament convex inferiorly.

Lateral to the pubic tubercle, the deep surface of the inguinal ligament extends posteriorly to the pecten pubis, forming the **lacunar ligament**. This triangular lacunar ligament [see Fig. 13.14] has an apex attached to the pubic tubercle, and a base which is sharp and curved. The free base of the lacunar ligament lies medial to the aperture, through which the femoral vessels enclosed in the femoral sheath enter the thigh.

Femoral sheath

To understand this region, you should appreciate certain general points. (1) At the inguinal ligament,

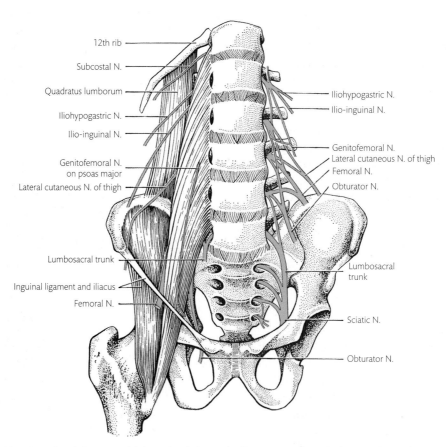

Fig. 13.11 Lumbar plexus (semi-diagrammatic) shown in relation to the iliopsoas muscles and other muscles on the posterior abdominal wall.

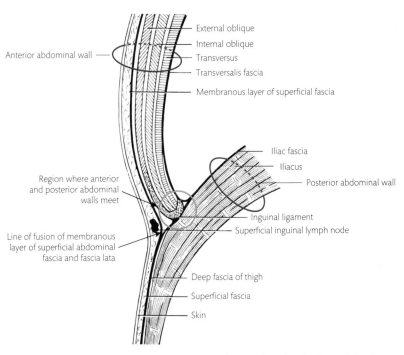

Fig. 13.12 Diagram of fasciae and muscles of the inguinal and subinguinal regions lateral to the femoral sheath.

the anterior and posterior abdominal walls come together. This means that the **transversalis fascia** lining the deep surface of the anterior abdominal wall and the **iliac fascia** covering the lower part of the posterior abdominal wall meet each other at the inguinal ligament [Fig. 13.12]. (2) Deep to the inguinal ligament and between it and the hip bone is a gap through which structures pass from the abdomen into the thigh. Here muscles (psoas and iliacus) and nerves (femoral and lateral cutaneous nerve of the thigh) of the posterior abdominal wall enter into the thigh behind the iliac fascia and the lateral part of the inguinal ligament [Fig. 13.11]. Also deep to the medial part of the inguinal ligament, the external iliac vessels in the abdomen become the femoral vessels in the thigh. They are covered by a funnel-shaped extension of the fascial lining of the abdomen, and carry with them the transversalis fascia anteriorly and the iliac fascia posteriorly [Fig. 13.13]. These coverings form the **femoral sheath** which lies immediately lateral to the lacunar ligament [Figs. 13.14, 13.15]. The femoral sheath has within it, from lateral to medial, the femoral artery and the **femoral branch of the genitofemoral nerve**, the **femoral vein** (in the middle), and a space called the **femoral canal**, medial to the vein. This canal allows for the expansion of the femoral vein within the sheath. It

narrows inferiorly and disappears where the sheath fuses with the adventitia of the vessels at the lower margin of the saphenous opening. The canal contains loose fatty tissue (the femoral septum), a small lymph node, and some lymph vessels.

Dissection 13.5 explores these features.

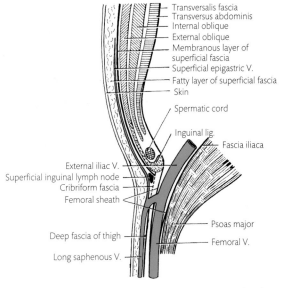

Fig. 13.13 Diagram of fasciae and muscles of the inguinal and subinguinal regions in the line of the femoral vein.

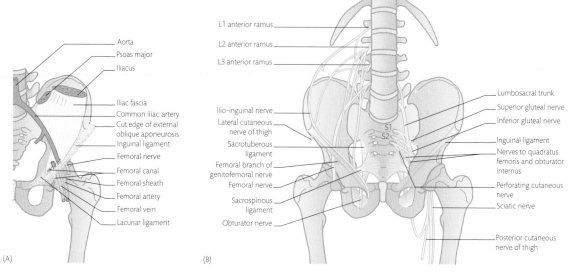

Fig. 13.14 (A) Diagram to show the routes of entry of femoral nerves and blood vessels into the lower limb. A portion of the aponeurosis of the external oblique muscle of the abdomen and the inguinal and lacunar ligaments are shown. (B) Diagram to show the course of sciatic, femoral and obturator nerves as they enter the lower limb.

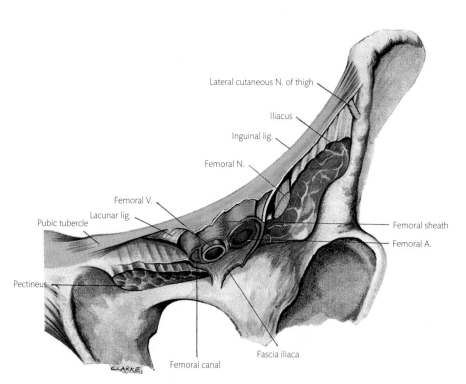

Fig. 13.15 Dissection to show the femoral sheath and structures which pass between the inguinal ligament and the hip bone. Seen from below and in front.

Objective

I. To clean and study the femoral sheath and its contents. II. To study the margins of the femoral ring.

Instructions

1. Follow the long saphenous vein through the anterior wall of the femoral sheath to the femoral vein, and expose the femoral vein.

2. Split the femoral sheath, lateral and medial to the vein, to expose the femoral artery and femoral canal, respectively. Note the septa of the sheath which separate the compartments in which the artery, vein, and canal lie.

3. Note that the canal is shorter than the spaces which contain the vessels. Introduce your little finger into the canal, and push it upwards. It is possible to enter the abdomen through the canal.

4. At the abdominal opening of the canal (the **femoral ring**), feel the edge of the lacunar ligament medially, the inguinal ligament anteriorly, and the pecten pubis posteriorly.

Femoral canal

As mentioned earlier, the femoral canal is the most medial compartment within the femoral sheath. This short fascial tube rapidly diminishes in width from above downwards and is closed inferiorly by fusion of its walls. The wide upper end is the **femoral ring**. It is separated from the abdominal cavity only by the smooth innermost lining of the abdominal wall—the peritoneum. The **boundaries of the femoral ring** are: the inguinal ligament anteriorly; the sharp edge of the lacunar ligament medially; the pecten of the pubic bone posteriorly; and the femoral vein laterally. Inferiorly, the canal lies posterior to the saphenous opening and cribriform fascia, and anterior to the fascia covering the pectineus muscle.

Femoral triangle

The femoral triangle is formed by the inguinal ligament (base) superiorly, the medial border of the sartorius laterally, and the medial border of the adductor longus medially. Inferiorly, the apex of the triangle is continuous with a narrow intermuscular space—the **adductor canal** [Fig. 13.16].

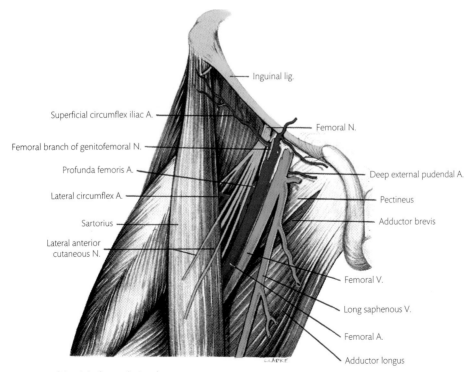

Inguinal lig.

Superficial circumflex iliac A.

Femoral N.

Femoral branch of genitofemoral N.

Profunda femoris A.

Deep external pudendal A.

Lateral circumflex A.

Pectineus

Sartorius

Adductor brevis

Lateral anterior
cutaneous N.

Femoral V.

Long saphenous V.

Femoral A.

Adductor longus

Fig. 13.16 Dissection of the right femoral triangle.

The roof, or **anterior wall**, of the triangle consists of the deep fascia, superficial inguinal lymph nodes and lymph vessels, the upper part of the long saphenous vein, the femoral branch of the genitofemoral nerve, branches of the ilio-inguinal nerve, and superficial branches and tributaries of the femoral vessels.

The floor or posterior wall is formed by the adductor longus, pectineus, psoas major, and iliacus, from the medial to lateral sides. The floor slopes posteriorly, and the femoral vessels lie in the central hollow.

Dissection 13.6 studies the femoral triangle.

Contents of the femoral triangle

Important blood vessels, nerves, lymph nodes, and lymphatics lie in the femoral triangle.

1. The **femoral vessels** traverse the triangle from the base to the apex. The vein is medial to the artery at the base, but behind it at the apex.

2. The **profunda femoris artery** is the main artery supplying the thigh. It arises from the posterolateral side of the femoral artery, curves down behind it, and goes posterior to the adductor longus. The profunda vein is anterior to its artery and ends in the femoral vein.

3. The **lateral** and **medial circumflex femoral arteries** arise from the profunda near its origin. The lateral circumflex femoral artery runs laterally among the branches of the femoral nerve and passes posterior to the sartorius. The medial circumflex femoral artery passes backwards between the psoas and pectineus muscles. The circumflex veins end in the femoral vein.

4. The **deep external pudendal** artery arises from the femoral artery near the base of the triangle. It runs medially to the scrotum in the male and to the labium majus in the female.

5. Three or four **deep inguinal lymph nodes** lie along the medial side of the femoral vein. They

---

DISSECTION 13.6 Femoral triangle

Objective

I. To identify the muscles, vessels, and nerves of the femoral triangle.

Instructions

1. Expose the sartorius and adductor longus muscles down to the apex of the triangle where they meet. Preserve the nerves close to the sartorius [Fig. 13.16].

2. Place a block under the knee to flex the hip joint, and relax the structures in the triangle. Find the femoral nerve lateral to the artery in the groove between the psoas and iliacus muscles.

3. Note that the femoral nerve divides almost immediately into a number of cutaneous and muscular branches.

4. Find the nerve to the pectineus passing medially behind the femoral artery.

5. Follow the other branches of the femoral nerve, till they leave the triangle. Avoid injury to the lateral circumflex artery which passes laterally among these nerves near their origin.

6. Remove the venae comitantes of the smaller arteries to get a clear picture of the arrangement of the vessels.

7. Clean the upper part of the femoral artery. Find the deep external pudendal artery which arises from the upper part of the femoral artery and runs medially.

8. Identify the root of the large profunda femoris artery which arises from the posterolateral surface of the femoral artery, about 5 cm below the inguinal ligament. Follow it downwards with the profunda vein behind the femoral vessels, until it leaves the triangle.

9. Find the lateral and medial circumflex femoral arteries which arise from the profunda near its origin or from the adjacent femoral artery. Trace the lateral artery as far as the sartorius, and the medial one backwards as far as possible behind the femoral vessels. Preserve the proximal parts of the circumflex veins which enter the femoral vein.

10. Trace the nerve to the pectineus behind the femoral vein.

11. Remove the fascia from the pectineus, and find the anterior branch of the obturator nerve in the interval between it and the adductor longus. The nerve descends behind both muscles in front of the adductor brevis.

12. Strip the fascia from the surface of the iliacus and psoas major. Place your finger on the anterior surface of the tendon of the psoas, and push it downwards and backwards, following the line of the tendon. It is usually possible to reach the lesser trochanter of the femur to which the tendon is attached.

13. The medial circumflex artery passes backwards between the psoas and pectineus muscles, parallel to your finger. Expose it as far as possible.

receive lymph vessels from the superficial inguinal and popliteal lymph nodes, and from the deep structures of the limb. Efferent lymph vessels pass from the deep inguinal nodes to the external iliac nodes on the external iliac vessels in the abdomen.

6. The **femoral branch of the genitofemoral nerve** [Fig. 13.9] supplies the skin over the femoral triangle.

7. The **lateral cutaneous nerve of the thigh** crosses the lateral angle of the triangle.

8. The **femoral nerve** ends in the femoral triangle.

Dissection 13.7 continues the dissection of the front of the thigh.

Sartorius

This long, strap-like muscle arises from the anterior superior iliac spine and runs across the front of the thigh to the posterior part of the medial side of the knee. In the leg, it forms a thin tendinous sheet which is inserted into the upper part of the medial surface of the tibia [see Fig. 18.13]. This tendon is separated by a bursa (**bursa anserina**) from the tendons of the gracilis and semitendinosus which are inserted on the tibia posterior to it.

The sartorius forms the lateral boundary of the femoral triangle, the roof of the adductor canal, and produces a vertical, fleshy ridge far back on the medial side of the extended knee. When the knee is flexed, the muscle slips backwards into the medial boundary of the popliteal fossa. **Nerve supply**: femoral nerve. **Actions**: it flexes the hip joint and the knee joint, and rotates the thigh laterally to bring the limb into the position adopted when sitting cross-legged (**sartorius** comes from the Latin word *sartor*, meaning tailor. This name was chosen in reference to the cross-legged position in which tailors once sat). When the knee is flexed, the sartorius medially rotates the tibia on the femur.

Adductor canal

The adductor canal is a deep furrow on the medial side of the thigh between the vastus medialis anteriorly and the adductor longus and magnus muscles posteriorly. The roof of the canal is formed by a strong fascia that stretches from the vastus medialis to the adductors and has the sartorius lying on it. The femoral vessels, the **saphenous nerve**, and the nerve to the vastus medialis lie in this canal. The roof is pierced inferiorly by the saphenous nerve. Inferiorly, there is an opening in the adductor magnus muscle—the tendinous (adductor) opening—through which the femoral vessels pass from the canal into the popliteal fossa. The

---

DISSECTION 13.7 Front of the thigh

Objective

I. To identify the tensor fasciae latae and the parts of the quadriceps femoris. II. To trace the medial and lateral circumflex femoral arteries and their branches. III. To demonstrate the boundaries and contents of the adductor canal.

Instructions

1. Expose the sartorius down to its insertion onto the tibia.

2. Make a vertical incision through the fascia lata from the tubercle of the iliac crest to the lateral margin of the patella. Remove the fascia lata between the incision and the sartorius. This uncovers the tensor fasciae latae and parts of the four elements of the quadriceps muscle but leaves the greater part of the iliotibial tract in position.

3. Find: (1) the rectus femoris in the middle of the front of the thigh; (2) part of the vastus lateralis lateral to the rectus femoris; (3) the vastus intermedius deep to the rectus femoris; and (4) part of the vastus medialis between the lower parts of the rectus femoris and sartorius [Fig. 13.17].

4. Lift the rectus femoris, and follow it to its origin on the hip bone.

5. Trace the lateral circumflex femoral artery behind the sartorius and the rectus femoris. Follow its three branches: (1) the descending branch along the anterior border of the vastus lateralis; (2) the ascending branch that runs between the sartorius and tensor fasciae latae on a deeper plane; and (3) a small transverse branch that enters the vastus lateralis.

6. Pull the middle third of the sartorius laterally. This exposes a narrow strip of the fascia, the roof of the adductor canal, between the vastus medialis and the adductor muscles. Divide the fascia longitudinally, and find the femoral vessels, the saphenous nerve, and the nerve to the vastus medialis in the canal [Fig. 13.18].

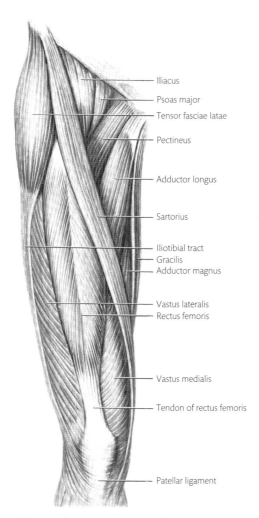

Iliacus
Psoas major
Tensor fasciae latae
Pectineus
Adductor longus
Sartorius
Iliotibial tract
Gracilis
Adductor magnus
Vastus lateralis
Rectus femoris
Vastus medialis
Tendon of rectus femoris
Patellar ligament

Fig. 13.17 Muscles of the front of the right thigh.

nerve to the vastus medialis descends in the canal and enters that muscle.

Femoral artery

The femoral artery is the main artery of the lower limb and is the continuation of the external iliac artery of the abdomen. As this vessel passes behind the inguinal ligament at the mid-inguinal point [Figs. 13.14, 13.15], its name changes to the femoral artery. At the mid-inguinal point, the femoral artery is medial to the femoral nerve, lateral to the femoral vein, and anterior to the psoas major and the hip bone. By compressing the artery against the bone, it is possible to control bleeding from a more distal point, when a distal branch of the artery is cut. The artery enters the femoral triangle, anterior to the head of the femur, and is covered only by skin and the fascia in the triangle. It leaves the triangle at its apex and runs through the adductor canal with the femoral vein, the saphenous nerve, and the nerve to the vastus medialis. Here it lies close to the shaft of the femur and receives a branch from the obturator nerve. It continues as the **popliteal artery** by passing through the tendinous opening in the adductor magnus. [Fig. 13.16].

Branches

The main branch and principal artery of the thigh is the **profunda femoris**. Three small superficial arteries of the groin (superficial circumflex iliac, superficial epigastric, and superficial external

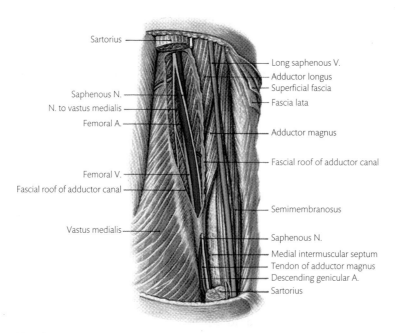

Sartorius
Saphenous N.
N. to vastus medialis
Femoral A.
Femoral V.
Fascial roof of adductor canal
Vastus medialis

Long saphenous V.
Adductor longus
Superficial fascia
Fascia lata
Adductor magnus
Fascial roof of adductor canal
Semimembranosus
Saphenous N.
Medial intermuscular septum
Tendon of adductor magnus
Descending genicular A.
Sartorius

Fig. 13.18 Dissection of the adductor canal in the right thigh. A portion of the sartorius has been removed.

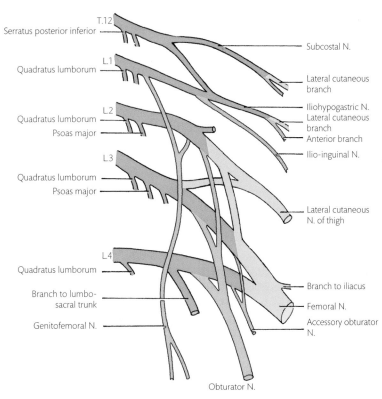

Front of the thigh

Fig. 13.19 Diagram of the lumbar plexus. Ventral divisions, light orange; dorsal divisions, yellow.

pudendal) and one deep artery (deep external pudendal) also arise in the femoral triangle. Muscular branches and the **descending genicular artery** arise in the adductor canal. The descending genicular artery supplies adjacent muscles and the knee joint, and sends a branch with the saphenous nerve to the medial side of the knee and leg [see Fig. 16.1].

Femoral vein

The femoral vein is the continuation of the popliteal vein. It begins at the opening in the adductor magnus and runs with the femoral artery to the inguinal ligament behind which it becomes the external iliac vein. The relationship between the femoral vein and artery changes—the vein is posterior to the artery in the lower part of the femoral triangle, and medial in the upper part [Fig. 13.16].

The femoral vein contains several **valves**. One is constantly present, proximal to the entry of the profunda vein. Open the vein, and examine the valve.

Tributaries

The tributaries in the thigh correspond to the branches of the arteries, with some exceptions.

The superficial veins of the groin end in the long saphenous vein, and the medial and lateral circumflex veins enter the femoral vein, though the corresponding arteries are usually branches of the profunda femoris artery.

Femoral nerve (L. 2, 3, 4)

The femoral nerve arises from the lumbar plexus in the abdomen [Figs. 13.11, 13.14, 13.19]. It descends between the iliacus and psoas major muscles behind the iliac fascia and enters the thigh, posterior to the inguinal ligament [Fig. 13.15]. It ends by dividing into branches 2 cm below the inguinal ligament. The branches are muscular, articular, or cutaneous. Muscular branches are to the pectineus, sartorius, and quadriceps femoris. Articular branches are to the hip and knee joints. Cutaneous branches include the anterior cutaneous nerves of the thigh (medial and lateral) and the saphenous nerve.

The innervation to the quadriceps femoris is by separate nerves to each of its four parts—the rectus femoris and the three vasti. The nerve to the rectus femoris sends a branch to the hip joint; the nerves to the vasti send branches to the knee joint. Thus, the nerves to the parts of the quadriceps which act only on the knee joint (vasti) send branches to that joint; the nerve to the part that acts also on the hip joint sends a branch to that joint.

The **lateral** and **medial anterior cutaneous nerves** (L. 2, 3) run along the medial margin of the sartorius and pierce the deep fascia to supply the skin and subcutaneous tissue.

The **saphenous nerve** (L. 3, 4) is the longest branch of the femoral nerve and the only one that has its main distribution in the leg and foot. It accompanies the femoral vessels in the adductor canal and pierces the fibrous roof of the canal and the deep fascia at the posterior border of the sartorius, medial to the knee [Fig. 13.9].

The **branch to the pectineus** runs medially and downwards behind the femoral vessels to the pectineus. Two or three **nerves to the sartorius** usually arise in common with the lateral anterior cutaneous nerve. The **nerves to the rectus femoris** (usually two) enter the deep surface of the muscle, and the upper one supplies the hip joint. The **nerve to the vastus medialis** enters the adductor canal and supplies the muscle at different levels. It sends a branch to the knee joint. The **nerve to the vastus lateralis** passes deep to the rectus femoris and accompanies the descending branch of the lateral circumflex artery to the anterior border of the muscle. It usually gives a branch to the knee joint. Two or three **nerves to the vastus intermedius** enter its anterior surface. The most medial nerve is a long, slender branch which runs along the medial edge of the vastus intermedius to the articularis genus muscle (for a description of the articularis genus, see Vastus intermedius, p. 181). Its terminal filaments pass to the knee joint.

Lateral circumflex femoral artery

The lateral circumflex femoral artery is the largest branch of the profunda femoris artery. It supplies structures on the lateral side of the hip and thigh. It arises from the profunda femoris artery near its origin and runs laterally among the branches of the femoral nerve, and then deep to the rectus femoris. It ends by dividing into ascending, transverse, and descending branches.

The **ascending branch** passes along the intertrochanteric line of the femur to the gluteal surface of the ilium. It supplies the surrounding muscles and the hip joint, and anastomoses with the **superior gluteal artery**. The small **transverse**

branch passes backwards through the vastus lateralis. It anastomoses with other arteries, posterior to the femur. The **descending branch** runs along the anterior border of the vastus lateralis. It supplies a large part of the quadriceps and sends a long branch through the vastus lateralis to the anastomosis at the knee joint.

Tensor fasciae latae

This muscle lies between the gluteal region and the front of the thigh [Fig. 13.17]. It arises from the anterior part of the iliac crest and is inserted into the iliotibial tract, 3–5 cm below the level of the greater trochanter. It is enclosed between two layers of the iliotibial tract. **Nerve supply**: superior gluteal nerve. **Actions**: flexion and medial rotation of the hip joint; extension of the knee through the iliotibial tract.

Iliotibial tract

The iliotibial tract is a thick band of fascia lata which runs vertically on the lateral side of the thigh from the iliac crest to the lateral condyle of the tibia [Fig. 13.20]. The greater part of the gluteus maximus and the tensor fasciae latae are inserted into it. These muscles, through their insertion into the tract, help to steady the pelvis on the thigh and

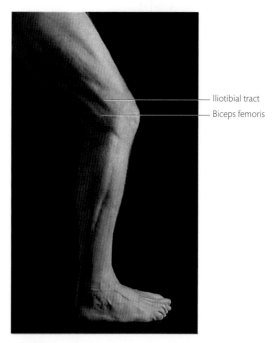

Iliotibial tract
Biceps femoris

Fig. 13.20 Lateral side of the knee, showing surface projection of the iliotibial tract and biceps tendon.

keep the knee extended in the erect position. While standing, the tensed iliotibial tract is readily felt on the lateral side of the thigh, immediately proximal to the lateral condyle of the femur. By comparison, the palpably relaxed quadriceps and mobile patella indicate that the quadriceps is not responsible for maintaining knee extension in standing.

Superiorly, most of the posterior part of the tract passes deep to the gluteus maximus. Its anterior part splits to enclose the tensor fasciae latae, and the intermediate part passes directly to the iliac crest. Inferiorly, the tract is continuous with the rest of the fascia lata and the lateral intermuscular septum.

Dissection 13.8 exposes the lateral intermuscular septum.

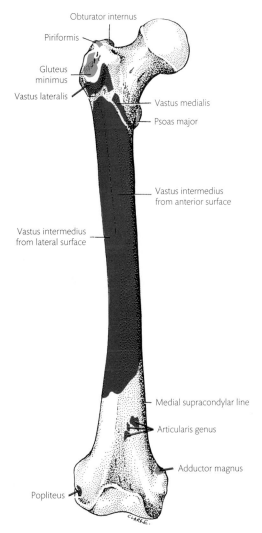

Fig. 13.21 Right femur (anterior aspect) to show muscle attachments.

Labels on figure:
- Obturator internus
- Piriformis
- Gluteus minimus
- Vastus lateralis
- Vastus medialis
- Psoas major
- Vastus intermedius from anterior surface
- Vastus intermedius from lateral surface
- Medial supracondylar line
- Articularis genus
- Adductor magnus
- Popliteus

DISSECTION 13.8 Lateral intermuscular septum

Objective

I. To expose the lateral intermuscular septum.

Instructions

1. Expose the lateral intermuscular septum by detaching the vastus lateralis from it, and reflecting the muscle forwards.

Intermuscular septa

There are three intermuscular septa in the thigh—lateral, medial, and posterior intermuscular septa [Fig. 13.10]. The lateral is strong; the others are thin fascial layers on the front and back of the adductor muscles. All three septa pass to the linea aspera (rough line) and the corresponding supracondylar line. All muscles attached to the body of the femur are attached only to these lines, except the vastus intermedius [Figs. 13.21, 13.22]. The order of attachment of the thigh muscles to the linea aspera is that of their position in the thigh, i.e. from medial to lateral—vastus medialis, the adductors, the short head of the biceps, and vastus lateralis.

The fibrous lateral intermuscular septum passes from the deep surface of the iliotibial tract to the lateral supracondylar line and the linea aspera between the vastus lateralis and the short head of biceps femoris.

Quadriceps femoris

The quadriceps femoris is the powerful extensor of the knee joint. The four muscles that contribute to it are the rectus femoris, vastus medialis, vastus intermedius, and vastus lateralis [Fig. 13.17]. All four parts are inserted into the patella and through it and the patellar tendon on the tibial tuberosity. The vastus medialis, intermedius, and lateralis arise from the femur and act solely on the knee joint. The rectus femoris arises from the hip bone and is also a flexor of the hip joint. It is more separate than the vasti and only fuses with them, as it approaches the insertion into the patella. Because of the wide range of movement possible at the knee joint, the tendon of the quadriceps, the patella, and the patellar tendon form the anterior part of the fibrous capsule of the joint and the suprapatellar bursa.

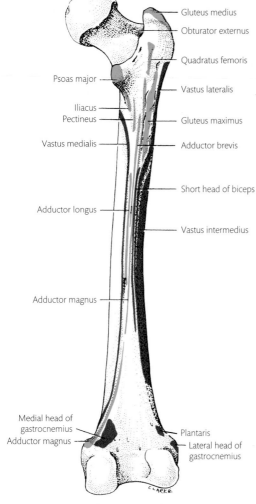

Fig. 13.22 Right femur (posterior aspect) to show muscle attachments.

Rectus femoris

This muscle arises by two heads from the anterior or inferior iliac spine (**straight head**) and from a groove immediately above the acetabulum (**reflected head**) [Fig. 13.23]. In varying degrees of flexion of the hip joint, one or other of these heads takes the major part of the strain. The muscle runs vertically down the front of the thigh in a groove between the iliopsoas and tensor fasciae latae superiorly, and between the vastus lateralis and vastus medialis inferiorly. It overlies the anterior part of the vastus intermedius.

Vastus lateralis

Together with the vastus intermedius with which it is partly fused, the vastus lateralis muscle covers the lateral aspect of the femur. It has a long linear origin from the root of the greater trochanter to the lateral supracondylar line [Fig. 13.22]. The muscle fibres run downwards and forwards to the patella and the anterolateral part of the fibrous capsule of the knee joint. The lowest fibres lie 3–4 cm proximal to the patella.

Vastus medialis

The vastus medialis muscle has a long linear origin from the intertrochanteric and spiral lines, the linea aspera, the medial supracondylar line [Figs. 13.4, 13.22], the medial intermuscular septum, and the tendons of the adductors longus and magnus. Most of its muscle bundles are directed downwards and forwards onto the proximal surface of the patella,

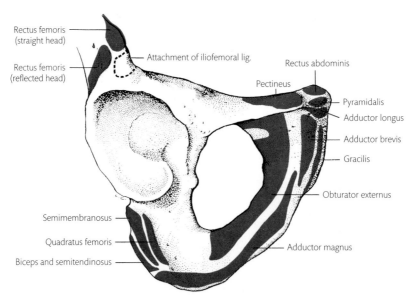

Fig. 13.23 Muscle attachments to the outer surface of the right pubis and ischium.

except the lowest fibres which run horizontally into the medial aspect of the upper half of the patella. These lowest fibres help to hold the patella medially (prevent lateral displacement of the patella) and form a prominent bulge, just proximal to the medial condyle of the femur [Fig. 13.5]. Some of the fibres of the vastus medialis are inserted into the anteromedial part of the fibrous capsule of the knee joint.

Vastus intermedius

The vastus intermedius takes origin from the lateral and anterior surfaces of the body of the femur [Fig. 13.21]. Some of the lowest fibres arise from the front of the femur and are inserted into the **suprapatellar bursa**. These fibres constitute the **articularis genus muscle** which pulls up the bursa during extension of the knee joint. The remainder of the vastus intermedius passes to the common tendon of the quadriceps which is inserted into the proximal surface of the patella. **Nerve supply**: femoral nerve. **Actions** of quadriceps: extension of the knee and flexion of the hip (rectus femoris).

Medial side of the thigh

The muscles on the medial side of the thigh produce adduction at the hip joint. These **adductor muscles** are arranged in three layers, from anterior to posterior. The anterior layer is composed of the pectineus and adductor longus. The middle layer is the adductor brevis. The posterior layer is the adductor magnus. These muscles are attached proximally to the hip bone [Fig. 13.23] and distally to the back of the femur [Fig. 13.22]. Medial to these is the gracilis muscle. It is long and slender (*gracilis* = slender), arises from the hip bone, and is the only member of the group which is inserted into the tibia. As a result, it acts on the knee joint, in addition to the hip joint.

The two branches of the **obturator nerve**, anterior and posterior divisions, descend between the muscles and are separated from each other by the adductor brevis. The nerve supplies these muscles and the obturator externus, but not the pectineus. The **profunda femoris artery** descends posterior to the adductor longus, close to the femur.

Adductor longus

This triangular muscle takes origin by a narrow tendon from the front of the body of the pubis, immediately below the pubic crest [Fig. 13.23]. It widens as it passes inferolaterally, and is inserted into the linea aspera of the femur, between the vastus medialis and the other adductors [Fig. 13.22]. **Nerve supply**: anterior branch of the obturator nerve. **Action**: adduction of the thigh.

Dissection 13.9 begins the dissection of the medial compartment of the thigh.

DISSECTION 13.9 Medial compartment of the thigh-1

Objectives

I. To study the adductor longus, gracilis, and obturator externus. II. To identify and trace the anterior and posterior divisions of the obturator nerve.

Instructions

1. Remove the fascia from the adductor longus, gracilis, and obturator externus and the nerves that supply them.

2. Divide the adductor longus transversely, 2–3 cm below its origin. Turn the distal part towards the femur.

3. Find the nerve supplying it, and trace it to the anterior branch of the obturator nerve.

4. Follow the anterior branch of the obturator nerve inferiorly to the gracilis, and find a small branch entering the adductor canal.

5. Trace the gracilis to its attachments.

6. Define the attachments of the pectineus [Figs. 13.22, 13.23]. Avoid injury to the branches of the obturator nerve behind it and the medial circumflex artery superolateral to it. Detach the pectineus from its origin, and turn it laterally.

7. Trace the anterior branch of the obturator nerve and the medial circumflex artery as far as possible.

8. Identify the obturator externus. It lies superior to the medial circumflex artery and has the anterior branch of the obturator nerve passing anterosuperior to it [Fig. 13.24].

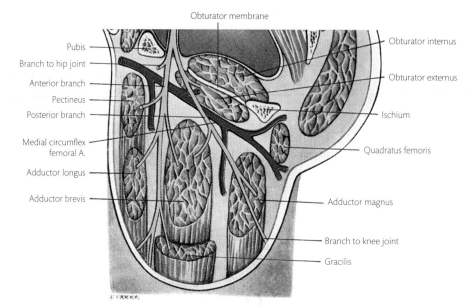

Fig. 13.24 Schematic diagram of the adductor muscles and obturator nerve.

Pectineus

The pectineus arises from the pectineal surface of the pubis [Fig. 13.23] and is inserted into the upper half of a line joining the lesser trochanter of the femur to the linea aspera [Fig. 13.22]. In the base of the femoral triangle, the pectineus lies between the adductor longus and the iliopsoas [Fig. 13.17]. **Nerve supply**: femoral nerve. **Action**: see Actions of the adductor muscles, p. 183.

Accessory obturator nerve

The accessory obturator nerve, when present, is a branch of either the lumbar plexus or the obturator nerve. It descends along the medial side of the psoas major and crosses the superior ramus of the pubis into the thigh (it does not pass through the obturator canal). It may end in the hip joint or in the pectineus, or it may pass between the psoas and the pectineus to replace part of the obturator nerve [Fig. 13.19].

Medial circumflex femoral artery

The medial circumflex femoral artery is a branch of the profunda femoris. It passes back superior to the pectineus and the adductor muscles, and inferior to the psoas, obturator externus, and quadratus femoris muscles [Fig. 13.24]. It gives branches to the adjacent muscles and supplies the hip joint through the acetabular notch. The terminal branches take part in the formation of the **cruciate anastomosis**, posterior to the adductor magnus.

Adductor brevis

The adductor brevis muscle arises from the pubis, inferior to the origin of the adductor longus. It lies behind the pectineus and adductor longus, and is inserted into the linea aspera in this position [Figs. 13.22, 13.23]. **Nerve supply**: obturator nerve. **Action**: see Actions of the adductor muscles, p. 183.

Dissection 13.10 continues the dissection of the medial compartment of the thigh.

DISSECTION 13.10 Medial compartment of the thigh-2

Objective

I. To expose and clean the adductor brevis and magnus, and the nerve which supplies them.

Instructions

1. Divide the adductor brevis close to its origin. Turn it laterally, preserving the anterior branch of the obturator nerve.

2. Find and trace the posterior branch of the obturator nerve behind the muscle.

3. Remove the fascia from the surface of the obturator externus and adductor magnus, without damaging the branches of the obturator nerve. Define the attachments of the adductor magnus.

Gracilis

The gracilis muscle arises from the lower half of the body of the pubis close to the symphysis, and from the anterior part of the inferior pubic ramus [Fig. 13.23]. It lies on the medial side of the thigh and is inserted into the upper part of the medial surface of the tibia, posterior to the sartorius. It is separated from the sartorius and the tibial collateral ligament of the knee by a complex bursa—the bursa anserina. **Nerve supply**: anterior branch of the obturator nerve. **Action**: see Actions of the adductor muscles, see below.

Adductor magnus

This muscle takes origin from the ischiopubic ramus and the lower part of the ischial tuberosity [Fig. 13.23]. It lies posterior to the other adductor muscles and is inserted into the back of the femur, from the gluteal tuberosity to the adductor tubercle [Fig. 13.22]. At intervals, the insertion to bone is interrupted, and muscle fibres are inserted instead to tendinous slips which arch over the **perforating arteries** on the surface of the femur. The opening through which the femoral vessels pass—the adductor hiatus—is the largest of these arches. It lies at the medial supracondylar line approximately at the junction of the middle and lower thirds of the thigh.

The adductor magnus is fan-shaped [see Fig. 16.1] with horizontal anterior fibres, oblique middle fibres, and nearly vertical posterior fibres. The vertical fibres pass from the ischial tuberosity to the adductor tubercle. At the adductor tubercle, the tendon is continuous with the medial intermuscular septum and gives attachment to the lower fibres of the vastus medialis. **Nerve supply**: (1) the part originating from the ischiopubic ramus is supplied by the posterior branch of the obturator nerve; (2) the part originating from the ischial tuberosity with the hamstring muscles is supplied by the tibial part of the sciatic nerve.

Actions of the adductor muscles

The adductor longus, brevis, magnus, pectineus, and gracilis adduct the thigh. In addition, the **gracilis** flexes the knee joint and medially rotates the leg when the knee is flexed. The ischial part of the adductor magnus acts with the hamstring muscles to extend the hip joint but has no action on the knee joint. One important action of the adductor muscles is to stabilize the hip bone on the femur. They prevent the hip bone from tilting laterally when standing on one leg. They are active in the supporting limb during the whole period in which it supports the body weight while walking (see also action of gluteal muscles: Gluteus maximus, p. 189; Actions of the gluteus medius and minimus, p. 196).

Obturator nerve (L. 2, 3, 4)

The obturator nerve arises from the lumbar plexus in the abdomen [Fig. 13.11]. It descends medial to the psoas muscle, on to the lateral wall of the lesser pelvis where it lies lateral to the **ovary**. Here it joins the obturator vessels and enters the **obturator canal**. In the obturator canal, it divides into anterior and posterior branches. The **anterior branch** descends in the thigh, anterior to the obturator externus and adductor brevis. It supplies the adductor longus, adductor brevis, gracilis, and the **hip joint** [Fig. 13.24]. Distal to the adductor longus, it enters the adductor canal and forms a plexus with branches from the medial anterior cutaneous nerve of the thigh and the saphenous nerve. Through this plexus, it may supply parts of the medial side of the thigh.

The **posterior branch** supplies and pierces the obturator externus and descends between the adductors brevis and magnus, supplying both. An **articular branch** passes through the lower part of the adductor magnus to the back of the knee joint.

Obturator externus

This fan-shaped muscle arises from the anterior half of the obturator membrane and from the anterior and inferior margins of the obturator foramen [Fig. 13.23]. It passes back curving upwards on the inferior and posterior surfaces of the neck of the femur, to be inserted into the trochanteric fossa [Fig. 13.4]. **Nerve supply**: posterior branch of the obturator nerve. **Actions**: flexion and lateral rotation of the thigh. Importantly, it functions as an extensile ligament of the hip joint.

Obturator artery

The obturator artery is a branch of the internal iliac artery. It accompanies the obturator nerve in the obturator canal. It divides into branches which form an arterial circle on the obturator membrane, deep to the obturator externus. It supplies the adjacent muscles, the bone, and the hip joint. Its **articular branch** runs through the acetabular notch and enters the ligament of the head of the femur, sometimes playing a minor role in the supply of the femoral head.

Psoas major and iliacus

The psoas major and iliacus arise within the abdomen and fuse with each other as they enter the thigh, posterior to the inguinal ligament [Fig. 13.14], the femoral nerve, and the lateral part of the femoral sheath. They are separated posteriorly from the capsule of the hip joint by a **bursa** which may communicate with the joint cavity. The muscles pass inferior to the neck of the femur and are inserted into the lesser trochanter (psoas) and the surface of the femur below it (iliacus).

Nerve supply: the ventral rami of L. 2 and L. 3.
Actions: the iliopsoas are the chief flexors of the hip joint. If the limb is fixed, it flexes the trunk on the thigh. It also produces medial rotation of the thigh, because its insertion is lateral to the axis of rotation of the femur.

❯ Its action is important clinically, because spasm of the psoas produces flexion and medial rotation of the hip joint—a position taken up by the right lower limb in appendicitis when the inflamed appendix causes spasm on the underlying right psoas.

When the neck of the femur is fractured, the iliopsoas produces marked lateral rotation of the distal segment of the femur (and of the distal part of the limb). As a result, the toes of the affected limb point laterally in the supine patient.

See Clinical Applications 13.1 and 13.2.

CLINICAL APPLICATION 13.1 Femoral hernia

In the erect position, the weight of the abdominal contents presses down on the inguinal region. The femoral ring forms a point of weakness and may allow the entry of a loop of intestine or other abdominal contents into the femoral canal. Such protrusion of abdominal contents into the thigh constitutes a femoral hernia. As the femoral ring is limited anteriorly by the inguinal ligament, any event which stretches the inguinal ligament enlarges the femoral ring. This could happen as a result of repeated pregnancies that weaken the abdominal muscles. Any other condition which chronically raises the intra-abdominal pressure, e.g. repeated coughing or straining, will also predispose to the development of such a hernia. Femoral hernias are more common in women.

When a loop of intestine enters the femoral ring, it carries the peritoneum covering of the abdominal opening of the canal in front of it. The peritoneum forms a hernial sac which descends in the femoral canal and bulges forwards through the cribriform fascia into the superficial fascia of the thigh. If the sac continues to enlarge, it expands superolaterally in the superficial fascia, so that the entire hernia becomes U-shaped. This course of the hernia should be kept in mind when external pressure is applied in an attempt to return the hernial sac and its contents to the abdomen. The sac should first be pushed down and medially towards the saphenous opening, then through the cribriform fascia, and only then should an attempt be made to return it through the distended femoral canal.

As the hernial sac expands in the subcutaneous tissue, the margins of the femoral ring may constrict the neck of the sac. This tends to obstruct the passage of intestinal contents in the loop of gut and occlude the blood vessels to it. This could lead to strangulation of the hernia, possibly resulting in gangrene and rupture. Surgical reduction of an obstructed or strangulated hernia commonly requires division of the lacunar ligament. Care should be taken in dividing the lacunar ligament, as an abnormal obturator artery may lie on it. When present, this abnormal artery arises from the inferior epigastric artery, instead of the internal iliac artery, and commonly crosses the abdominal aspect of the lacunar ligament.

The patellar tendon reflex is a deep tendon reflex routinely done to test L. 3 and L. 4 segments of the spinal cord. The patient sits at the edge of the examination table, with his legs hanging freely. The physician strikes the patellar tendon sharply with a reflex hammer. This causes the leg to extend at the knee. Mostly, the response is evaluated visually by watching for the extension of the knee. The contraction of the quadriceps muscle can be evaluated by palpation as well.

The impact of the reflex hammer stretches the patellar tendon. This triggers sensory nerves that innervate the quadriceps to send information from the tendon to the spinal cord—segments L. 3 and L. 4. In the spinal cord, small internuncial neurons are activated which, in turn, stimulate the motor neurons supplying the quadriceps. This leads to contraction of the quadriceps and extension of the knee

Some important points about the deep tendon reflexes are:

1. Sensory fibres relaying the stimulus to the spinal cord form the afferent limb of the reflex arc (see the black somatic efferent fibre in Fig. 1.5).

2. The motor fibres supplying the quadriceps form the efferent limb (see the blue somatic afferent fibre in Fig. 1.5).

3. Deep tendon reflexes are withdrawal reflexes involving the spinal cord (no involvement from the higher centres).

4. Both afferent and efferent nerves have to be intact for the reflex action to occur.

5. Abnormal reflexes include reflexes that are lost, diminished, or heightened (of increased power and/or speed).

6. Responses are graded using standard criteria.

Medial side of the thigh

185

CHAPTER 14
The gluteal region

Surface anatomy

The gluteal region is bound by the iliac crest superiorly, the **gluteal fold** of the round **buttock** inferiorly, a line joining the anterior superior iliac spine to the front of the greater trochanter laterally, and the **natal cleft** between the buttocks medially [Fig. 14.1]. The horizontal gluteal fold is due to adherence of the skin to the deep fascia over the gluteus maximus, the large buttock muscle [Fig. 14.2]. Deep to the lower part of this muscle is the **ischial tuberosity** [Fig. 14.1]. This can be felt by pressing your fingers upwards into the medial part of the gluteal fold but is most easily identified as the rounded bony mass on which you sit.

The natal cleft begins near the third sacral spine. The lower part of the sacrum and the coccyx are in its floor. Palpate your own sacrum and coccyx. The **coccyx** can be identified by its relative mobility. Between the lower part of the sacrum and the ischial tuberosity, a deep resistance can be felt through the posterior part of the gluteus maximus. This is the **sacrotuberous ligament**. It holds the lower part of the sacrum and prevents the upper part from being pushed down by the weight of the body.

Trace your iliac crest forwards to the anterior superior iliac spine and backwards to the **posterior superior iliac spine**. The posterior superior iliac spine lies in a skin dimple at the level of the second sacral spine. The posterior surface of the sacrum lies between the right and left posterior superior iliac spines.

Dissection 14.1 looks at the cutaneous nerves in the gluteal region.

Superficial fascia

This is dense and contains a lot of fat, especially at the upper and lower margins of the gluteus maximus.

Cutaneous nerves

These reach the gluteal region from all four directions—above, below, laterally, and medially.

1. From above: the **lateral cutaneous branches** of the **subcostal** (T. 12) and **iliohypogastric** (L. 1) nerves pass downwards, anterior and posterior to the tubercle of the iliac crest. They supply the skin down to the level of the greater trochanter.
2. From below: branches of the **posterior cutaneous nerve of the thigh** curve over the lower border of the gluteus maximus to the posteroinferior part of the gluteal region.
3. From the lateral side: the posterior branch of the **lateral cutaneous nerve of the thigh** (L. 2, 3) supplies the anteroinferior part.
4. From the medial side: cutaneous branches of the **dorsal rami** of L. 1–3, S. 1–3 and the **perforating cutaneous nerve** (S. 2, 3 ventral rami) supply the medial and intermediate part. The lumbar nerves are long and descend obliquely across the region almost to the gluteal fold. The sacral branches are short. The perforating cutaneous nerve

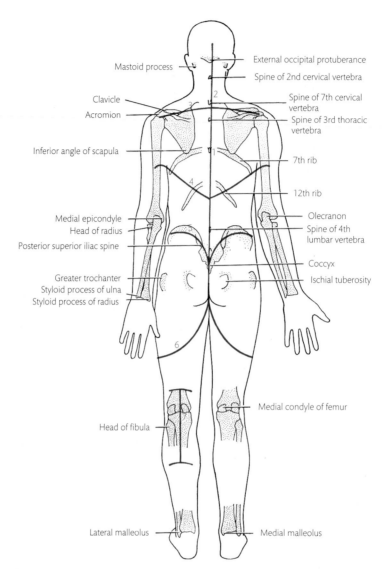

Mastoid process
External occipital protuberance
Spine of 2nd cervical vertebra
Clavicle
Acromion
Spine of 7th cervical vertebra
Spine of 3rd thoracic vertebra
Inferior angle of scapula
7th rib
12th rib
Medial epicondyle
Head of radius
Posterior superior iliac spine
Olecranon
Spine of 4th lumbar vertebra
Greater trochanter
Styloid process of ulna
Styloid process of radius
Coccyx
Ischial tuberosity
Head of fibula
Medial condyle of femur
Lateral malleolus
Medial malleolus

Fig. 14.1 Landmarks and incisions.

DISSECTION 14.1 Skin reflection and cutaneous nerves-1

Objective

I. To reflect the skin and identify the cutaneous nerves.

Instructions

1. Make skin incisions 5 and 6 [Fig. 14.1]. Reflect the flap of skin and superficial fascia laterally.

2. Attempt to find the cutaneous nerves of the gluteal region. They are difficult to find because of the dense superficial fascia, but it is usually possible to identify the branches of the lumbar nerves [Fig. 14.2].

pierces the sacrotuberous ligament and the gluteus maximus midway between the coccyx and the ischial tuberosity [Fig. 14.2].

Deep fascia

The deep fascia is thick over the anterior border of the gluteus maximus where the iliotibial tract splits to enclose the muscle. Everywhere else, the fascia is thin over the muscle and thick deep to it.

Dissection 14.2 looks at the gluteus maximus.

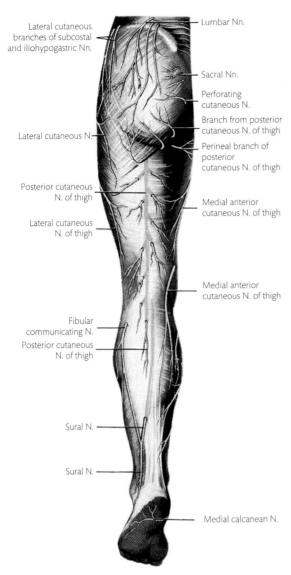

Lateral cutaneous branches of subcostal and iliohypogastric Nn.

Lumbar Nn.

Sacral Nn.

Perforating cutaneous N.

Branch from posterior cutaneous N. of thigh

Lateral cutaneous N.

Perineal branch of posterior cutaneous N. of thigh

Posterior cutaneous N. of thigh

Medial anterior cutaneous N. of thigh

Lateral cutaneous N. of thigh

Medial anterior cutaneous N. of thigh

Fibular communicating N.

Posterior cutaneous N. of thigh

Sural N.

Sural N.

Medial calcanean N.

Fig. 14.2 Cutaneous nerves on the back of the lower limb.

DISSECTION 14.2 Gluteus maximus

Objective

I. To define the extent of the gluteus maximus.

Instructions

1. If any branches of the posterior cutaneous nerve of the thigh have been found, follow them back to the trunk of the nerve.

2. Remove the thin deep fascia from the gluteus maximus, and define the attachments of the muscle. (Leave the insertion of the muscle into the iliotibial tract intact.)

Gluteus maximus

This powerful muscle takes origin from: (1) the external surface of the ilium behind the posterior gluteal line [Fig. 14.3]; (2) the back of the sacrum and coccyx; and (3) the sacrotuberous ligament. Its fibres run downwards and laterally, and abruptly become aponeurotic. This abrupt thinning produces the hollow of the hip, posterior to the greater trochanter of the femur. Fibres of the deeper one-fourth of the muscle are inserted into the **gluteal tuberosity** of the femur [see Fig. 13.22]. The remainder are inserted into the iliotibial tract. Aponeurotic fibres passing to the iliotibial tract run superficial to the greater trochanter and the upper part of the vastus lateralis, while the lower part of the muscle crosses the ischial tuberosity. The gluteus maximus is separated from all three deeper structures (greater trochanter, vastus lateralis, and ischial tuberosity) by large **bursae**. **Nerve supply**: inferior gluteal nerve. **Actions**: it is a powerful extensor of the hip joint used when strength is required, e.g. when the erect position has to be regained while lifting heavy weights from the floor. It is also used in running and climbing, more especially in achieving full extension of the hip joint. It acts jointly with the tensor fasciae latae to stabilize the pelvis on the thigh (supporting the trunk) in an anteroposterior plane. With the tensor fascia latae, it extends the knee through the iliotibial tract.

Dissection 14.3 looks at some of the structures deep to gluteus maximus.

Structures deep to the gluteus maximus

Begin by studying an articulated pelvis, preferably one with the sacrotuberous and sacrospinous ligaments attached [Fig. 14.4]. The **sacrotuberous ligament** passes from the medial side of the ischial tuberosity to the posterior iliac spines. The sacrospinous ligament runs from the ischial spine to the side of the lower part of the sacrum and coccyx, deep to the sacrotuberous ligament. These two ligaments convert the two sciatic notches into foramina—an upper **greater sciatic foramen** and a lower **lesser sciatic foramen**. The sacrospinous ligament lies edge to edge with the levator ani muscle. Together with the muscle of the opposite side, the levator ani forms the muscular floor

189

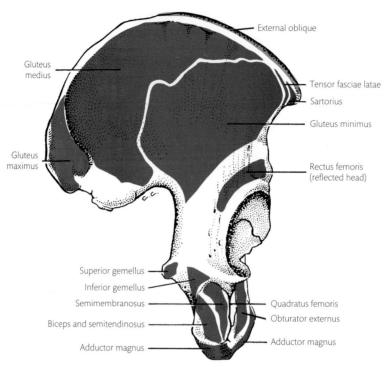

Fig. 14.3 Muscle attachments to the outer surface of the right hip bone.

DISSECTION 14.3 Structures deep to gluteus maximus-1

Objectives

I. To expose piriformis.   II. To identify and trace the superior and inferior gluteal vessels and nerves and the posterior cutaneous nerve of thigh.

Instructions

1. Cut across the gluteus maximus from its inferior margin upwards, 2–3 cm medial to its femoral insertion, and reflect it. This is difficult because the vessels (superior and inferior gluteal) and the inferior gluteal nerve enter its deep surface and are easily destroyed before they are seen. Avoid this by passing two fingers deep to the lower edge of the muscle and cutting upwards between the fingers to the upper border at a point directly superior to the greater trochanter.

2. As you reflect the lateral part of the muscle to its insertion, identify the bursae which separate it from the greater trochanter and the upper part of the vastus lateralis.

3. Reflect the medial part of the muscle. Keep close to the deep surface of the muscle to avoid injury to the posterior cutaneous nerve of the thigh [Fig. 14.2].

4. Find the inferior gluteal vessels and nerve entering the lower part of the muscle.

5. As the ischial tuberosity is uncovered, look for the bursa superficial to the origin of the hamstring muscles.

6. Identify the piriformis muscle.

7. Trace the branch of the superior gluteal artery to where it emerges between the gluteus medius superiorly and the piriformis inferiorly.

8. Remove the fascia from the piriformis muscle, and trace it to its attachment to the greater trochanter.

9. Find and follow the posterior cutaneous nerve of the thigh upwards to the point where it emerges at the lower border of the piriformis. A perineal branch of this nerve curves medially, below the ischial tuberosity, towards the perineum.

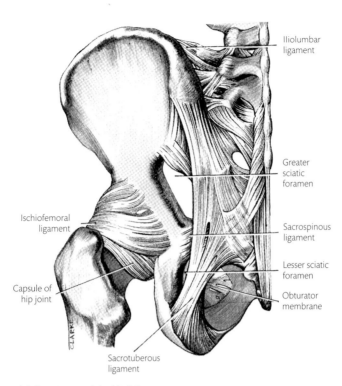

Iliolumbar ligament

Greater sciatic foramen

Ischiofemoral ligament

Sacrospinous ligament

Lesser sciatic foramen

Capsule of hip joint

Obturator membrane

Sacrotuberous ligament

Fig. 14.4 Dorsal view of the pelvic ligaments and the hip joint.

of the pelvis and separates the pelvis above from the perineum below. The greater sciatic foramen (which lies superior to the ischial spine) leads from the gluteal region into the pelvis. The lesser sciatic foramen (which lies inferior to the ischial spine) leads from the gluteal region into the perineum. This arrangement allows for structures to pass between the gluteal region and the pelvis through the greater sciatic foramen, and between the gluteal region and the perineum through the lesser sciatic foramen.

Vessels and nerves which enter the gluteal region from the pelvis may: (1) remain in the gluteal region; (2) descend into the back of the thigh; or (3) enter the perineum by turning forwards through the lesser sciatic foramen. Structures remaining in the gluteal region include the gluteal vessels and nerves. Structures descending to the back of the thigh include the sciatic nerve, the posterior cutaneous nerve of the thigh, and branches of the inferior gluteal vessels. Structures entering the perineum are the internal pudendal vessels, the pudendal nerve, and the nerve to the obturator internus. The lesser sciatic foramen also allows passage of the **obturator internus** from the lateral wall of the perineum into the gluteal region.

Sacrotuberous ligament

The sacrotuberous ligament passes upwards from the medial side of the ischial tuberosity to the margins of the sacrum and coccyx, and to the posterior superior and inferior iliac spines of the hip bone. The lateral edge of the ligament forms the posteromedial border of the greater and lesser sciatic foramina. The medial edge forms the posterior boundary of the perineum. The ligament holds down the posterior part of the sacrum and prevents the weight of the body from depressing the anterior part [Fig. 14.5]. When the loading on the anterior part of the sacrum is severe, e.g. in landing on the feet when jumping from a height, the ligament gives resilience by allowing slight movement at the sacro-iliac joint.

Sacrospinous ligament

This thick, triangular band is the aponeurotic posterior surface of the coccygeus muscle. It passes from the spine of the ischium to the margin of the coccyx and of the last piece of the sacrum, deep to the sacrotuberous ligament.

Dissection 14.4 continues to explore the gluteal region.

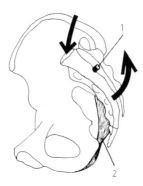

Fig. 14.5 Diagram to show the forces applied to the sacrum due to the weight of the body acting through the vertebral column (thick straight arrow). Note how the sacrotuberous ligament (2) will act as a shock absorber, permitting only slight movement of the sacrum at the sacro-iliac joint around its axis of movement (1). This causes the lower part of the sacrum to swing upwards (thick curved arrow).

Inferior gluteal nerve (L. 5; S. 1, 2)

This branch of the sacral plexus enters the gluteal region with the posterior cutaneous nerve of the thigh, inferior to the piriformis. It breaks into a number of nerves which enter the deep surface of the gluteus maximus—the only structure it supplies [Figs. 14.6, 14.8].

Inferior gluteal artery

This branch of the internal iliac artery emerges from the pelvis below the piriformis. It sends large branches into the deep surface of the gluteus maximus and cutaneous branches to the buttock and to the back of the thigh with the posterior cutaneous nerve of the thigh. The artery also gives rise to the slender **companion artery of the sciatic nerve** and anastomoses with the circumflex femoral arteries.

DISSECTION 14.4 Structures deep to gluteus maximus-2

Objectives

I. To expose the sciatic nerve and its branches. II. To identify the nerve to the obturator internus, the internal pudendal artery, pudendal nerve, nerve to the quadratus femoris and gemelli, and the medial circumflex femoral artery. III. To identify the tendon of the obturator internus, superior and inferior gemelli, quadratus femoris, and adductor magnus.

Instructions

1. Find the large sciatic nerve, as it emerges from the pelvis at the lower border of the piriformis. Carefully split the fascia surrounding the nerve. Trace the nerve downwards to where it gives branches to the hamstring muscles near the ischial tuberosity. The vessels running with these branches arise from the medial circumflex femoral artery [Figs. 14.6, 14.7].

2. Push the upper part of the sciatic nerve laterally to expose the posterior surface of the acetabulum.

3. Find the slender nerve to the quadratus femoris.

4. Medial to the upper part of the sciatic nerve, identify the ischial spine and the sacrospinous ligament. The ligament can be felt as a tough resistance medial to the spine. On the surface of the spine and ligament, find the nerve to the obturator internus, the internal pudendal vessels, and the pudendal nerve.

5. Remove the fascia from the muscles deep to the sciatic nerve. From above downwards, these are [Figs. 14.6, 14.7]: (1) the tendon of the obturator internus overlapped by the superior and inferior gemelli; separate the gemelli, and expose the tendon; follow the tendon to the greater trochanter; (2) the quadratus femoris passing from the ischial tuberosity to the back of the femur; and (3) the posterior surface of the adductor magnus.

6. Find and trace the branches of the medial circumflex femoral artery which appear both above and below the quadratus femoris [see Figs. 13.24, 14.6].

7. Inferior to this, the first perforating artery (a branch of the profunda femoris) may be found piercing the adductor magnus, close to the gluteal tuberosity of the femur [Fig. 14.7].

8. Separate the gemellus inferior from the quadratus femoris.

9. Lift the gemelli and obturator internus, and cut across them, lateral to the nerve to the quadratus femoris.

10. Follow the nerve to the quadratus femoris and its branch to the inferior gemellus.

11. Separate the quadratus femoris from the adductor magnus, and remove the quadratus femoris to expose the lesser trochanter of the femur, the medial circumflex femoral artery, the posterior part of the capsule of the hip joint, and the tendon of the obturator externus.

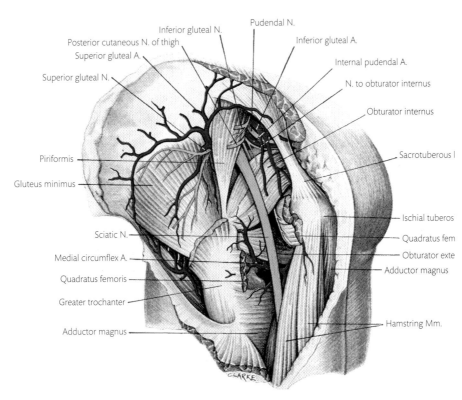

Inferior gluteal N.
Pudendal N.
Posterior cutaneous N. of thigh
Inferior gluteal A.
Superior gluteal A.
Internal pudendal A.
Superior gluteal N.
N. to obturator internus
Obturator internus
Piriformis
Sacrotuberous l
Gluteus minimus
Ischial tuberos
Sciatic N.
Quadratus fem
Medial circumflex A.
Obturator exte
Adductor magnus
Quadratus femoris
Greater trochanter
Hamstring Mm.
Adductor magnus

Fig. 14.6 Dissection of the left gluteal region. The gluteus maximus and gluteus medius have been removed, and the quadratus femoris has been reflected. In the specimen, the inferior gluteal artery was medial to the internal pudendal, instead of lateral to it.

Sciatic nerve (L. 4, 5; S. 1, 2, 3)

This is the thickest nerve in the body. It arises from the sacral plexus and passes through the lower part of the greater sciatic foramen into the gluteal region. It lies deep to the gluteus maximus. From above downwards, it lies on the: (1) ischial wall of the acetabulum and the nerve to the quadratus femoris; (2) obturator internus muscle with the two gemelli; (3) quadratus femoris [Fig. 14.6]. At this level, one or more nerves leave its medial side to supply the hamstring muscles. The sciatic nerve then enters the thigh on the posterior surface of the adductor magnus [Fig. 14.7] and descends between it and the hamstring muscles. The sciatic nerve usually ends halfway down the back of the thigh by dividing into the **common fibular** and **tibial nerves**. The point of division of the sciatic nerve is variable. If it occurs before the nerve leaves the pelvis, the tibial nerve emerges below the piriformis while the common fibular nerve pierces that muscle.

Pudendal nerve, internal pudendal artery, and nerve to the obturator internus

These three structures enter the gluteal region through the lowest part of the greater sciatic foramen. They lie on the posterior surface of the junction of the ischial spine and the sacrospinous ligament, with the pudendal nerve most medial, lateral to it the artery and the nerve to the obturator internus. They turn forwards immediately and enter the perineum through the lesser sciatic foramen [Fig. 14.6].

Small muscles on the back of the hip joint

The **piriformis** takes origin from the pelvic surface of the middle three pieces of the sacrum. It passes through the greater sciatic foramen and is inserted into the upper border of the greater trochanter of the femur [see Fig. 13.21], immediately

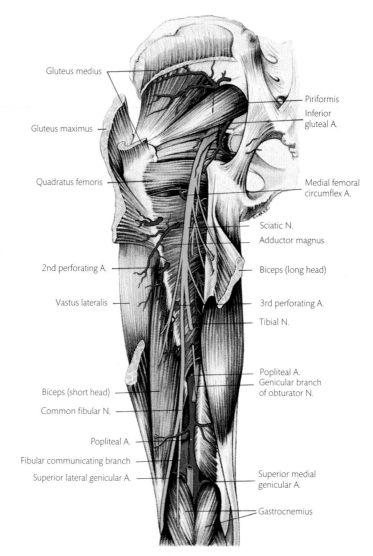

Gluteus medius

Gluteus maximus

Quadratus femoris

2nd perforating A.

Vastus lateralis

Biceps (short head)

Common fibular N.

Popliteal A.

Fibular communicating branch

Superior lateral genicular A.

Piriformis

Inferior gluteal A.

Medial femoral circumflex A.

Sciatic N.

Adductor magnus

Biceps (long head)

3rd perforating A.

Tibial N.

Popliteal A.
Genicular branch of obturator N.

Superior medial genicular A.

Gastrocnemius

Fig. 14.7 Dissection of the gluteal region and the back of the thigh.

lateral to the tendon of the obturator internus. **Nerve supply**: branches of the first and second sacral nerves in the pelvis.

The **obturator internus** is a large, fan-shaped muscle which arises from the pelvic surface of the obturator membrane and most of the bone surrounding the foramen [Fig. 14.9]. The muscle fibres converge posteriorly to the lesser sciatic foramen, turn sharply over the lesser sciatic notch, and run laterally to be inserted into the upper medial part of the greater trochanter [see Fig. 13.21]. The tendon is separated from the notch by a bursa. The **levator ani muscle**—which separates the pelvis from the perineum—arises from the fascia covering the pelvic surface of the obturator internus. As such, the obturator internus is in the lateral wall of

both the pelvis and the perineum. **Nerve supply**: nerve to the obturator internus (L. 5; S. 1, 2).

The **gemelli** are continuations of the muscular part of the obturator internus on either side of its tendon. They arise from the superior and inferior margins of the lesser sciatic notch and are inserted into the posterior surface of the tendon. **Nerve supply**: superior gemellus from the nerve to the obturator internus; inferior gemellus from the nerve to the quadratus femoris.

The **quadratus femoris** originates from the lateral margin of the ischial tuberosity and is inserted into the back of the greater trochanter of the femur in the region of the quadrate tubercle [see Fig. 13.22]. The muscle lies between the inferior gemellus and the superior margin of the adductor

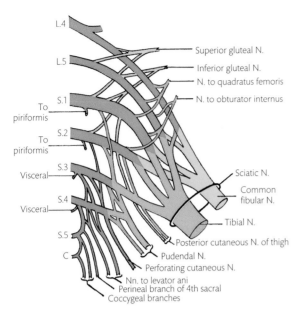

Fig. 14.8 Diagram of the sacral plexus. Ventral divisions, light orange; dorsal divisions, yellow.

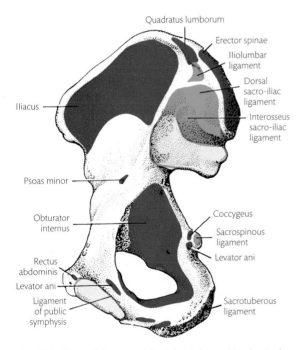

Fig. 14.9 The medial aspect of the right hip bone. Muscle attachments, red; ligament attachments and cartilage, blue.

magnus. **Nerve supply**: nerve to the quadratus femoris (L. 4, 5; S. 1).

Medial circumflex femoral artery

This artery arises from the profunda femoris (or femoral) artery in the femoral triangle. It passes backwards between the pectineus and iliopsoas, and then inferior to the obturator externus and the hip joint, above the adductor muscles [see Fig. 13.24]. It sends muscular branches down between the adductor muscles, a branch to the acetabulum, and anastomoses with the obturator artery. Posteriorly, the artery divides into an **ascending branch** which runs to the trochanteric fossa with the tendon of the obturator externus and a **transverse branch** to the hamstring muscles. The transverse branch anastomoses with: (1) the terminal part of the transverse branch of the lateral femoral circumflex artery; (2) the inferior gluteal artery; and (3) the first perforating artery to take part in the **cruciate anastomosis**. The ascending branch anastomoses with branches of both gluteal arteries and sends branches to the neck of the femur. These branches supply a large part of the **femoral head**.

Dissection 14.5 continues with dissection of the gluteal region.

Gluteus medius

This powerful muscle arises from the ilium between the anterior and posterior gluteal lines [Fig. 14.3]. It is overlapped posteriorly by the gluteus maximus and anteriorly by the tensor fasciae latae. Between these muscles, it is felt in the living through the skin and iliotibial tract. To check this on yourself, feel it contracting when the opposite foot is raised from the ground. The flattened tendon is inserted into the posterosuperior angle of the greater trochanter and the oblique ridge on its lateral surface [see Fig. 13.22]. A small bursa lies between the tendon and the trochanter in front of the insertion. **Nerve supply**: superior gluteal nerve.

Gluteus minimus

This thick muscle arises from the ilium between the anterior and inferior gluteal lines [Fig. 14.3]. It is inserted into the front of the greater trochanter [see Fig. 13.21] and fuses with the fibrous capsule of the hip joint. A bursa separates the tendon from the upper anterior part of the trochanter. **Nerve supply**: superior gluteal nerve.

Objectives

I. To expose the gluteus medius and minimus muscles.

II. To identify and trace the superior gluteal nerves and vessels.

Instructions

1. Remove the fascia from the superficial surface of the gluteus medius, and define its attachments.

2. Lift the inferior border of the gluteus medius away from the piriformis, and define the plane of separation between it and the gluteus minimus beneath. Separate the muscles from behind forwards by pushing your fingers between them.

3. Cut across the gluteus medius, 5 cm above the greater trochanter, and reflect its parts. Confirm its insertion. Find the bursa between the tendon of insertion and the greater trochanter.

4. Find the branches of the superior gluteal vessels and nerve, deep to the upper part of the muscle. Trace these between the gluteus medius and minimus to the deep surface of the tensor fasciae latae. Here the artery anastomoses with the ascending branch of the lateral femoral circumflex artery, and the nerve enters and supplies the tensor.

Actions of the gluteus medius and minimus

These muscles abduct the thigh when the limb is free to move. When the limb is supporting the weight of the body, their action is reversed, and they tilt the pelvis on the hip joint, so that the opposite foot can be raised from the ground. While walking, their contraction prevents the pelvis from sagging to the unsupported side when that foot is raised from the ground. When the glutei are paralysed and the opposite foot is raised from the ground, the weight of the body has to be moved laterally on the supporting limb by flexing the trunk to that side. ➲ Bilateral paralysis of these muscles (or bilateral congenital dislocation of the hip joints which prevents the muscles from acting) produces a waddling gait, in which the trunk is flexed from side to side with each step. See Clinical Application 14.2. The anterior fibres of both these muscles are also medial rotators of the thigh.

Superior gluteal nerve (L. 4, 5; S. 1)

This branch of the sacral plexus enters the gluteal region through the greater sciatic foramen above the piriformis [Figs. 14.6, 14.8]. It runs between the gluteus medius and minimus, and divides into a number of branches. The upper branches enter the gluteus medius. The lowest branch crosses the

minimus, gives small branches to the gluteus medius and minimus, and supplies the tensor fasciae latae.

Superior gluteal artery

This artery arises from the posterior division of the internal iliac artery and enters the gluteal region with the corresponding nerve. Here it divides into a superficial and deep branch. The **superficial branch** passes between the gluteus medius and piriformis to supply the gluteus maximus. The **deep branch** divides and runs with the branches of the superior gluteal nerve to supply the gluteus medius and minimus, the hip joint, and the tensor fasciae latae. It ends by anastomosing with the ascending branch of the lateral circumflex femoral artery. Together, they give branches to the neck and greater trochanter of the femur.

Anastomosis between branches of the internal and external iliac arteries

The many anastomoses between branches of the internal iliac and external iliac (or femoral) arteries are listed: (1) The important cruciate anastomosis occurs between the medial femoral circumflex artery, the obturator artery, the superior and inferior gluteal arteries, the lateral circumflex femoral artery, and the perforating branches of the profunda femoris. (2) The superior gluteal artery anastomosis with the lateral femoral circumflex artery, and the superficial circumflex iliac artery. (3) In the perineum, the internal pudendal artery anastomosis with the deep and superficial external pudendal branches of the femoral artery. (4) In the abdomen, the external iliac artery may anastomose with, or form, the obturator artery. In addition, the external iliac artery may communicate with the subclavian artery through an anastomosis between the superior and inferior epigastric arteries in the anterior abdominal wall.

Dissection 14.6 provides instruction on exposure of the capsule of the hip joint..

See Clinical Applications 14.1 and 14.2 for the practical implications of the anatomy discussed in this chapter.

DISSECTION 14.6 Capsule of hip joint

Objective

I. To complete exposure of the capsule of the hip joint.

Instructions

1. Detach the gluteus minimus from its origin, and turn it downwards. Separate it inferiorly from the fibrous capsule of the hip joint, and examine this part of the capsule.

2. Find the tendon of the rectus femoris attached to the anterior inferior iliac spine. Follow the tendon to its reflected head. Trace the reflected head to its attachment on a groove immediately above the margin of the acetabulum.

CLINICAL APPLICATION 14.1 Intragluteal injection

A 39-year-old man with a respiratory infection was given an intragluteal injection of penicillin on the right side. The next day, he developed numbness and tingling in his right leg down to the toes, and later the same day he developed a foot drop (inability to dorsiflex his foot). On examination, he was found to have significant sensory and motor loss in his right leg.

Study question 1: what is the most likely cause for the neurological symptom? (Think of the nerves supplying the lower limb and the likely nerve affected, given this history.) (Answer: injury to the sciatic nerve sustained during the intragluteal antibiotic injection.)

Study question 2: What is the surface marking of the sciatic nerve in the gluteal region? (Answer: a line joining two points: (1) the midpoint between the ischial tuberosity and the posterior inferior iliac spine; and (2) a point 1 cm medial to the midpoint of a line joining the ischial tuberosity to the greater trochanter.)

Study question 3: what is the standard rule for intragluteal injections, and was it followed in this case? (Answer: intragluteal injections should be given in the upper lateral quadrant of the buttocks. The rule was not followed in this case.)

CLINICAL APPLICATION 14.2 Gluteus medius gait

Stabilizing the hip, when one foot is off the ground, requires abduction of the opposite (supporting) hip. When the left foot is raised off the ground, the right abductors act to: (1) prevent the pelvis from sagging to the left side; and (2) create space to swing the left foot in taking a forward step. If the hip abductors—gluteus medius and minimus—are weak or paralysed, the patient is unable to stabilize the hip when standing on one leg or in walking.

Trendelenburg's sign: is elicited by asking the patient to stand on one leg. When the sign is positive, the pelvis sags to the unsupported side. It indicates damage to

the superior gluteal nerve or to the gluteus medius and minimus.

Trendelenburg's gait: is an abnormal gait adopted by a patient who is unable to abduct the hip. When the opposite foot is off the ground, the patient compensates for the tendency to fall on the unsupported side (due to lack of stability in the supporting hip) by leaning laterally to the affected side. A person with this gait will be seen lurching towards the weakened side every time the opposite foot is raised. If both hips are affected, the person will have a 'waddling gait'.

CHAPTER 15
The popliteal fossa

Surface anatomy

The popliteal fossa is an intermuscular space behind the knee, posterior to the lower third of the femur, the knee joint, and the upper part of the tibia. It forms a hollow when the knee is flexed, as the tendons which form its boundaries stand out from the femur. The fossa bulges slightly when the knee is straight.

Review the major palpable structures around the knee joint by examining your own knee. Find the **tendon of the biceps femoris** behind the lateral condyle of the femur. With the knee extended, press your finger against the posterior surface of the lateral condyle, immediately medial to the biceps tendon, and move the finger from side to side. The **common fibular nerve** can be felt in this location as a rounded cord. Follow the tendon of the biceps to the head of the fibula, and repeat the process on the back of the head. The same nerve can be felt again. Slide the finger down to the posterolateral side of the neck of the fibula. Move the finger up and down, maintaining some pressure to feel the nerve on the fibular neck. In all these positions, the common fibular nerve may be damaged by an injury to the bone.

With the knee flexed and the lateral side of the foot pressed against the floor, feel the **fibular collateral ligament** of the knee joint—a firm resistance between the head of the fibula and the lateral femoral condyle.

Place a finger in the middle of the popliteal fossa, with the knee bent. Press firmly, and feel the pulsations of the popliteal artery. In the lower part of the fossa, the two heads of the gastrocnemius form rounded swellings which merge inferiorly in the calf.

Immediately above the popliteal fossa, the back of the thigh is smooth and rounded. But the distal part of the belly of the semimembranosus may be seen to bulge near the midline, as it contracts in walking [Fig. 15.1].

Dissection 15.1 explores the popliteal region.

DISSECTION 15.1 Skin reflection, and cutaneous nerves and vessels of the popliteal region

Objective

I. To identify and trace the posterior cutaneous nerve of the thigh, the short saphenous vein, and the sural nerve in the roof of the popliteal fossa.

Instructions

1. Make skin incision 7 [see Fig. 14.1], and reflect the skin flaps, leaving the superficial fascia intact. Strip the superficial fascia from the deep fascia, starting proximally.

2. Look for branches of the posterior cutaneous nerve of the thigh piercing the deep fascia in the proximal part of the fossa.

3. Look for the short saphenous vein, with the terminal part of the posterior cutaneous nerve in the distal part of the fossa.

4. Follow the medial anterior cutaneous nerve of the thigh downwards in the posteromedial part of the calf [see Fig. 14.2].

5. The fibular communicating nerve (a branch of the common fibular nerve) may be found in the lower lateral part of the popliteal area. It may pierce the deep fascia at a much lower level, in which case it will be found later.

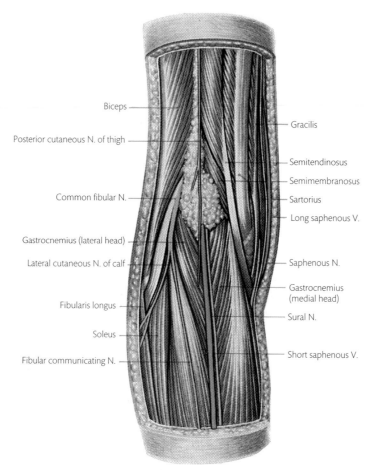

Biceps

Posterior cutaneous N. of thigh

Common fibular N.

Gastrocnemius (lateral head)

Lateral cutaneous N. of calf

Fibularis longus

Soleus

Fibular communicating N.

Gracilis

Semitendinosus

Semimembranosus

Sartorius

Long saphenous V.

Saphenous N.

Gastrocnemius (medial head)

Sural N.

Short saphenous V.

Fig. 15.1 Left popliteal region after removal of the deep fascia.

Fascia of the popliteal region

There is relatively little fat in the superficial fascia. The deep fascia, though thin, is strong and firmly bound to the tendons which form the boundaries of the popliteal fossa.

Boundaries of the popliteal fossa

The popliteal fossa is a narrow space between the diverging hamstring muscles superiorly and the converging heads of the gastrocnemius inferiorly. When dissected, the popliteal fossa is a diamond-shaped space. The fossa has four boundaries: upper lateral, upper medial, lower lateral, and lower medial. The biceps femoris forms the upper lateral boundary. The semimembranosus and semitendinosus form the upper medial boundary. The gracilis, sartorius,

and tendon of the adductor magnus lie close to the semimembranosus and semitendinosus as they approach the knee. The two lower boundaries are the two heads of the gastrocnemius. The space between the boundaries is narrow, and only a small part of the popliteal vessels just above the knee joint is not covered by muscles. The posterior wall of the fossa is the deep fascia. Its anterior wall is the popliteal surface of the femur, the capsule of the knee joint, and the fascia covering the popliteus.

Dissection 15.2 describes the dissection of the popliteal fossa.

Contents of the popliteal fossa

The popliteal fossa has the branches of the sciatic nerve and the popliteal vessels running through it. These vessels lie close to the posterior surface of the knee joint and are minimally affected by its

DISSECTION 15.2 Popliteal fossa

Objectives

I. To identify and define the muscles and tendons forming the boundaries of the popliteal fossa.   II. To identify the plantaris.   III. To identify and trace the tibial nerve, common fibular nerve, posterior cutaneous nerve of the thigh, and the popliteal artery and its branches. IV. To trace the short saphenous vein to the popliteal vein.

Instructions

1. Cut through the deep fascia along the biceps femoris. Expose the muscle and its tendon to the insertion.

2. Make a similar incision over the semitendinosus and semimembranosus. Follow the tendon of the semitendinosus to the medial surface of the tibia, then lift the semimembranosus, and follow it distally to the tibia. Find the bursa between the semimembranosus and the medial head of the gastrocnemius.

3. Find and follow the gracilis and its tendon. As you free the gracilis from the posterior surface of the sartorius, look for the saphenous nerve which emerges between them. Follow the nerve down with the long saphenous vein.

4. Follow the posterior cutaneous nerve of the thigh upwards to the upper angle of the popliteal fossa. Strip the deep fascia from the posterior surface of the popliteal fossa, and remove the fat from its upper angle to expose the tibial nerve. Follow this large nerve down.

5. Find the branches of the tibial nerve [Figs. 15.2, 15.3]. The cutaneous branch—the sural nerve—lies between the two heads of the gastrocnemius. There are three articular branches to the knee joint—superior medial, inferior medial, and middle genicular. The superior arises near the upper angle of the fossa, and the others below this. Trace them as far as possible. The muscular branches to the gastrocnemius, plantaris, soleus, and popliteus arise near the middle of the fossa. Separate the heads of the gastrocnemius, and follow these branches as far as possible.

6. Find the common fibular nerve, medial to the tendon of the biceps femoris. Trace the nerve proximally to the upper angle of the fossa and distally to the back of the head of the fibula. Find the superior lateral and inferior lateral genicular branches. They arise near the upper limit of the fossa. The superior lateral genicular leaves the fossa above the lateral femoral condyle. The inferior lateral genicular accompanies the trunk of the nerve. The fibular communicating nerve and the lateral cutaneous nerve of the calf arise near the lateral angle of the fossa. Follow these branches downwards.

7. Remove the fascia from the heads of the gastrocnemius. Identify and separate the plantaris from the posteromedial surface of the lateral head, but avoid injury to the nerve to the lateral head of the gastrocnemius which passes between them.

8. Lift the upper part of the tibial nerve from the popliteal vessels. The vein is posterolateral to the artery, with the genicular branch of the obturator nerve in the groove between them. If this nerve is found, trace it proximally and distally.

9. Remove the fascia from the popliteal vein, the popliteal artery, and the venous channels which run on it. Remove these venous channels to expose the artery, but retain the short saphenous vein.

10. Find the large muscular branches of the popliteal artery, and divide these. They pass with the nerves to the muscles. Gently scrape the fat from the popliteal surface of the femur, and find the genicular branches of the artery [Fig. 15.4]. Follow the lateral and medial superior and inferior genicular arteries and the middle genicular artery piercing the posterior capsule of the knee joint.

movements. They are the continuation of the femoral vessels which enter or leave the fossa through the tendinous opening in the adductor magnus. In the fossa, the tibial nerve runs with the vessels in the centre of the fossa. The common fibular nerve deviates laterally and runs along the medial side of the biceps femoris. The fossa also contains the popliteal lymph nodes close to the vessels. They drain the deep tissues of the leg, foot, and knee. They also receive superficial lymph vessels from the lateral side of the foot, heel, and back of the calf, and lymph vessels that run along the short saphenous vein. These lymph vessels pierce the deep fascia over the lower part of the popliteal fossa.

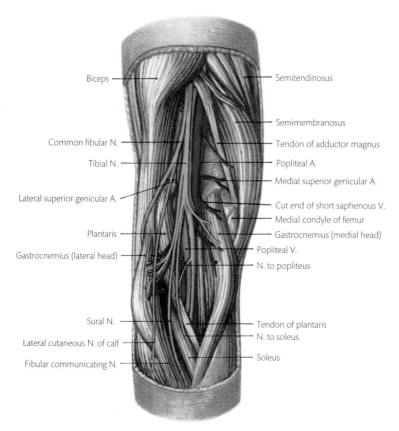

Fig. 15.2 Dissection of the left popliteal fossa. The boundaries have been pulled apart and separated.

Biceps
Semitendinosus
Semimembranosus
Common fibular N.
Tendon of adductor magnus
Tibial N.
Popliteal A.
Medial superior genicular A.
Lateral superior genicular A.
Cut end of short saphenous V.
Medial condyle of femur
Plantaris
Gastrocnemius (medial head)
Gastrocnemius (lateral head)
Popliteal V.
N. to popliteus
Sural N.
Tendon of plantaris
N. to soleus
Lateral cutaneous N. of calf
Fibular communicating N.
Soleus

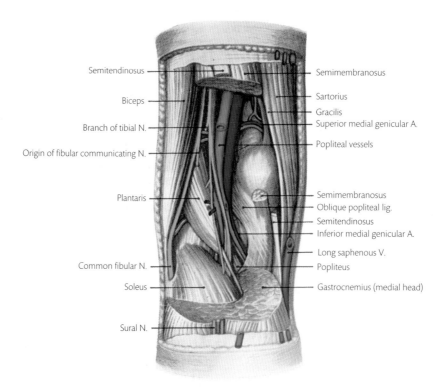

Fig. 15.3 Dissection of the left popliteal fossa. The two heads of the gastrocnemius and portions of the semimembranosus and semitendinosus have been removed.

Semitendinosus
Semimembranosus
Biceps
Sartorius
Gracilis
Superior medial genicular A.
Branch of tibial N.
Origin of fibular communicating N.
Popliteal vessels
Plantaris
Semimembranosus
Oblique popliteal lig.
Semitendinosus
Inferior medial genicular A.
Long saphenous V.
Common fibular N.
Popliteus
Soleus
Gastrocnemius (medial head)
Sural N.

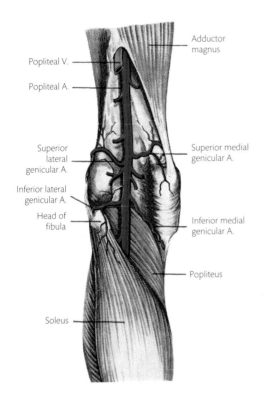

Popliteal V.

Popliteal A.

Adductor magnus

Superior lateral genicular A.

Superior medial genicular A.

Inferior lateral genicular A.

Head of fibula

Inferior medial genicular A.

Popliteus

Soleus

Fig. 15.4 Left popliteal artery and its branches.

Muscular branches arise in the distal part of the fossa and pass to the gastrocnemius, plantaris, soleus, and popliteus. The nerve to the soleus passes between the lateral head of the gastrocnemius and the plantaris to enter the superficial surface of the soleus. The nerve to the popliteus descends over the muscle and curves around its inferior border to reach its anterior surface. This nerve also supplies the **superior tibiofibular joint** and sends branches to the **interosseous membrane**.

Articular branches arise in the upper part of the fossa. They descend to join the corresponding arteries [Fig. 15.4]. The **superior medial genicular nerve** runs above the medial condyle of the femur, deep to the muscles. The **middle genicular nerve** pierces the posterior capsule of the knee joint and supplies the structures in the intercondylar notch of the femur. The **inferior medial genicular nerve** runs inferomedially on the upper border of the popliteus and forwards, deep to the superficial part of the tibial collateral ligament of the knee.

The **posterior cutaneous nerve of the thigh** passes through the fossa, immediately deep to the deep fascia. It gives branches to the overlying skin and enters the superficial fascia with the short saphenous vein.

Tibial nerve (L. 4, 5; S. 1, 2, 3)

The tibial nerve is the larger of the two terminal branches of the sciatic nerve and arises in the middle of the back of the thigh. It runs vertically through the popliteal fossa, posterior to the popliteal vessels [Fig. 15.2]. The tibial nerve supplies the muscles of the back of the leg and the sole of the foot, and the skin of the lower half of the back of the leg and the lateral side and sole of the foot.

Branches in the popliteal fossa

The **sural nerve** is a cutaneous nerve. It arises in the middle of the fossa and descends between the heads of the gastrocnemius. It pierces the deep fascia about the middle of the back of the leg, and supplies the skin on the back of the leg and along the lateral side of the dorsum of the foot up to the little toe.

Common fibular nerve (L. 4, 5; S. 1, 2)

The common fibular nerve is the smaller of the two terminal branches of the sciatic nerve [Figs. 15.2, 15.3]. It supplies the muscles on the lateral and anterior sides of the leg and the dorsum of the foot, and the skin on the lateral side of the leg and the greater part of the dorsum of the foot. The common fibular nerve runs along the medial border of the biceps femoris to the back of the head of the fibula and curves around the neck of the fibula, deep to the upper fibres of the fibularis longus muscle. At the neck of the fibula, it ends by dividing into **superficial** and **deep fibular nerves**.

Branches in the popliteal fossa

Cutaneous branches: the **fibular communicating nerve** arises in the upper part of the popliteal fossa. It joins the sural nerve at a variable level [see Fig. 14.2]. The **lateral cutaneous nerve of the calf** arises on the lateral head of the gastrocnemius. It supplies the skin on the lateral side of the upper half of the leg.

Articular branches: the **superior** and **inferior lateral genicular nerves** are small. They accompany the corresponding arteries to the knee joint [Fig. 15.4]. The **recurrent genicular nerve** also supplies the knee joint.

Genicular branch of the obturator nerve

This slender continuation of the posterior branch of the obturator nerve pierces the distal part of the adductor magnus, descends on the popliteal artery, and pierces the posterior surface of the fibrous capsule of the knee joint to supply it.

Popliteal artery

The popliteal artery begins at the tendinous opening in the adductor magnus and is the continuation of the femoral artery. It ends at the lower border of the popliteal artery by dividing into **anterior** and **posterior** tibial arteries. The artery lies on the anterior wall of the popliteal fossa. From above downwards, it is anterior to the semimembranosus, popliteal vein, tibial nerve, gastrocnemius, and plantaris [Figs. 15.2, 15.3, 15.4].

Branches

Muscular branches pass to the lower parts of the hamstring muscles and to the upper parts of the muscles of the calf. These are large and give rise to cutaneous branches, one of which accompanies the sural nerve. The hamstring branches anastomose superiorly with the perforating branches of the profunda femoris artery.

The **superior**, **inferior**, and **middle genicular arteries** lie on the anterior wall of the popliteal fossa [Fig. 15.4]. The popliteal artery is the only significant route through which blood can reach the leg and foot from the thigh. It may be compressed when sitting on a hard edged seat or with the legs crossed. ➲ When obliterative arterial disease affects the popliteal artery, blood supply to the large muscles of the leg is seriously compromised. This results in ischaemic pain in muscles on exercise, which is relieved by rest—a condition known as intermittent claudication.

Popliteal vein

The popliteal vein is formed by the union of the anterior and posterior tibial veins at the lower border of the popliteus. The vein ascends on the posterior surface of the popliteal artery. The tributaries of the popliteal vein correspond to the branches of the artery. It also receives the short saphenous vein. Open the popliteal vein, and note its numerous **valves**. Fig. 15.5 is a cross-section through the lower part of the thigh, showing the upper boundaries and contents of the popliteal fossa.

Clinical Applications 15.1 and 15.2 demonstrate the practical implications of the anatomy described in this chapter.

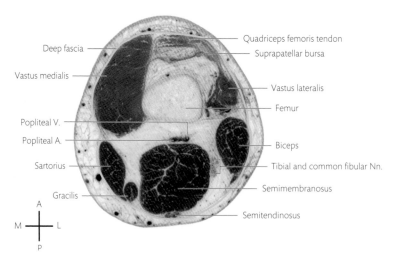

Fig. 15.5 Transverse section through the proximal part of the popliteal region of the thigh. A = anterior; P = posterior; M = medial; L = lateral.

Image courtesy of the Visible Human Project of the US National Library of Medicine.

CLINICAL APPLICATION 15.1 Closed supracondylar femoral fracture

A 25-year-old man suffered a closed supracondylar fracture of the femur. Because the popliteal artery is closely applied to the popliteal surface of the femur and the joint capsule, fractures of the distal femur may rupture the artery, resulting in haemorrhage. A computed tomography angiography was done to rule out damage to the popliteal artery and its branches [Fig. 15.6].

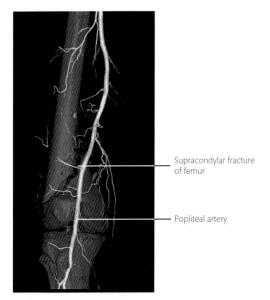

Supracondylar fracture of femur

Popliteal artery

Fig. 15.6 Computed tomography angiogram of the popliteal artery showing the undamaged artery close to the fracture.

CLINICAL APPLICATION 15.2 Popliteal pulse and popliteal aneurysm

The rhythmical throbbing of arteries produced by the regular contractions of the heart can be felt at a number of peripheral locations. The popliteal pulse is palpable in the popliteal fossa by pressing the artery against the anterior surface of the fossa. It is especially important, as a strong popliteal pulse is an indicator of good blood flow to the distal parts of the lower limb. Because the popliteal artery is deep, it may be difficult to feel the pulsations. Palpation is commonly performed with the person in the prone position, with the knee flexed to relax the popliteal fascia and hamstrings.

A popliteal aneurysm is an abnormal thinning of the wall of the popliteal artery and dilatation of the vessel. It presents as a pulsatile swelling and should be differentiated from a popliteal cyst or a Baker's cyst. A popliteal cyst is an outpouching of the synovial membrane from the bursa between the medial head of the gastrocnemius and the semimembranosus tendon.

CHAPTER 16
The back of the thigh

Introduction

This chapter begins with Dissection 16.1.

Posterior cutaneous nerve of the thigh (S. 1, 2, 3)

The posterior cutaneous nerve leaves the pelvis through the lower part of the greater sciatic foramen, close to the inferior gluteal vessels and nerve. In the gluteal region, it is deep to the gluteus maximus and lies on the sciatic nerve. It then runs down the middle of the back of the thigh, immediately deep to the deep fascia, and is separated from the sciatic nerve by the long head of the biceps. It pierces the deep fascia at the back of the knee and supplies the skin as far as the middle of the back of the calf [see Fig. 14.2].

Branches

All branches are cutaneous: (a) in the gluteal region—it gives (1) the gluteal branches which curve around the lower border of the gluteus maximus and supply a small area of skin in the lower part of the buttock; and (2) a perineal branch which turns medially across the back of the hamstring muscles to the perineum. The perineal branch supplies the skin on the upper medial side of the thigh and the

---

DISSECTION 16.1 Back of the thigh-1

Objectives

I. To reflect the skin and deep fascia on the back of the thigh. II. To expose the sciatic nerve and trace its branches. III. To identify and study the semimembranosus, semitendinosus, and biceps femoris.

Instructions

1. Make a vertical incision through the skin remaining on the back of the thigh. Strip the skin and superficial fascia from the deep fascia by blunt dissection. Look for the branches of the posterior cutaneous nerve of the thigh as you do so.

2. Find and follow the branches of the medial anterior and lateral cutaneous nerves of the thigh into this region [see Fig. 14.2].

3. Divide the deep fascia vertically. Find the posterior cutaneous nerve of the thigh, and trace it to the gluteal region.

4. Remove the fascia from the posterior surfaces of the hamstring muscles.

5. Follow the sciatic nerve down from the gluteal region. Trace its branches into the hamstring muscles, including the short head of the biceps and adductor magnus. Find the branches of the perforating arteries which run with the nerves.

6. Separate the hamstring muscles from each other, and trace them to their attachments.

external genital organs; (b) in the thigh and leg: numerous small branches to the medial side and back of the thigh, and the upper half of the posterior surface of the leg [see Fig. 14.2].

Flexor muscles

These muscles form a mass on the back of the thigh and have their tendons in the back of the knee. The tendons of these muscles in the popliteal region, or back of the thigh, give them the name **hamstrings** (ham = Old English word for the depression behind the knee). The muscles—semitendinosus, semimembranosus, and long head of the biceps femoris—arise from the ischial tuberosity and are inserted into the bones of the leg. They extend the hip and flex the knee.

Biceps femoris

This muscle has two heads. The **long head** arises with the semitendinosus from the medial part of the ischial tuberosity [see Fig. 14.3]. It is partly continuous with the sacrotuberous ligament. The **short head** arises from the linea aspera and the upper half of the lateral supracondylar line. The two heads unite and are inserted into the head of the fibula [see Figs. 15.1, 18.13]. Near its insertion, the tendon of the biceps overlies the **fibular collateral ligament** of the knee joint. This ligament passes obliquely through the tendon, dividing it into two unequal parts. **Nerve supply**: the long head is supplied by the tibial part of the sciatic nerve, and the short head by the common fibular part. Thus, each head may be separately paralysed as a result of a wound. **Actions**: it extends the hip joint, flexes the knee joint, and rotates the leg laterally when the knee is flexed. The short head acts only on the knee joint.

Semitendinosus

The semitendinosus originates with the long head of the biceps from the medial part of the ischial tuberosity [see Fig. 14.3]. In the distal third of the thigh, the muscle forms a cylindrical tendon. On the medial side of the knee, the tendon turns forwards and spreads out to be inserted into the upper part of the medial surface of the tibia, posterior to the tendons of the gracilis and sartorius. A complex **bursa** separates these tendons from one another and communicates with a

bursa between the semitendinosus and the tibial collateral ligament of the knee. **Nerve supply**: branches from the tibial part of the sciatic nerve. **Actions**: it extends the hip joint, flexes the knee, and medially rotates the leg when the knee is flexed.

Semimembranosus

The semimembranosus arises from the lateral part of the ischial tuberosity [see Fig. 14.3]. The broad tendon of origin passes down and medially deep to the biceps and semitendinosus. At the back of the knee, it forms a thick, flattened tendon which is inserted chiefly into the groove on the posteromedial surface of the medial condyle of the tibia [see Fig. 18.20]. The tendon also has extensions which form: (1) the **oblique popliteal ligament** of the knee joint; and (2) the **fascia covering the popliteus**, through which it is inserted into the soleal line of the tibia. The semimembranosus bursa lies between the tendon and the medial head of the gastrocnemius. It is often continuous with the bursa between that head and the back of the knee joint. **Nerve supply**: tibial part of the sciatic nerve. **Actions**: like the semitendinosus, the semimembranosus extends the hip, flexes the knee, and medially rotates the leg when the knee is flexed.

Sciatic nerve (L. 4, 5; S. 1, 2, 3)

The sciatic nerve leaves the pelvis through the greater sciatic foramen. It descends through the inferomedial part of the gluteal region between the gluteus maximus posteriorly and the ischium, obturator internus and gemelli, and quadratus femoris anteriorly. In the back of the thigh, the nerve lies deep to the long head of the biceps on the posterior surface of the adductor magnus. It ends by dividing into the tibial and common fibular nerves midway down the thigh.

Branches

Branches from the trunk of the nerve (tibial part) supply the **ischial** (hamstring) **part of the adductor magnus** and the **hamstrings**, except the short head of the biceps femoris which is supplied by the common fibular nerve.

Dissection 16.2 continues to look at the back of the thigh.

Objectives

I. To expose the adductor magnus and adductor longus.
II. To identify and trace the profunda femoris artery and vein. III. To identify and trace the perforating arteries.

Instructions

1. Detach the hamstring muscles from the ischial tuberosity, and turn them aside. This exposes the posterior surface of the adductor magnus.

2. Remove the fascia from this muscle, but preserve the branch of the sciatic nerve which enters it near its medial border.

3. Explore the insertion of the adductor magnus and the perforating arteries which pass between the muscle and the femur. Trace the perforating arteries laterally into the vastus lateralis.

4. From the front, identify the adductor longus, and follow it to its insertion into the linea aspera.

5. Turn the muscle forwards, and follow the profunda vessels which pass downwards behind it. They lie close to the femur.

6. Remove the fascia from the profunda vein, which is anterior to the artery, then cut its tributaries to expose the artery and its branches.

7. Divide the muscular branches of the profunda femoris artery, but preserve the perforating arteries which lie close to the femur. Demonstrate their continuity with the vessels found on the posterior surface of the adductor magnus.

Profunda femoris artery

This is the chief artery to the muscles of the thigh. It arises from the lateral side of the femoral artery in the femoral triangle and curves medially behind the femoral vessels, giving off the lateral and medial circumflex femoral arteries. It then passes posteriorly between the pectineus and adductor longus, and descends close to the femur, posterior to the adductor longus. Here it gives off the first three perforating arteries. A little below the middle of the thigh, the profunda femoris continues as the fourth perforating artery [Fig. 16.1].

Branches

The medial and lateral circumflex femoral arteries have been seen already. The muscular branches of the profunda supply the adductor muscles. The four perforating arteries arise in series from the profunda femoris [Fig. 16.1]. They wind round the back of the femur to the vastus lateralis [see Fig. 13.22]. They give branches to the adductor and hamstring muscles, and the second or third forms the nutrient artery to the femur.

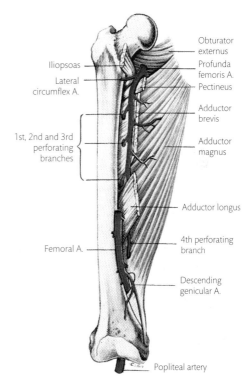

Fig. 16.1 Profunda femoris artery and its branches. The upper part of the adductor longus has been removed to expose the artery.

Arterial anastomoses

There is a longitudinal anastomosis between branches of the internal iliac, femoral, and popliteal arteries in the back of the thigh. From above down, this anastomosis is formed by communication between the inferior gluteal artery, terminal branches of the circumflex femoral arteries, perforating arteries, arteries on the hamstring muscles, and branches of the popliteal artery. An alternative supply to the distal part of the limb is established by this route.

Clinical Application 16.1 looks at the condition sciatic neuritis.

CLINICAL APPLICATION 16.1 Sciatic neuritis

A 45-year-old woman consulted her neurologist for low back pain which radiated to the hip and back of the thigh. The neurologist investigated her complaints and diagnosed her to have a 'lumbar radiculopathy' leading to 'sciatic neuritis'.

Study question 1: which lumbar nerves contribute to the formation of the sciatic nerve? (Answer: L. 4 and L. 5.)

Study question 2: using your knowledge of the parts of the typical spinal nerve, deduce which part/parts are involved in a 'radiculopathy'. (Answer: the root of the nerves. *Radicle* = roots.)

Using Fig. 13.11, review the proximity of the intervertebral discs to the spinal nerve roots. The sciatic neuritis seen in this patient could well be the result of a spinal disc herniation pressing on one of the lumbar roots of the sciatic nerve.

The doctor tests to see if the pain is worse on stretching the sciatic nerve. Study question 3: what movement of the hip would stretch the sciatic nerve? (Answer: flexion of the hip.) This forms the basis for the 'straight leg raising' test. The patient lies supine, and the doctor lifts the patient's leg while the knee is straight. The patient experiences sciatic pain when the leg is raised to 30 to 40 degrees.

CHAPTER 17
The hip joint

Introduction

The hip joint is a good example of a ball-and-socket joint, in which the head of the femur articulates with the acetabulum of the hip bone. Compared to the shoulder joint, the range of movement is less, but strength and stability are much greater. The strength and stability is due to: (1) the greater depth of the **acetabulum** which is further increased by the **acetabular labrum**; and (2) the strength of the ligaments and surrounding muscles. The reduced range of movements is offset, to some extent, by the long, narrow **neck of the femur**.

Articular capsule and extracapsular ligaments

Articular capsule

The fibrous capsule surrounds the joint on all sides. It is strong anteriorly, and thin posteriorly. Proximally, it is attached to the margin of the acetabulum and to the transverse ligament of the acetabulum. Distally, it is attached anteriorly to the intertrochanteric line of the femur and to the root of the greater trochanter. Posteriorly, it is attached to the neck of the femur, about 1.5 cm medial to the intertrochanteric crest.

The fibres which comprise the capsule run in two different directions. The majority run obliquely downwards and laterally from the acetabulum to the femur. The oblique fibres are best seen on the anterior surface. Other bundles encircle the capsule approximately parallel to the margin of the acetabulum. These circular bundles form the **zona orbicularis** and are best seen on the posterior and inferior parts of the fibrous capsule. The fibrous membrane has three thickenings that form ligaments on the capsule—the iliofemoral, pubofemoral, and ischiofemoral ligaments.

Iliofemoral ligament

This ligament lies on the front of the joint. It forms the thickest and most powerful part of the articular capsule. Proximally, it is attached to the inferior part of the anterior inferior iliac spine and to the surface of the ilium, immediately lateral to the spine. Distally, it widens to be attached to the intertrochanteric line of the femur. It is thicker at the sides than in the middle and has the appearance of an inverted Y [Fig. 17.1].

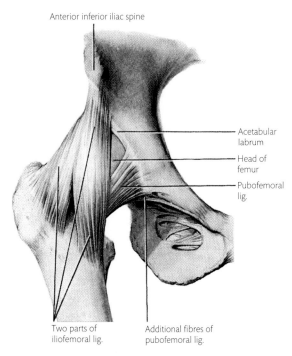

Anterior inferior iliac spine

Acetabular labrum

Head of femur

Pubofemoral lig.

Two parts of iliofemoral lig.

Additional fibres of pubofemoral lig.

Fig. 17.1 Dissection of the hip joint from the front.

The iliofemoral ligament is more than 0.5 cm thick. It is one of the strongest ligaments in the body—its only rival being the interosseous sacroiliac ligament. It is rarely torn. ◑ In hip dislocation, the surgeon may use the iliofemoral ligament as a support to lever the head of the femur back into the acetabulum.

In the erect posture, the centre of gravity of the body falls slightly behind a line joining the centres of the two hip joints. As such, there is a natural tendency for the body to fall backwards on the hip joints. This is resisted by the iliofemoral ligaments, which maintain the erect posture without muscular activity at these joints. Dissection 17.1 exposes this ligament.

Pubofemoral ligament

This ligament arises from the pubic bone and the obturator membrane [Fig. 17.1]. It lies in the lower and anterior parts of the fibrous capsule.

Ischiofemoral ligament

This is a weak band which arises from the ischium below the acetabulum. It passes upwards and laterally into the fibrous capsule.

Intracapsular structures

Transverse ligament of the acetabulum

This strong band of fibres bridges across the acetabular notch. It completes the rim of the acetabulum and converts the notch into a foramen, through which vessels and nerves enter the acetabular fossa. It gives attachment to the ligament of the head of the femur.

Acetabular labrum

This fibrocartilaginous ring is attached to the rim of the acetabulum and the transverse ligament. It deepens the cavity of the acetabulum and narrows its mouth by sloping inwards. The labrum is a tight fit on the head of the femur and plays an important function in maintaining the head of the femur in the acetabulum. Both surfaces of the labrum are covered by synovial membrane. The free margin is relatively thin, and the attached margin is much thicker.

Ligament of the head of the femur

The ligament of the head of the femur extends from the transverse ligament of the acetabulum to the pit on the head of the femur [Fig. 17.2]. Its narrow, cylindrical end is implanted into the **pit on the head of the femur**, and its broad, flattened end is attached to the transverse ligament of the acetabulum and the adjacent margins of the acetabular fossa. It is a weak band of connective tissue surrounded by a synovial membrane. The ligament is too weak to play a part in strengthening the hip joint. Sometimes it transmits a small blood vessel to the head of the femur.

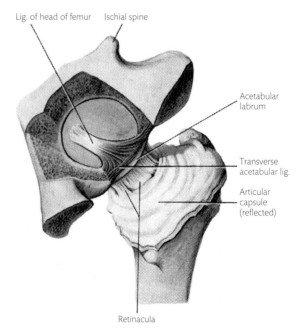

Fig. 17.2 Dissection of the right hip joint from the pelvic side. The floor of the acetabulum has been removed, and the articular capsule of the joint drawn laterally towards the trochanters.

Synovial membrane and retinacula

The synovial membrane lines the inner surface of the fibrous capsule and covers the neck of the femur as far as the margin of the articular cartilage of the head. From the attachment of the fibrous capsule to the femur, a number of fibre bundles turn back on the neck of the femur. These are called **retinacula**. Small arteries and veins pass along the retinacula to supply the neck and head of the femur (note the multiple foramina in the bone, especially on the posterosuperior surface of the neck). ⊃ When the neck of the femur is fractured within the capsule, the retinacula help to hold the fragments together. If the retinacula are torn when the neck is fractured, the blood supply of the head of the femur may be destroyed and affect repair of the fracture.

At the acetabular attachment of the articular capsule, the synovial membrane is reflected on to the acetabular labrum, the transverse ligament, and the ligament of the head of the femur.

A mass of fat occupies the non-articular fossa of the acetabulum. It is covered by the synovial membrane which extends from the inner margin of the lunate surface of the acetabulum and is reflected on to the ligament of the head of the femur at the acetabular notch. Acetabular branches from the obturator and medial circumflex femoral arteries, and obturator nerve enter the ligament through the acetabular notch.

Blood vessels and nerves

The hip joint is supplied by arterial anastomosis formed around the neck of the femur between the following pairs of vessels: (1) ascending branches of the medial and lateral circumflex femoral arteries; (2) acetabular branches of the obturator and medial circumflex femoral arteries; and (3) branches of the superior and inferior gluteal arteries. Arteries which run in the ligament of the head of the femur sometimes enter the head of the femur, but they do not form a significant part of its blood supply.

Nerves enter the joint from: (1) the nerve to the quadratus femoris; (2) the femoral nerve through the nerve to the rectus femoris; and (3) the anterior division of the obturator nerve, and occasionally the accessory obturator nerve.

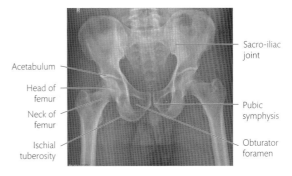

Fig. 17.3 Anteroposterior radiograph of the adult pelvis.

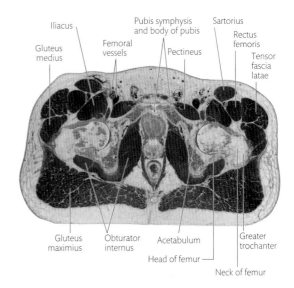

Fig. 17.4 Section through the pubic symphysis and the two hip joints.

Image courtesy of the Visible Human Project of the US National Library of Medicine.

Identify the hip joint and the important bony landmarks on the radiograph of the pelvis [Fig. 17.3]. The important muscles surrounding the hip joint and acting on it are seen in sectional images [Figs. 17.4, 17.5].

Movements of the hip joint

The movements possible at the hip joint are **flexion**, **extension**, **abduction**, **adduction**, and **medial** and **lateral rotation**. Test the range of movements of your own joint. **Flexion** is very free, and limited only when the thigh comes into contact with the anterior abdominal wall. **Extension** from the anatomical position is restricted by the iliofemoral ligament. Extending the limb posteriorly to the horizontal plane is only possible

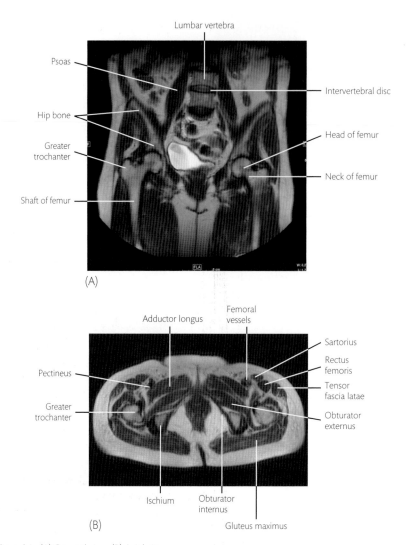

Fig. 17.5 MRI of the pelvis. (A) Coronal view. (B) Axial view.

by tilting the pelvis forwards on the opposite limb. **Abduction** is restricted by the pubofemoral ligament. **Adduction** (as in crossing one thigh over the other) is limited by the lateral part of the iliofemoral ligament and the upper part of the fibrous capsule. **Medial rotation** tightens the ischiofemoral ligament and is limited by it. **Lateral rotation** is limited by the pubofemoral ligament and the lateral parts of the iliofemoral ligament.

Movements of the hip joint are brought about by muscles which cross the joint. Table 17.1 lists the muscles which act on the hip joint, together with the origin, insertion, relation to the hip joint, nerve supply, and action of each muscle. In Table 17.2, the muscles are grouped according to the actions which they produce on the hip joint, and the nerve supply of each muscle is repeated. This allows for easy assessment of the degree of

impairment of a particular movement following destruction of a particular nerve.

In movements of the hip, as in all movements in the joints of the lower limb, it should be remembered that, when the foot is on the ground, the muscles of that limb are being used in a reversed manner, i.e. the trunk and proximal parts of the limb are moving while the distal part is stationary.

➲ From this table, it is obvious that medial rotation and abduction are seriously disturbed by injuries to the superior gluteal nerve. Adduction is severely impaired when the obturator nerve is damaged. Extension is most usually produced by the hamstrings, the gluteus maximus being used mainly when extra power is required or in extremes of extension when the hamstrings may be actively insufficient to produce the movement.

See Clinical Application 17.1 for a practical application of the anatomy discussed in this chapter.

Table 17.1 Muscles acting on the hip joint

Muscle	Origin	Insertion	Relation to hip joint	Action	Nerve supply
Adductor longus	Pubis, body	Femur, linea aspera	Medial	Adduction	Obturator nerve
Adductor brevis	Pubis, body and inferior ramus	Femur, linea aspera	Medial	Adduction	Obturator nerve
Adductor magnus	Pubis, inferior ramus Ischium, ramus and tuberosity	Femur, linea aspera, medial supracondylar line, adductor tubercle	Medial and posterior	Adduction, extension (medial rotation)	Obturator nerve
Psoas major	Lumbar vertebrae	Femur, lesser	Anterior	Flexion (medial rotation)	Lumbar plexus
Iliacus	Iliac fossa	Femur, line inferior to lesser trochanter	Anterior	Flexion	Lumbar plexus
Pectineus	Pubis, body and superior ramus	Femur, back of lesser trochanter to linea aspera	Anterior and medial	Adduction, flexion	Femoral nerve
Gluteus minimus	Ilium between anterior and inferior gluteal lines	Femur, greater trochanter, anterior surface	Lateral and anterolateral	Abduction, medial rotation, fixes pelvis on thigh*	Superior gluteal nerve
Gluteus medius	Ilium between anterior and posterior gluteal lines	Femur, greater trochanter, lateral surface	Lateral and anterolateral	Abduction, medial rotation, fixes pelvis on thigh*	Superior gluteal nerve
Gluteus maximus, deep one-fourth	Sacrum, posterior surface, sacrotuberous lig.	Femur, gluteal tuberosity	Posterior	Extension, lateral rotation	Inferior gluteal nerve
Gluteus maximus, superficial three-fourths	Ilium posterior to posterior gluteal line. Sacrum posterior aspect. Sacrotuberous ligament	Tibia lateral condyle, via iliotibial tract	Posterior	Extension, lateral rotation	Inferior gluteal nerve
Piriformis	Sacrum pelvic surface, middle three pieces	Femur, greater trochanter	Posterior and lateral	Abduction, lateral rotation	Sacral nerves
Obturator externus	Hip bone, obturator membrane external surface, margin of obturator foramen	Femur, trochanteric fossa	Inferior	Lateral rotation (flexion)	Obturator nerve
Obturator internus	Internal surfaces of ilium, pubis, and ischium and obturator membrane	Femur, greater trochanter, medial surface	Inferior	Lateral rotation	Nerve to obturator internus

(Continued)

Movements of the hip joint

Table 17.1 Muscles acting on the hip joint (*Continued*)

Muscle	Origin	Insertion	Relation to hip joint	Action	Nerve supply
Gemelli	Ischium, each side of lesser sciatic notch	With obturator internus	Posterior	Lateral rotation	Nerve to obturator internus Nerve to quadratus femoris
Biceps femoris long head	Ischial tuberosity	Head of fibula	Posterior	Extension	Tibial branch of sciatic nerve
Semimembranosus	Ischial tuberosity	Tibia, medial condyle, posteromedial surface	Posterior	Extension	Tibial branch of sciatic nerve
Semitendinosus	Ischial tuberosity	Tibia, medial surface, upper one-fourth	Posterior	Extension	Tibial branch of sciatic nerve
Gracilis	Pubis body and inferior ramus	Tibia, medial surface, upper one-fourth	Posterior and medial	Adduction	Obturator nerve
Sartorius	Ilium anterior superior iliac spine	Tibia, medial surface, upper one-fourth	Anterior	Flexion, lateral rotation	Femoral nerve
Tensor fasciae latae	Iliac crest anterior one-fourth	Tibia lateral condyle, via iliotibial tract	Anterior	Flexion, abduction. Stabilizes pelvis on thigh	Superior gluteal nerve
Rectus femoris	Ilium anterior inferior iliac spine and area above acetabulum	Patella through quadriceps tendon	Anterior	Flexion	Femoral nerve

*This action prevents the pelvis from sagging towards the opposite side when the opposite lower limb is raised from the ground.

Table 17.2 Movements at the hip joint

Movement	Muscles	Nerve supply
Flexion	Iliacus and psoas major	Lumbar ventral rami
	Rectus femoris	Femoral
	Sartorius	Femoral
	Tensor fasciae latae	Superior gluteal
	Pectineus	Femoral
	Adductors longus and brevis	Obturator
Extension	Gluteus maximus	Inferior gluteal
	Semimembranosus	Sciatic (tibial part)
	Semitendinosus	Sciatic (tibial part)
	Biceps femoris, long head	Sciatic (tibial part)
	Adductor magnus, ischial part	Sciatic (tibial part)
Adduction	Adductors longus, brevis, and magnus	Obturator
	Gracilis	Obturator
	Pectineus	Femoral
	Quadratus femoris	L. 4, 5 and S. 1 ventral rami
Abduction	Gluteus medius and minimus	Superior gluteal
	Tensor fasciae latae	Superior gluteal
	Piriformis, in flexion	L. 5, S. 1 and 2 ventral rami
	Obturator internus in flexion	L. 5, S. 1 and 2 ventral rami
Medial rotation	Tensor fasciae latae	Superior gluteal
	Gluteus minimus	Superior gluteal
	Gluteus medius, anterior fibres	Superior gluteal
	Adductors	Obturator
	Iliopsoas	L. 1, 2 ventral rami
Lateral rotation	Sartorius	Femoral
	Gluteus maximus	Inferior gluteal
	Obturator internus and gemelli	L. 5, S. 1 and 2 ventral rami
	Obturator externus	Obturator
	Quadratus femoris	L. 4 and 5, S. 1 ventral rami
	Piriformis, in extension	L. 5, S. 1 and 2 ventral rami

CLINICAL APPLICATION 17.1 Fractured neck of femur with partial hip replacement

A 72-year-old man slipped and fell in the bathroom. He had severe pain in his left hip and was unable to stand up. On examination, his left leg was laterally rotated, and he was unable to lift his left heel off the bed. The greater trochanter on the left side appeared to be higher than on the right. On palpation, there was tenderness in the femoral triangle in front of the hip joint. A diagnosis of fractured neck of femur was made. An X-ray confirmed the diagnosis and showed a fracture just below the head of the femur [Fig. 17.6A].

Study question 1: what are the attachments of the fibrous capsule? Are all neck fractures intracapsular? (Answer: the fibrous capsule is attached to the margin of the acetabulum. On the femur, it is attached anteriorly to the intertrochanteric line, and posteriorly 1 cm medial to the intertrochanteric crest. Fractures of the lateral most part of the neck are extracapsular.)

One cause for concern in a fractured neck of femur is the possibility of inadequate blood supply. Study question 2: what is the most important blood vessel supplying the head and neck of femur? (Answer: the most important source of blood supply to the femoral head and neck is the medial circumflex femoral artery. Vessels which arise from it pierce the capsule and run medially on the posterior and superior aspects of the neck.)

The patient was operated upon, with removal of the femoral head and replacement with an artificial prosthesis. He had an uneventful recovery. An X-ray after hip replacement is shown in Fig. 17.6B.

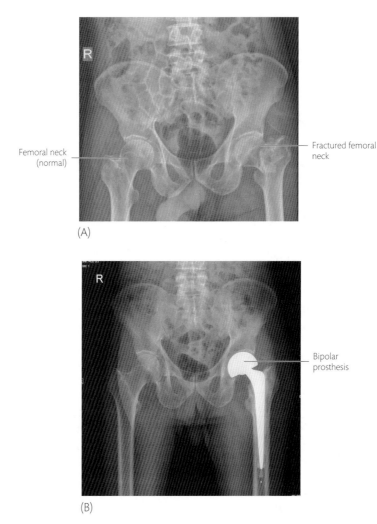

(A)

(B)

Fig. 17.6 (A) Plain X-ray of the hip showing fracture of the neck of femur. (B) Hip X-ray after hemiarthroplasty (different patient).

CHAPTER 18
The leg and foot

Introduction

Bones and surface anatomy of the leg

The leg bones are the tibia medially and the fibula laterally [Figs. 18.1, 18.2]. Make use of a set of leg bones to confirm the following points, and identify the palpable parts in your own leg. The shaft of the **tibia** is roughly triangular in transverse section, with medial, posterior, and lateral surfaces. The medial surface is subcutaneous, except in its upper quarter where the tendons of the sartorius, gracilis, and semitendinosus are inserted into it. The superficial part of the tibial collateral ligament of the knee is attached to the upper part of the tibia immediately in front of the medial border. Inferiorly, the medial surface is continuous with the medial surface of the medial malleolus—a thick downwards projection of the distal end of the tibia.

The expanded upper end of the tibia is flattened to form the medial and lateral **condyles**. The condyles are limited inferiorly by an almost horizontal line. Anteriorly, this line curves down to the junction of the smooth and rough parts of the **tibial tuberosity**. The patellar tendon is attached to the smooth part of the tibial tuberosity. Inferiorly, the tibial tuberosity is continuous with the sharp **anterior border of the tibia** [Fig. 18.1]. This border is palpable throughout its length, though it becomes less sharp in the lower third of the bone, and deviates medially to the anterior surface of the medial malleolus. The posteromedial surface of the medial condyle has a long, horizontal groove, with a roughened area below it for the attachment of the semimembranosus [see Fig. 18.20]. In a similar,

but slightly lower, position, the inferior surface of the lateral condyle has a smooth area for articulation with the **head of the fibula**. The upper surfaces of the medial and lateral tibial condyles have smooth, oval, concave areas for articulation with the corresponding condyles of the femur. Between these condyles is the **intercondylar area** which is divided into anterior and posterior parts by an **intercondylar eminence**. On the intercondylar eminence are the medial and lateral **intercondylar tubercles**.

The interosseous border of the tibia begins immediately inferior to the articular area for the fibula. The interosseous membrane between the tibia and fibula is attached to this border. At the distal end of the tibia, the interosseous border becomes continuous with a rough, triangular, concave area for the thickened part of the interosseous membrane—the interosseous tibiofibular ligament. The interosseous tibiofibular ligament binds the tibia to the fibula above the ankle joint. The interosseous border separates the lateral surface of the shaft of the tibia from the posterior surface, and hence the areas from which the anterior (extensor) muscles and posterior (flexor) muscles of the leg arise. On the posterior surface of the tibia, an oblique ridge—the **soleal line** [Fig. 18.2]—passes from just below the articular surface for the head of the fibula to the medial border of the tibia, at the junction of the upper and middle thirds of the shaft. This line gives attachment to the tibial head of the soleus muscle and to the popliteal fascia on the posterior surface of the **popliteus muscle**. The popliteus is attached on the tibia to the triangular area, proximal to the soleal line. The nutrient artery to the shaft of the tibia enters the bone

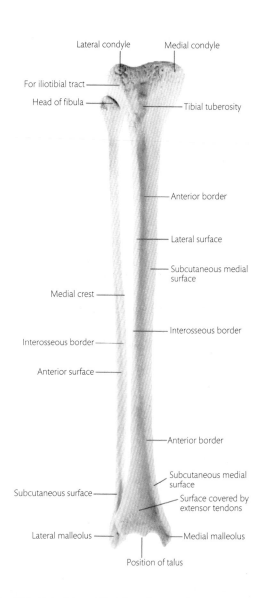

Lateral condyle
Medial condyle
For iliotibial tract
Head of fibula
Tibial tuberosity
Anterior border
Lateral surface
Subcutaneous medial surface
Medial crest
Interosseous border
Interosseous border
Anterior surface
Anterior border
Subcutaneous medial surface
Subcutaneous surface
Surface covered by extensor tendons
Lateral malleolus
Medial malleolus
Position of talus

Fig. 18.1 Right tibia and fibula (anterior aspect).

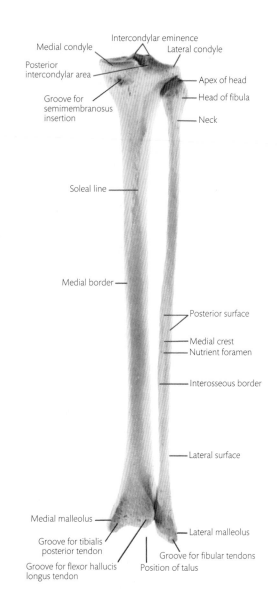

Intercondylar eminence
Medial condyle
Lateral condyle
Posterior intercondylar area
Apex of head
Head of fibula
Groove for semimembranosus insertion
Neck
Soleal line
Medial border
Posterior surface
Medial crest
Nutrient foramen
Interosseous border
Lateral surface
Medial malleolus
Lateral malleolus
Groove for tibialis posterior tendon
Groove for fibular tendons
Groove for flexor hallucis longus tendon
Position of talus

Fig. 18.2 Right tibia and fibula (posterior aspect).

midway between the distal part of the soleal line and the interosseous border. Medial to the nutrient foramen is a **vertical ridge** which joins the middle of the soleal line to the interosseous border distally. The area between the soleal line, interosseous border, and vertical ridge gives attachment to the **tibialis posterior** [see Fig. 18.20].

The **medial border** of the tibia is sharp and continues distally with the medial edge of a groove for the tendon of the tibialis posterior, on the posterior surface of the medial malleolus [Fig. 18.2].

The **inferior surface** on the distal end of the tibia is concave anteroposteriorly, with a slight, central anteroposterior ridge. It is an articular

surface and is continuous medially with the articular surface on the lateral aspect of the medial malleolus. Both surfaces articulate with the body of the talus at the ankle joint.

The **medial malleolus** projects inferiorly as the apex and has a smooth notch on its posterior aspect. The notch and apex give attachment to the powerful **medial** (deltoid) **ligament of the ankle joint**.

The **fibula** has an expanded head at its proximal end, and a narrow **neck** below the head. On the superomedial surface of the head is the area for articulation with the tibia, and the **apex of the head** lateral to it. The distal end of the fibula is expanded to form the **lateral malleolus**. The lateral malleolus projects beyond the medial malleolus and has a larger triangular surface on its medial aspect for articulation with the body of the talus. The tibial and fibular malleoli hold the body of the talus between them. Posterior to the articular area on the lateral malleolus is the **malleollar fossa**. The **shaft** of the fibula is covered with muscles, and its shape varies considerably with the degree of muscularity.

The anterolateral surface of the lateral malleolus is continuous above with a rough, triangular **subcutaneous area**. This is continuous superiorly with the **anterior border** of the fibula which marks the attachment of an intermuscular septa separating the muscles of the anterior compartment of the leg (extensors) from those of the lateral compartment (fibular muscles). Superior to the articular surface of the lateral malleolus is a rough triangular area for attachment of the **interosseous tibiofibular ligament**. This triangular area is continuous above with the **interosseous border** of the fibula. This border bends forwards as it ascends, so that it comes close to the anterior border. A narrow **medial surface** between the anterior and interosseous borders gives attachment to the extensor muscles. Posterior to the interosseous border is the **posterior surface** of the fibula. This posterior surface has a curved vertical ridge—the **medial crest**—which separates it into medial and posterior parts. The strong intermuscular septum posterior to the tibialis posterior muscle is attached to the medial crest. Behind the medial crest, the posterior surface gives rise to the soleus and flexor hallucis longus [see Fig. 18.20].

The fibular muscles arise from the lateral surface of the fibula. Inferiorly, they pass behind the subcutaneous triangular area to run over the posterior surface of the lateral malleolus.

On your own leg, identify the head of the fibula, and the condyles and tuberosity of the tibia. Feel the anterior and medial borders of the tibia and the subcutaneous medial surface between them. Follow this surface to the **medial malleolus**. The **long saphenous vein** and the **saphenous nerve** run along the upper two-thirds of the medial border of the tibia.

Find the **neck of the fibula**, and roll the common fibular nerve on its posterolateral surface. Trace the fibula downwards, feeling it through the muscles. Press on the middle of the bone, and note that it can be pushed inwards to a slight extent, like a firm spring. Find the **lateral malleolus**, and confirm that it projects further distally than the medial malleolus.

On the back of your leg, feel the fleshy mass of the **gastrocnemius** and **soleus**. These two muscles can be made to contract by standing on your toes. When this is done, the two heads of the superficial gastrocnemius stand out. Deep to the gastrocnemius, the soleus bulges laterally, medially, and inferiorly. Trace these muscles to the **tendo calcaneus**—the thick tendon through which they are inserted into the tip of the heel. Note that the tendo calcaneus lies more than 2 cm posterior to the bones of the leg. Place your fingers in the depressions anterior to the tendo calcaneus, and press forwards. The malleoli are felt indistinctly through the tendons which cover their posterior surfaces. On the back of the medial malleolus, feel the pulsations of the **posterior tibial artery**.

Bones and surface anatomy of the foot

The general arrangement of the bones of the foot is described below and shown in Figs. 18.3 and 18.4. Make use of a set of foot bones to confirm the following points, and identify the palpable parts in your own foot.

The **talus** consists of a cuboidal **body**, with a **neck** and **head** projecting forwards and slightly medially from it. The **trochlea tali** is the articular surface on the superior aspect of the body. Posterior to the trochlea, the lower part of the talus projects backwards as the **posterior process**. This process is grooved by the tendon of the flexor hallucis longus, resulting in the formation of the lateral and medial **tubercles of the posterior process**. (The posterior process ossifies from a separate centre. Rarely, it fails to fuse with the remainder of the talus and remains in the adult as the **os trigonum**.) The talus forms numerous joints with adjacent bones: (1) the superior surface of the body—the trochlea tali—articulates with the distal end of the tibia; (2) the medial surface of the body articulates with the medial malleolus through a flat, comma-shaped surface; (3) the lateral surface of the body articulates with the lateral malleolus through a large, triangular area. On the inferior surface, the body of the talus articulates with the calcaneus at the (4) cylindrical **subtalar joint**. Anterior to this, but separated from it by the groove of the talus—the **sulcus tali**—there is a long, oblique articular

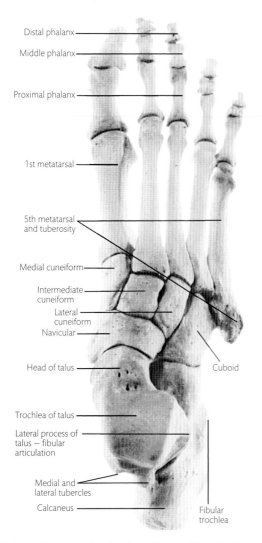

Fig. 18.3 Superior or dorsal surface of bones of the right foot.

Labels (Fig. 18.3):
Distal phalanx
Middle phalanx
Proximal phalanx
1st metatarsal
5th metatarsal and tuberosity
Medial cuneiform
Intermediate cuneiform
Lateral cuneiform
Navicular
Head of talus
Trochlea of talus
Lateral process of talus — fibular articulation
Medial and lateral tubercles
Calcaneus
Cuboid
Fibular trochlea

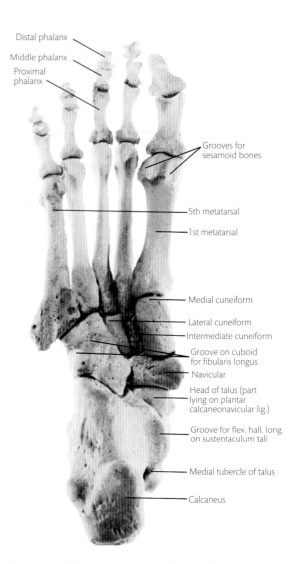

Fig. 18.4 Inferior or plantar surface of bones of the right foot.

Labels (Fig. 18.4):
Distal phalanx
Middle phalanx
Proximal phalanx
Grooves for sesamoid bones
5th metatarsal
1st metatarsal
Medial cuneiform
Lateral cuneiform
Intermediate cuneiform
Groove on cuboid for fibularis longus
Navicular
Head of talus (part lying on plantar calcaneonavicular lig.)
Groove for flex. hall. long. on sustentaculum tali
Medial tubercle of talus
Calcaneus

surface on the body, neck, and lateral part of the inferior surface of the head [Fig. 18.5]. The posterior part of this surface articulates with a (5) medial projection of the calcaneus—the **sustentaculum tali**. The anterior part of this articular surface articulates with (6) a separate area on the distal superior surface of the calcaneus. These two surfaces on the talus are angled to each other but are continuous. Medial to, and between, them is (7) another articular area on the inferomedial part of the head which articulates with the powerful **plantar calcaneonavicular** (spring) **ligament**. The plantar calcaneonavicular ligament binds the sustentaculum tali to the navicular and supports the head of the talus. (8) The distal surface of the head of the talus forms a shallow ball for the ball-and-socket joint with the navicular. The complex consisting of

the talus, calcaneus, spring ligament, and navicular is the **talocalcaneonavicular** joint.

The talus is firmly held between the tibia and fibula at the ankle joint. Only movements in the transverse plane (**dorsiflexion** and **plantar flexion**) are possible here. Note that the **malleolar surfaces on the talus** are wider apart anteriorly than posteriorly. Thus, in dorsiflexion, the talus is more firmly held between the bones than in plantar flexion. The flexibility which is present in the shaft of the fibula allows the lateral malleolus to move outwards to a slight degree in dorsiflexion. ⊃ If the talus is twisted in the ankle joint in dorsiflexion, the lateral malleolus may be forced so far laterally that the resilience of the body of the fibula is overcome and it is fractured. The fulcrum for this movement is the thick interosseous tibiofibular ligament.

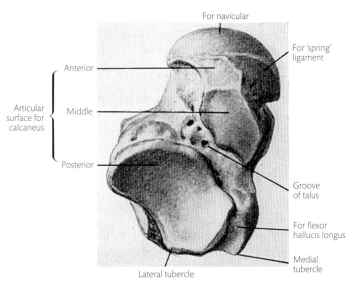

Fig. 18.5 Right talus (inferior surface). The groove of the talus is the sulcus tali.

The complex joints between the talus, calcaneus, and navicular permit the calcaneus and navicular to move round a relatively fixed talus on an almost horizontal axis. During this movement, the remaining bones of the foot are carried with the calcaneus and navicular. Movement of the calcaneus and navicular medially around this axis turns the foot, so that the sole faces medially (**inversion**). The opposite movement is **eversion** and is more limited [Fig. 18.6].

The **cuboid** articulates with the distal end of the calcaneus by a curved, saddle-shaped joint which permits a moderate amount of movement. It also articulates medially with the navicular and the lateral cuneiform bone. The inferior surface of the cuboid is grooved by the **tendon of the fibularis longus** which passes transversely across the

foot. The remaining intertarsal and tarsometatarsal joints are all flat surfaces. These include joints between the navicular and the three cuneiform bones, between the cuneiform bones, between the cuneiforms and the medial three metatarsals, and between the cuboid and the lateral two metatarsals. These joints permit relatively little movement.

Certain unique features of the joint surfaces make the foot a relatively rigid, yet resilient, structure. The first metatarsal articulates with the medial cuneiform bone by two surfaces angled to one another. The second metatarsal is inserted between the medial and lateral cuneiform bones. The principal movements in the foot occur at the subtalar and talocalcaneonavicular joint complex.

Note that the foot may be considered in lateral and medial parts. The lateral part consists of the

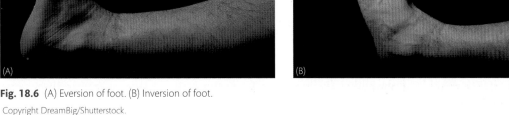

Fig. 18.6 (A) Eversion of foot. (B) Inversion of foot.
Copyright DreamBig/Shutterstock.

calcaneus, the cuboid, and the lateral two metatarsals. These together form a relatively flat **lateral longitudinal arch**, with the cuboid at the highest point. The medial part of the foot consists of the calcaneus, the talus, the navicular, the cuneiform bones, and the medial three metatarsals. These together form a high **medial longitudinal arch**. The head of the talus is at the summit of the arch and rests on the plantar calcaneonavicular ligament. The anterior pillar of the medial longitudinal arch is the powerful **first metatarsal** bone. The head of the first metatarsal rests on the ground through two **sesamoid bones**. The sesamoid bones transmit the pull of the short muscles of the big toe and form a tunnel through which the long tendon passes. This arrangement prevents compression of the tendon and small muscles when the full weight of the body is thrust forwards on the head of the first metatarsal in walking or running. The other **metatarsals** are relatively thin and weak. A **transverse arch** is formed by the metatarsals and the distal row of the tarsal bones. The fifth metatarsal forms the lateral end of this arch. The half dome-shaped arched arrangement of the foot protects structures in the sole of the foot from being compressed. This no longer holds when the arches sag in 'flat foot'.

On your own foot, identify the following structures.

Grip the posterior part of the **calcaneus**. Feel its lateral and medial **processes**. These are blunt prominences on each side of the plantar surface of the calcaneus. Feel the subcutaneous lateral surface of the calcaneus and the resistance of the fibular tendons, immediately posteroinferior to the lateral malleolus. Follow the tendons inferiorly.

Find the **tuberosity on the base of the fifth metatarsal**. It lies midway between the point of the heel and the little toe. The **head of the fifth metatarsal** is felt as a rounded bulge at the root of the little toe.

Extend the toes firmly. A bulge appears on the lateral side of the dorsum of the foot, a thumb-breadth anterior to the lateral malleolus. This is the **extensor digitorum brevis** muscle which arises from the dorsal surface of the distal part of the calcaneus.

Repeatedly plantar flex and dorsiflex the foot. The anterior part of the **trochlea tali** can be felt under the anterior part of the distal end of the tibia in plantar flexion. Invert the foot. The **tendon of the tibialis anterior** becomes prominent, as it passes to the junction of the medial cuneiform and the base of the first metatarsal. Appreciate the bony prominence on the dorsum of the foot, distal to the lateral malleolus. This is the lateral part of the **head of the talus**. Confirm that it disappears on eversion.

On the medial side of the ankle, feel the sustentaculum tali below the medial malleolus. Note that this moves with the posterior part of the calcaneus, as the foot is inverted and everted. Evert the foot as far as possible, and feel the bony prominence anteroinferior to the medial malleolus. This is the medial surface of the head of the talus. Keep your finger on it, and invert the foot. Note that it disappears and that the proximal edge of the **navicular** becomes prominent, distal to it. Follow the navicular to its **tuberosity** on the plantar aspect. The tendon which passes forwards to this tuberosity is the **tendon of the tibialis posterior**.

Note the parts of the foot which are normally in contact with the ground. Note also that it is the head of the first metatarsal which takes the pressure when you push off to take a step.

The arrangement of the phalanges and their joints with each other and with the metatarsals (metatarsophalangeal and interphalangeal joints) is similar to that in the fingers. The main difference lies in the massive phalanges in the big toe and the relatively small phalanges in the others. The appearance of these bones indicates that the major stresses to the foot are carried by the big toe.

Intermuscular septa

These intermuscular septa have been mentioned in connection with the bones. They separate the various groups of muscles, give attachments to muscle fibres proximally, and hold the muscle groups tightly within a fascial space. Due to this arrangement, when the muscles contract, they are compressed by the fascia, and the blood within them is pumped upwards in the veins. This is an essential part of the mechanism of venous return from the lower limb. ➲ Extensive division of the fascia or wasting of the muscles within the fascial compartments impair venous return and lead to swelling of the limb (oedema).

There are three named intermuscular partitions in the leg: (1) the interosseous membrane between B and E in Fig. 18.7; (2) the anterior septum between A and B; and (3) the posterior septum

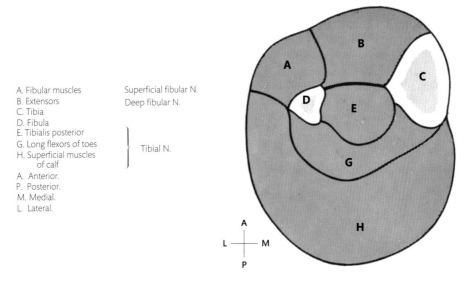

A. Fibular muscles
B. Extensors
C. Tibia
D. Fibula
E. Tibialis posterior
G. Long flexors of toes
H. Superficial muscles
    of calf
A. Anterior.
P. Posterior.
M. Medial.
L. Lateral.

Superficial fibular N.
Deep fibular N.

Tibial N.

Fig. 18.7 Diagram of osteofascial compartments of the leg. The interosseus membrane lies between B and E.

between A and H. In addition, the muscles of the back of the leg are divided into three layers by two coronal sheets of fascia between E and G, and between G and H.

Front of the leg and dorsum of the foot

See Dissection 18.1.

Superficial veins of the front of the leg and dorsum of the foot

There are two **dorsal digital veins** in each toe. Each joins the corresponding vein from the adjacent toe to form a **dorsal metatarsal vein**. The dorsal metatarsal vein drains into the **dorsal venous arch**. The dorsal digital veins on the medial side of the big toe and the lateral side of the little toe join the ends of the arch to form the long and short saphenous veins, respectively. The dorsal

DISSECTION 18.1 Skin reflection, and cutaneous nerves and vessels

Objectives

I. To reflect the skin.   II. To identify and trace the lateral cutaneous nerve of the calf, sural nerve, superficial fibular nerve, dorsal digital nerves, and long and short saphenous veins in the leg.

Instructions

1. Place the limb in a convenient position, e.g. with a block under the knee and the foot bent down (plantar flexed). Make incision 11 [see Fig. 13.6]. Reflect the skin from the front of the leg and the dorsum of the foot, but retain the superficial fascia so as not to destroy the veins.

2. Find the lateral cutaneous nerve of the calf and the long saphenous vein, with the saphenous nerve beside

it. Follow all three to the foot [see Fig. 13.9]. Note the branches of the nerves and the tributaries of the vein.

3. Establish the continuity of the long saphenous vein with the medial extremity of the dorsal venous arch of the foot. This arch lies transversely on the anterior parts of the metatarsals. Follow the arch to the lateral side of the foot, finding its dorsal metatarsal tributaries. Laterally, the arch is continuous with the short saphenous vein.

4. Trace the beginning of the short saphenous vein to a point below the lateral malleolus, and find the sural nerve beside it. Follow the sural nerve along the lateral side of the foot to the little toe. It gives a communicating branch to the superficial fibular nerve.

5. Find the superficial fibular nerve, as it pierces the deep fascia at the junction of the middle and distal thirds of the leg. Trace the nerve and its branches into the dorsum of the foot. Note that the most medial branch is to the medial side of the big toe and that a branch does not pass to the first interdigital cleft.

6. Find the dorsal digital nerves of the adjacent sides of the big and second toes. Follow them proximally. They arise from a branch of the deep fibular nerve, proximal to the cleft.

venous arch lies on the distal parts of the shafts of the metatarsals. It drains the dorsum of the foot and toes.

The **short saphenous vein** runs back inferior and posterior to the lateral malleolus. It ascends to the popliteal fossa in the back of the leg [Fig. 18.8].

The **long saphenous vein** passes posteriorly on the medial side of the foot. It ascends anterior to the medial malleolus, obliquely across the distal third of the medial surface of the tibia [Fig. 18.9]. The further course and termination are described in Chapter 13.

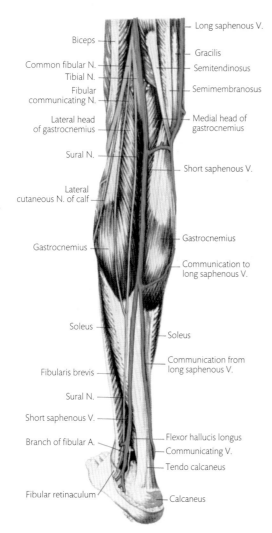

Fig. 18.8 Superficial dissection of the leg, viewed from the posterolateral side, showing veins and nerves. (Usually the short saphenous vein ends in the popliteal fossa.)

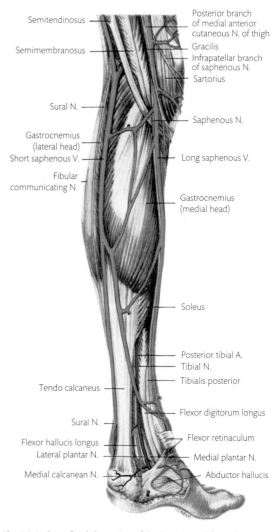

Fig. 18.9 Superficial dissection of the leg, viewed from the posteromedial side, showing veins and nerves.

Cutaneous nerves of the front of the leg and dorsum of the foot

The upper two-thirds of the **front of the leg** are supplied by two nerves—the **saphenous nerve** (L. 3, 4) medially, and the **lateral cutaneous nerve of the calf** laterally. The lower third is supplied by the **superficial fibular** and **saphenous nerves**.

The dorsum of the foot is supplied mainly by the medial and intermediate cutaneous branches of the **superficial fibular nerve**. The lateral margin is supplied by the **sural nerve,** and the medial margin by the **saphenous nerve** proximally and the **superficial fibular** nerve distally. The first interdigital cleft and the skin immediately proximal to it are supplied by the **deep fibular nerve**. The **dorsum of the toes** is supplied by the digital branches of these nerves [see Figs. 13.9, 20.1]. On the terminal phalanges, the supply is from the plantar nerves.

Superficial fibular nerve (L. 4, 5; S. 1)

The superficial fibular nerve arises from the common fibular nerve on the lateral side of the neck of the fibula. It descends between the fibularis longus and brevis supplying them. It enters the superficial fascia at the junction of the middle and distal thirds of the leg and branches into the **medial** and **intermediate dorsal cutaneous nerves**. Each of these supplies the skin in the lower part of the front of the leg and the dorsum of the foot, and divides into two **dorsal digital nerves** of the foot. Those from the medial nerve pass to the medial side of the big toe and the adjacent sides of the second and third toes. Those from the intermediate nerve pass to the adjacent sides of the third and fourth, and fourth and fifth toes [see Fig. 20.1]. All dorsal digital nerves lie deep to the dorsal venous arch.

Sural nerve (S. 1, 2)

The sural nerve arises from the tibial nerve in the popliteal fossa and descends in the back of the leg to the posterior surface of the lateral malleolus. It lies with the short saphenous vein in the superficial fascia of the lower leg and supplies the overlying skin. It is joined by the **fibular communicating** branch of the common fibular nerve [see Fig. 14.2]. It turns forwards along the lateral border of the foot and little toe, supplying the skin of both.

Dissection 18.2 looks at the deep fascia of the leg.

Deep fascia of the front of the leg

The deep fascia of the leg is very strong. It is fused with the periosteum where the bones are subcutaneous. At the ankle, it forms thickened bands (retinacula) which hold the tendons close to the joint and prevent them from springing forwards in dorsiflexion of the ankle.

Retinacula

The **superior extensor retinaculum** is a broad band between the triangular subcutaneous area of the fibula and the anterior border of the tibia.

The **inferior extensor retinaculum** is Y-shaped. The stem of the Y is attached to the upper surface of the anterior part of the calcaneus [Fig. 18.10]. Medially, the limbs of the Y separate. The upper limb is attached to the medial malleolus; the lower fuses with the fascia of the sole on the medial side of the foot. The deep fibres of the retinaculum form two loops around the tendons—one around the extensor digitorum longus and fibularis tertius, and another around the extensor hallucis longus. The retinacula prevent the tendons from slipping medially when the foot is inverted. When the foot is inverted, there is a marked medial angulation of the tendon of the extensor hallucis at the retinaculum. The superior and inferior **fibular retinacula** hold the tendons of the fibularis longus and brevis in position, as they pass postero-inferior to the lateral malleolus and on the lateral surface of the calcaneus [Fig. 18.4]. A similar **flexor retinaculum**, posteroinferior to the medial malleolus, holds the tendons of the deep muscles of the back of the leg in position, as they pass into the foot [see Fig. 18.17].

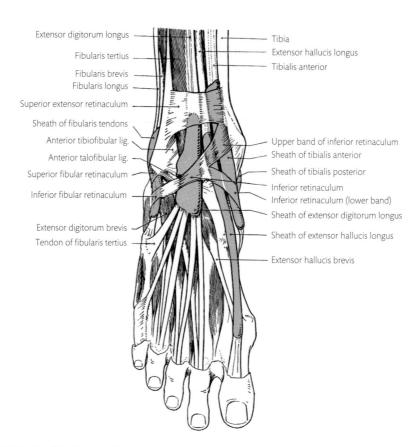

Extensor digitorum longus
Fibularis tertius
Fibularis brevis
Fibularis longus
Superior extensor retinaculum
Sheath of fibularis tendons
Anterior tibiofibular lig.
Anterior talofibular lig.
Superior fibular retinaculum
Inferior fibular retinaculum
Extensor digitorum brevis
Tendon of fibularis tertius

Tibia
Extensor hallucis longus
Tibialis anterior

Upper band of inferior retinaculum
Sheath of tibialis anterior
Sheath of tibialis posterior
Inferior retinaculum
Inferior retinaculum (lower band)
Sheath of extensor digitorum longus
Sheath of extensor hallucis longus
Extensor hallucis brevis

Fig. 18.10 Synovial sheaths of the dorsum of the foot.

See Dissection 18.3.

Synovial sheaths of extensor tendons

There are three synovial sheaths [Fig. 18.10] in the front of the ankle: (1) the synovial sheath surround-ing the tendon of the **tibialis anterior** extends from the upper border of the superior extensor retinaculum almost to the insertion of the tendon; (2) that on the **extensor hallucis longus** begins between the retinacula and reaches to the proximal

---

DISSECTION 18.3 Front of the leg-1

Objectives

I. To study the tibialis anterior, extensor hallucis longus, extensor digitorum longus, fibularis tertius, and extensor digitorum brevis.   II. To identify and trace the deep fibular nerve and anterior tibial vessels in the leg and foot.   III. To dissect the extensor expansion.

Instructions

1. Divide the deep fascia of the front of the leg longitudinally between the tibia and fibula. Extend the incision onto the dorsum of the foot. Leave the superior and inferior extensor retinacula intact. Near the superior retinaculum, pass a blunt seeker deep to these retinacula. This will allow you to define their margins more easily. Avoid injury to the synovial

sheaths of the tendons which lie deep to the reti-nacula [Fig. 18.10].

2. Turn the deep fascia medially and laterally, and con-firm its attachments to the bones. Open the synovial sheaths of the tendons, proximal to the superior ex-tensor retinacula, and pass a blunt probe along them to define their extent.

3. Follow the tendons upwards and downwards.

4. Define the individual muscles and their attachments to the bones. Separate the tibialis anterior from the other three muscles down to the interosseous membrane.

5. Find the anterior tibial vessels and the deep fibular nerve on the membrane. Trace these upwards and downwards.

6. Pull the fibularis tertius muscle aside, and find the perforating branch of the fibular artery, as it pierces the lower part of the interosseous membrane. Follow it into the foot [Fig. 18.11].

7. Find the extensor digitorum brevis muscle on the dorsum of the foot. Trace its tendons to the medial four toes [Fig. 18.12].

8. Follow the anterior tibial artery and the deep fibular nerve into the foot. Here the artery is known as the dorsalis pedis artery [Fig. 18.12].

9. On the second or third toe, clean the extensor expansion formed by the extensor tendons. Trace the expansion (which is similar to that in fingers) to the distal phalanx.

phalanx of the big toe; (3) the third surrounds the tendons of the **extensor digitorum longus** and **fibularis tertius**. It extends from the lower part of the superior extensor retinaculum to the middle of the dorsum of the foot.

Contents of the anterior compartment of the leg

The anterior compartment of the leg contains the tibialis anterior, extensor digitorum longus, extensor hallucis longus, and fibularis tertius. The compartment also contains the anterior tibial vessels and the deep fibular nerve which supply these muscles and continue into the dorsum of the foot [Figs. 18.11, 18.12].

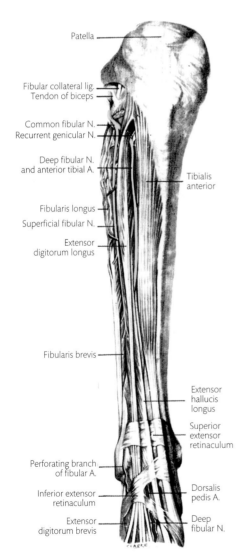

Fig. 18.11 Dissection of the front and lateral sides of the leg.

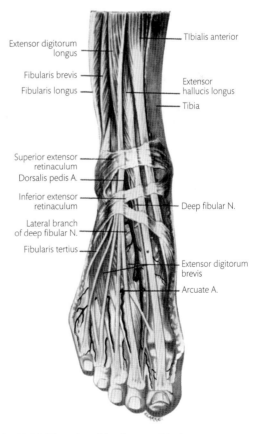

Fig. 18.12 Dissection of the dorsum of the foot.

Tibialis anterior

The tibialis anterior takes origin from the upper half of the lateral surface of the tibia and from the interosseous membrane [Fig. 18.13]. The tendon passes deep to the retinacula, bends medially, and is inserted into the medial surface of the medial cuneiform and adjacent part of the first metatarsal close to their plantar aspects. This insertion is almost continuous with that of the **fibularis longus** (see later). **Nerve supply**: deep fibular nerve and recurrent genicular nerves. **Actions**: it is a dorsiflexor and powerful invertor of the foot when the foot is raised from the ground. When the foot is on the ground, the muscle helps to balance the leg and talus on the other tarsal bones, so that the leg is kept vertical, even when walking on uneven ground.

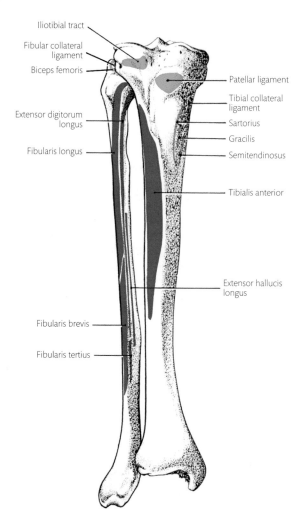

Fig. 18.13 Anterior aspect of bones of the leg to show attachments of muscles.

Labels on figure:
Iliotibial tract
Fibular collateral ligament
Biceps femoris
Extensor digitorum longus
Fibularis longus
Patellar ligament
Tibial collateral ligament
Sartorius
Gracilis
Semitendinosus
Tibialis anterior
Extensor hallucis longus
Fibularis brevis
Fibularis tertius

Extensor digitorum longus

The extensor digitorum longus is a long, thin muscle that arises mainly from the upper part of the medial surface of the fibula [Fig. 18.13]. The tendon passes deep to the retinacula. Anterior to the ankle joint, it divides into four parts which pass to the lateral four toes. As each tendon approaches the metatarsophalangeal joint, it forms an **extensor expansion**, similar to that in the fingers. Each extensor expansion fuses with the fibrous capsule on the dorsal surface of the metatarsophalangeal joint and extends on each side of the joint to the deep transverse metatarsal ligament. The thick central part of the expansion continues on the dorsal surface of the proximal phalanx and is inserted into the base of the middle phalanx. On the second to fourth toes, it is joined by the greater part of the tendon of the **extensor digitorum brevis**. The lateral and medial parts of the expansion continue distally, fused to the median portion. They cross the dorsolateral surfaces of the distal interphalangeal joint and are inserted into the base of the distal phalanx. The tendons of the **lumbricals** may join the medial side of the expansion in each toe; the interossei may send delicate extensions into it, although, in the foot, interossei are principally inserted into the proximal phalanx. The little toe has only the long extensor tendon, but the expansion is otherwise the same as in the second to fourth toes. **Nerve supply**: deep fibular nerve. **Actions**: it extends the interphalangeal and metatarsophalangeal joints of the lateral four toes. When the metatarsophalangeal joints of the foot are extended, extension of the interphalangeal joints depends solely on the **lumbricals**. This is because the interossei are not inserted to a significant degree into the extensor expansion. The extensor digitorum longus also dorsiflexes the ankle joint and acts with the fibular muscles to evert the foot. ➲ If lumbricals weaken or fail to join the extensor expansion, the toes tend to be pulled into extension at the metatarsophalangeal joints (extensor digitorum longus and brevis) with flexion at the interphalangeal joints—a condition known as 'hammer toe'.

Fibularis tertius

This small muscle is continuous at its origin with the extensor digitorum longus and appears to be a part of it [Fig. 18.13]. It arises from the distal part of the medial surface of the fibula and the adjacent interosseous membrane. It is inserted into the base of the fifth metatarsal bone. Frequently, it is partly fused with the tendon of the extensor digitorum longus to the fifth toe. **Nerve supply**: deep fibular nerve. **Actions**: it everts the foot and dorsiflexes the ankle.

Extensor hallucis longus

It arises from the middle of the medial surface of the fibula, medial to the extensor digitorum longus [Fig. 18.13]. The tendon passes deep to the retinacula and crosses in front of the anterior tibial artery. The inferior retinaculum holds the tendon laterally, so that it inclines forwards and medially to the big toe. On the head of the metatarsal, the tendon forms an **extensor expansion**. The central part of the expansion passes to the distal phalanx. The lateral part of the expansion passes to the deep transverse metatarsal ligament; the medial part joins the tendon of the **abductor hallucis** (see later). It is this part of the expansion which is stretched over the head of the first metatarsal when the big toe deviates laterally in 'hallux valgus'. **Nerve supply**: deep fibular nerve. **Actions**: it extends the phalanges of the big toe and dorsiflexes the ankle joint. It is used in inversion when the big toe is extended.

Deep fibular nerve

The deep fibular nerve is a branch of the common fibular nerve. It arises between the neck of the fibula and the fibularis longus muscle. It pierces the anterior intermuscular septum to enter the anterior compartment of the leg and descends with the anterior tibial vessels [Fig. 18.11]. It lies on the interosseous membrane between the tibialis anterior and the long extensors of the toe. Near the ankle joint, it is crossed superficially by the extensor hallucis longus tendon [Fig. 18.12] and enters the dorsum of the foot midway between the medial and lateral malleoli. It lies between the tendons of the extensor digitorum longus and extensor hallucis longus and the dorsalis pedis artery. It almost immediately divides into two branches: (1) A medial branch that continues towards the first interdigital space, it supplies the adjacent joints and the first dorsal interosseous muscle and ends by forming the **dorsal digital nerves** for the adjacent sides of the big and second toes. (2) The lateral branch supplies the **extensor digitorum brevis** and the surrounding joints. The deep fibular nerve supplies all the muscles of the anterior compartment of the leg and the extensor digitorum brevis. ◆ If the nerve is destroyed, dorsiflexion of the ankle and extension of the metatarsophalangeal joints are lost, and inversion is weakened. This condition is known as 'drop foot'.

Anterior tibial artery

This artery arises from the popliteal artery at the lower border of the popliteus. It enters the anterior compartment of the leg above the interosseous membrane, and runs on the anterior surface of that membrane with the deep fibular nerve. It becomes progressively more superficial, as it descends and forms the dorsalis pedis artery, midway between the medial and lateral malleoli [Fig. 18.12]. The anterior tibial veins are closely applied to the artery.

Branches

It supplies the muscles of the anterior compartment of the leg and sends an anterior tibial recurrent artery upwards to the knee joint [see Fig. 18.23]. Other branches, medial and lateral anterior malleolar arteries help to form a rete on each malleolus. The lateral one anastomoses with the perforating branch of the fibular artery.

Dorsalis pedis artery

The dorsalis pedis artery is the continuation of the anterior tibial artery [Fig. 18.12]. It begins on the anterior surface of the ankle joint and runs with the deep fibular nerve, deep to the inferior extensor retinaculum, to the proximal end of the first intermetatarsal space. Here it divides into the **arcuate artery** and the **first dorsal metatarsal artery**. On the dorsum of the foot, it lies on the tarsal bones and is readily palpated against them between the tendons of the extensor hallucis longus and extensor digitorum longus.

Branches

It gives medial and lateral **tarsal branches** to the tarsal bones and extensor digitorum brevis. The **arcuate artery** runs laterally across the base of the metatarsals, deep to the extensor tendons. It gives dorsal metatarsal arteries to the second, third, and fourth intermetatarsal spaces. Each of these communicates with the plantar arch in the sole of the foot through perforating branches at the proximal end of the intermetatarsal space. The perforating artery in the first space, the **deep plantar branch** of the arcuate artery, is larger than the others and carries blood to the medial end of the plantar arch [see Figs. 18.30, 18.31]. Each dorsal metatarsal artery runs forwards over the corresponding dorsal interosseous muscle and gives dorsal digital arteries to two adjacent toes. The first and last of these dorsal metatarsal arteries send branches to the medial side of the big toe and the lateral side of the little toe.

Extensor digitorum brevis

The extensor digitorum brevis originates from the anterior part of the dorsal surface of the calcaneus and from the stem of the inferior extensor retinaculum. It forms four tendons; the most medial is the **extensor hallucis brevis**. This tendon runs obliquely across the dorsum of the foot to the base of the proximal phalanx of the big toe. It extends the metatarsophalangeal joint of the big toe. The remaining three tendons join the long extensor tendons of the second to fourth toes. They are inserted into the middle and terminal phalanges of these toes through the extensor expansions. **Nerve supply**: deep fibular nerve. **Action**: extension of the metatarsophalangeal and interphalangeal joints of the second, third, and fourth toes.

Dissection 18.4 continues with the dissection of the front of the leg.

Lateral side of the leg

The fibularis longus and brevis muscles lie on the lateral surface of the fibula in the lateral compartment of the leg. They lie between the anterior and posterior intermuscular septa and take partial origin from them [Fig. 18.7].

Fibular muscles

The **fibularis longus** takes origin from the upper two-thirds of the lateral surface of the fibula

DISSECTION 18.4 Front of the leg-2

Objective

I. To study the extensor retinacula.

Instructions

1. Cut through the extensor retinacula, and reflect their attachments.

2. Note the extensions from the deep surface that hold the tendons in place.

[Fig. 18.13]. It lies over the **fibularis brevis** which arises from the lower two-thirds of the same surface. They descend together, closely applied to the lateral surface of the fibula, with the longus lying superficially. They pass behind the triangular subcutaneous area of the fibula to reach the posterior border of the lateral malleolus. (The lateral malleolus is slightly grooved near its tip by them.) They lie in a **common synovial sheath** and are held in position by the **superior fibular retinaculum**—a thickened part of deep fascia between the fibula and the calcaneus [Fig. 18.14]. The tendons emerge from the retinaculum and run anteroinferiorly below the lateral malleolus, on the lateral surfaces of the calcaneus and cuboid, with the fibularis brevis superior to the fibularis longus. On the lateral surface of the calcaneus, the tendons are separated by the **fibular trochlea**, to which the inferior fibular retinaculum is attached [Fig. 18.14]. At the lateral border of the foot, the fibularis brevis is attached to the base of the fifth metatarsal. Just proximal to this, the fibularis longus turns over the lateral margin of the cuboid, runs obliquely across the sole of the foot in a groove on the plantar surface of the cuboid, and is inserted into the medial cuneiform and the base of the first metatarsal. **Nerve supply**: superficial fibular nerve. **Actions**: the fibularis longus and brevis are both evertors of the foot and plantar flexors of the ankle joint. The fibularis longus also helps to maintain the transverse arch of the foot by pulling the lateral and medial borders of the foot together as it runs transversely across the sole.

Dissection 18.5 looks at the fibular compartment of the leg.

Terminal branches of the common fibular nerve

The common fibular nerve turns round the lateral surface of the neck of the fibula. It gives off a small recurrent genicular branch to the knee joint and the superior tibiofibular joint. The common fibular nerve then divides into the superficial and deep fibular nerves. The deep fibular nerve pierces the extensor digitorum to enter the anterior compartment of the leg.

Superficial fibular nerve (L. 4, 5; S. 1)

The superficial fibular nerve descends in the lateral compartment. It pierces the deep fascia in the distal third of the leg and divides into **medial** and

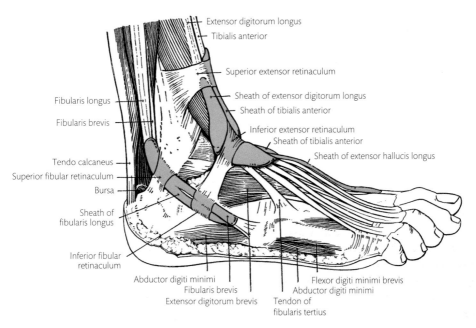

Extensor digitorum longus
Tibialis anterior
Superior extensor retinaculum
Sheath of extensor digitorum longus
Sheath of tibialis anterior
Inferior extensor retinaculum
Sheath of tibialis anterior
Sheath of extensor hallucis longus
Fibularis longus
Fibularis brevis
Tendo calcaneus
Superior fibular retinaculum
Bursa
Sheath of fibularis longus
Inferior fibular retinaculum
Abductor digiti minimi
Fibularis brevis
Extensor digitorum brevis
Flexor digiti minimi brevis
Abductor digiti minimi
Tendon of fibularis tertius

Fig. 18.14 Dissection showing the synovial sheaths of tendons of the lateral aspect of the foot.

intermediate dorsal cutaneous nerves. It supplies the fibularis longus and brevis, the skin of the lower part of the front of the leg, the large part of the dorsum of the foot, and most of the dorsal surfaces of the toes.

Medial side of the leg

This consists of the medial surface of the tibia. It is subcutaneous, except for a small part at the upper end which is covered by the tibial collateral ligament of the knee joint and the tendons of the sartorius, gracilis, and semitendinosus [Fig. 18.13].

Long saphenous vein

This important vein begins at the medial border of the foot by the union of the **dorsal venous arch** and the **medial dorsal digital vein** of the big toe. It ascends in front of the medial malleolus, obliquely backwards across the distal third of the medial surface of the tibia, along the medial border

DISSECTION 18.5 Fibular compartment of the leg

Objectives

I. To expose and study the fibularis longus and brevis.
II. To identify and trace the superficial fibular nerve.

Instructions

1. Divide the deep fascia over the fibular muscles by a longitudinal incision. Turn the flaps aside, and demonstrate their continuity with the anterior and posterior intermuscular septa. Retain the fibular retinacula.

2. Separate the muscles from each other. Determine their attachments, and find the nerves supplying them.

3. Trace the common fibular nerve to the fibularis longus, and divide the muscle to follow the nerve between

the muscle and the fibula. Trace the superficial fibular nerve downwards. Follow the deep fibular nerve into continuity with the part already found in the anterior compartment of the leg.

4. Find and open the common **synovial sheath of the fibular muscles**. It begins 3–5 cm above the superior fibular retinaculum. Pass a blunt seeker into it, and try to define its extent. Distally, it divides to surround each tendon separately and continues into the sole of the foot around the tendon of the fibularis longus.

5. Do not follow the latter tendon into the sole, but follow the tendon of the fibularis brevis to its insertion, and define the inferior fibular retinaculum.

of the tibia to the posteromedial side of the knee. The further course and termination of this vein is described in Chapter 13. In the leg, the long saphenous vein lies between two layers of membranous fascia and is crossed by a more superficial plexus of veins which tend to join it near the knee. The long saphenous vein receives many tributaries throughout its length and communicates through them with the short saphenous vein.

The long saphenous vein communicates through valved perforating veins with the deep veins of the leg. Communications between the long saphenous vein and deep veins include those with: (1) the medial plantar veins on the medial surface of the foot; (2) the anterior tibial veins anterior to the ankle; (3) tributaries of the posterior tibial veins behind the medial margin of the tibia; and (4) continuation with the femoral vein at the saphenous opening.

The clinical importance of the saphenous veins is discussed in Clinical Application 18.1.

Saphenous nerve (L. 3, 4)

The saphenous nerve arises from the femoral nerve in the femoral triangle and accompanies the femoral artery into the adductor canal. It leaves the canal through the roof and lies deep to the sartorius. Here it gives off the **infrapatellar branch**, which pierces the sartorius to reach the patellar plexus. The nerve then emerges between the sartorius and the tendon of the gracilis a little above the knee. The saphenous nerve lies posteromedial to the knee and pierces the deep fascia inferior to it. In the leg and foot, it accompanies the long saphenous vein and ends in the skin of the medial side of the foot. It supplies the skin on the medial side of the knee, leg, and proximal part of the dorsum of the foot [see Fig. 13.9].

Dissection 18.6 looks at the medial side of the leg.

Back of the leg

The muscles of the back of the leg are divided into three layers by two sheets of fascia [Fig. 18.7]. The superficial layer of muscles is inserted into the heel by the large **tendo calcaneus**, which can be felt behind the lower part of the leg and ankle. This layer consists of the gastrocnemius, soleus, and plantaris—muscles that are powerful plantar flexors of the ankle joint. They raise the weight of the body

DISSECTION 18.6 Medial side of the leg

Objectives

I. To expose and clean the tendons of the sartorius, gracilis, semitendinosus. II. To study the medial (tibial) collateral ligament.

Instructions

1. Trace the tendons of the sartorius, gracilis, and semitendinosus to their attachments.

2. Turn them forwards, and note the complex bursa which lies between them and the tibial collateral ligament of the knee joint.

3. Turn the tendons forwards, and clean the surface of the ligament. Note that the tendon of the semimembranosus and the inferior medial genicular vessels and nerves pass deep to the superficial part of the ligament.

4. The deep part of the ligament is attached to the margin of the tibial condyle, superior to the insertion of the semimembranosus.

on to the toes, using the heads of the metatarsals as a fulcrum, e.g. in the push-off phase of walking. These muscles move independently of the middle layer of muscles. The middle layer of muscles in the back of the leg consist of the long flexors of the toes—the flexor hallucis longus and flexor digitorum longus. They are separated from the superficial muscles by a well-defined fascial layer which stretches from the medial border of the tibia to the posterior border of the fibula. This fascia encloses the muscles, together with their vessels and nerve, and is attached above to the soleal line on the tibia. At the ankle, this fascia is thickened to form part of the **flexor retinaculum** [see Fig. 18.17].

The deepest layer consists of the tibialis posterior which lies on the interosseous membrane between the tibia and fibula (E in Fig. 18.7). The fascia covering the posterior surface of the tibialis posterior is attached above to the soleal line, laterally to the medial crest of the fibula, and medially to the vertical ridge on the tibia.

Dissection 18.7 looks at the cutaneous vessels and nerves of the back of the leg.

Short saphenous vein

The short saphenous vein is formed by the union of the medial end of the dorsal venous arch of the

Objectives

I. To reflect the skin. II. To identify and trace the cutaneous nerves and veins on the back of the leg.

Instructions

1. Make a transverse incision through the skin on the distal part of the heel. Carry the incision along the borders of the foot to join the previous incisions.

2. Find the sural nerve and the short saphenous vein below the lateral malleolus. Then strip the skin and superficial fascia upwards from the back of the leg, retaining the nerve and vein. Small medial calcanean nerves may be found, as the skin is removed from the medial side of the heel [Fig. 18.9].

3. Find the meeting point of the sural and fibular communicating nerves. Follow both upwards through the deep fascia to the tibial and common fibular nerves.

4. Trace the short saphenous vein into the popliteal vein.

foot and the dorsal digital vein of the lateral side of the little toe. It passes backwards, inferior to the lateral malleolus, and ascends in the back of the leg. It pierces the deep fascia at the lower border of the popliteal fossa and enters the popliteal vein. It drains the lateral side of the foot, ankle, and back of the leg.

Sural nerve (S. 1, 2)

The sural nerve arises from the tibial nerve in the popliteal fossa. It descends on the posterior surface of the gastrocnemius and enters the superficial fascia at the middle of the back of the leg. It is then joined by the **fibular communicating nerve** [see Fig. 14.2] and accompanies the short saphenous vein to the lateral side of the foot. The sural nerve supplies the skin on the lower lateral side of the back of the leg, the lateral border and lateral part of the dorsum of the foot, and the lateral side of the little toe.

Fibular communicating nerve (L. 5; S. 1, 2)

The fibular communicating nerve arises from the common fibular nerve in the popliteal fossa. It pierces the deep fascia over the lateral head of the

gastrocnemius and descends to join the sural nerve [see Fig. 14.2]. Area of supply: the skin on the proximal two-thirds of the posterolateral surface of the leg and the territory of the sural nerve.

The posterior branch of the **medial anterior cutaneous nerve of the thigh** (L. 2, 3) descends into the calf and supplies the skin in the upper posteromedial part of the leg.

Lymph vessels and lymph nodes of the lower limb

Very little of this system can be demonstrated by dissection as the lymph nodes are poorly seen, unless enlarged by disease. However, knowledge of the course of the lymph vessels, and the location of the nodes to which they drain, is essential in determining the possible site of disease when an enlarged lymph node is found. It follows that this important vascular system has to be understood principally from diagrams and from the text.

The student should study Figs. 18.15 and 18.16, and note the following points.

1. **Superficial lymph vessels and nodes** drain the skin and subcutaneous tissues. They lie superficial to the deep fascia, which separates them from the **deep lymph vessels** and **nodes**. The superficial and deep systems communicate with each other only at certain points. In the lower limb, such communications occur through the cribriform fascia in the thigh and the popliteal fascia. (In the upper limb, it occurs in the axilla and where the basilic vein pierces the deep fascia of the arm.)

2. The superficial vessels are much more numerous than the deep vessels. There are few lymph vessels in muscle, but very many in skin, synovial membranes, synovial sheaths, and bursae.

3. Superficial lymph vessels take a direct course to the superficial lymph nodes. Deep lymph vessels run with the deep blood vessels and enter the deep nodes.

4. **Superficial nodes** in the lower limb are virtually restricted to the inguinal region. These drain almost all the superficial tissues of the lower limb, perineum, and trunk below the level of the umbilicus. The only exception is the superficial tissue of the lateral side of the foot and the back of the leg, which drains to the popliteal nodes by lymph vessels that accompany the short saphenous vein.

5. The **superficial inguinal lymph nodes** are arranged in the shape of a T. The nodes forming the stem of the T drain the lower limb. The lateral nodes of the horizontal part of the T drain the upper lateral gluteal region and the posterior and

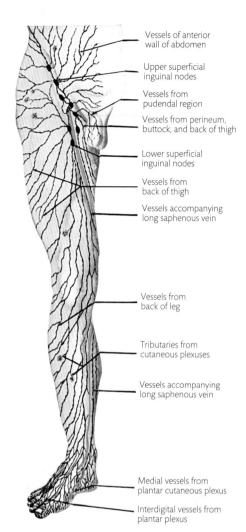

Vessels of anterior wall of abdomen

Upper superficial inguinal nodes

Vessels from pudendal region

Vessels from perineum, buttock, and back of thigh

Lower superficial inguinal nodes

Vessels from back of thigh

Vessels accompanying long saphenous vein

Vessels from back of leg

Tributaries from cutaneous plexuses

Vessels accompanying long saphenous vein

Medial vessels from plantar cutaneous plexus

Interdigital vessels from plantar plexus

Fig. 18.15 Superficial lymph vessels of the anterior surface of the lower limb.

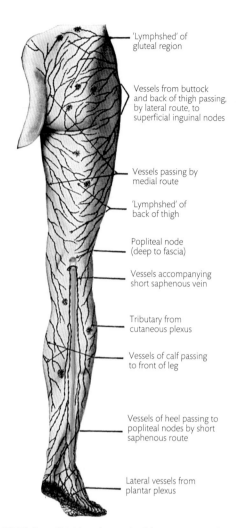

'Lymphshed' of gluteal region

Vessels from buttock and back of thigh passing, by lateral route, to superficial inguinal nodes

Vessels passing by medial route

'Lymphshed' of back of thigh

Popliteal node (deep to fascia)

Vessels accompanying short saphenous vein

Tributary from cutaneous plexus

Vessels of calf passing to front of leg

Vessels of heel passing to popliteal nodes by short saphenous route

Lateral vessels from plantar plexus

Fig. 18.16 Superficial lymph vessels of the posterior surface of the lower limb.

lateral parts of the trunk. The medial nodes in the horizontal part of the T drain the upper medial part of the thigh, the perineum, the medial gluteal region, and the anteromedial part of the abdominal wall below the umbilicus.

6. There is a 'lymphshed' along the back of the lower limb. (The term lymphshed refers to the imaginary line which separates areas draining medially and laterally.) Vessels from the medial half of the limb pass round the medial surface of the limb, and those from the lateral half pass round the lateral surface of the limb to converge on the inguinal lymph nodes [Fig. 18.16]. This 'lymphshed' is split distally by the vessels flowing to the popliteal nodes.

7. **Deep lymph vessels** of the leg and foot enter the **popliteal nodes**. The lymph from the popliteal nodes drains into the deep inguinal lymph nodes through lymphatics that run along the femoral ves-

sels. The deep inguinal lymph nodes also receive the efferent vessels from the superficial inguinal lymph nodes. They drain lymph to the **external iliac nodes** by passing behind the inguinal ligament.

8. Deep lymph vessels of the perineum and gluteal region drain with the corresponding blood vessels (gluteal and internal pudendal) through the greater sciatic foramen into the pelvis (**internal iliac nodes**).

Deep fascia

The importance of the dense deep fascia of the leg has already been mentioned in connection with venous drainage. At the ankle, the deep fascia is thickened to form the fibular and flexor retinacula [Figs. 18.14, 18.17] on the lateral and medial sides, respectively. The **flexor retinaculum** stretches

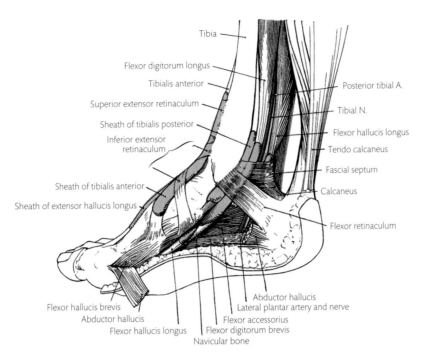

Tibia
Flexor digitorum longus
Tibialis anterior
Superior extensor retinaculum
Sheath of tibialis posterior
Inferior extensor retinaculum
Sheath of tibialis anterior
Sheath of extensor hallucis longus

Posterior tibial A.
Tibial N.
Flexor hallucis longus
Tendo calcaneus
Fascial septum
Calcaneus
Flexor retinaculum

Flexor hallucis brevis
Abductor hallucis
Flexor hallucis longus
Navicular bone
Flexor digitorum brevis
Flexor accessorius
Lateral plantar artery and nerve
Abductor hallucis

Fig. 18.17 Dissection of the leg and foot, showing the synovial sheaths.

from the calcaneus to the medial malleolus. It covers the tendons of the deep flexor muscles of the back of the leg, the tibial nerve, and posterior tibial vessels as they pass into the foot, posterior and inferior to the medial malleolus. Distally, the flexor retinaculum gives partial attachment to the abductor hallucis muscle of the foot.

Dissection 18.8 describes the dissection of the back of the leg.

Superficial muscles of the calf

Gastrocnemius

Gastrocnemius takes origin by two heads from the femur—the **lateral head** from the lateral surface of the lateral condyle, and the **medial head** from the popliteal surface above the medial condyle [Fig. 18.18]. The medial head is separated from the tendon of the semimembranosus and

DISSECTION 18.8 Back of the leg-1

Objectives

I. To dissect the flexor retinaculum. II. To study the gastrocnemius, soleus, plantaris, and tendo calcaneus. III. To identify and trace the tibial nerve and posterior tibial vessels.

Instructions

1. Define the flexor retinaculum posteroinferior to the medial malleolus. The medial calcanean nerves and vessels may be found passing through it to the skin.

2. Extend the division of the deep fascia (which was made when the sural nerve was followed) down to the calcaneus. Reflect the fascia.

3. Identify and follow the bellies of the gastrocnemius to their attachments. Lift the muscle from the

underlying soleus, and cut across the medial head, close to its attachment to the femur. Turn the medial head laterally to expose the lower part of the popliteal vessels and tibial nerve in the popliteal fossa. Find the large muscular branches to the gastrocnemius.

4. Lift the tendon of the semimembranosus from the proximal part of the medial head of the gastrocnemius, and find the bursa which separates them. Lift this part of the medial head of the gastrocnemius, and find the bursa which separates it from the fibrous capsule of the knee joint. This bursa may be continuous with the bursa under the semimembranosus and with the joint cavity through the articular capsule.

5. Trace the nerve to the soleus from the tibial nerve.

6. Find the plantaris, a small muscle posteromedial to the lateral head of the gastrocnemius. Follow its tendon between the gastrocnemius and soleus to the medial side of the tendo calcaneus.

7. Remove the fatty connective tissue in front of the tendo calcaneus. This uncovers the lower part of the intermuscular fascial septum which is close to the deep fascia here.

8. Cut across the lateral head of the gastrocnemius at the level of the knee joint. Turn its proximal part

9. Turn both bellies of the gastrocnemius downwards, and note their insertion into the tendo calcaneus.

10. Expose the posterior surface of the soleus, and define its attachments.

11. Note the tibial nerve and popliteal vessels passing deep to a tendinous arch, from which the intermediate fibres of the soleus arise.

upwards. A small sesamoid bone may be felt within the head.

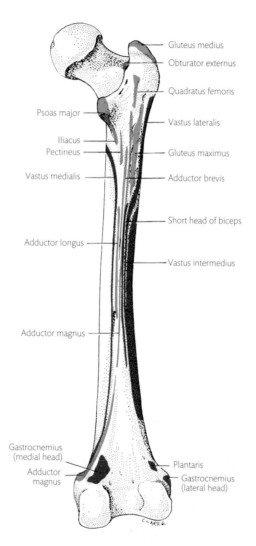

Fig. 18.18 Right femur to show muscles attached to the posterior aspect.

remain separate. They end near the middle of the leg on the posterior surface of a thin common tendon. This tendon fuses with the superficial surface of the tendon of the soleus to form the **tendo calcaneus**.

Soleus

This powerful, flat muscle arises from the: (a) posterior surface of the head and upper third of the shaft of the fibula; (b) soleal line and middle third of the medial border of the tibia; and (c) tendinous arch posterior to the popliteal vessels and tibial nerve. The thick tendon fuses with that of the gastrocnemius to form the tendo calcaneus [Figs. 18.19, 18.20].

Plantaris

This small muscle (8–10 cm long) arises from the popliteal surface of the femur [Fig. 18.18] and is partly hidden by the lateral head of the gastrocnemius. The long, slender tendon passes between the gastrocnemius and soleus and along the medial side of the tendo calcaneus to the calcaneus. The plantaris is occasionally absent (compare with the palmaris longus).

Nerve supply: these three muscles are supplied by the tibial nerve.

Actions: the gastrocnemius and soleus are powerful plantar flexors of the ankle. They act around the fulcrum of the heads of the metatarsals, mainly the first, to raise the weight of the body onto the toes—a position which the soleus maintains in running. They are responsible for the powerful push-off in running, jumping, and walking. They also act with the dorsiflexors of the ankle joint to stabilize the ankle.

The gastrocnemius also flexes the knee joint, but it becomes ineffective as a plantar flexor of the ankle when the knee is bent. ➲ If the femur is fractured

the articular capsule of the knee joint by bursae. The lateral head frequently contains a small sesamoid bone (the **fabella**). The two fleshy bellies

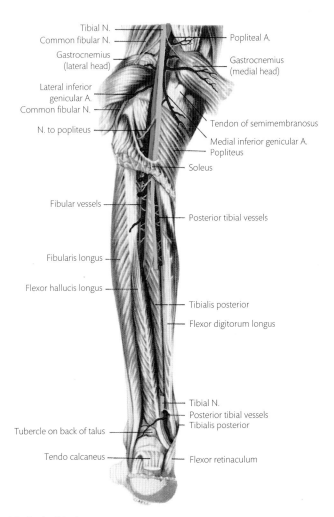

Tibial N.
Common fibular N.
Gastrocnemius (lateral head)
Lateral inferior genicular A.
Common fibular N.
N. to popliteus
Fibular vessels
Fibularis longus
Flexor hallucis longus
Tubercle on back of talus
Tendo calcaneus

Popliteal A.
Gastrocnemius (medial head)
Tendon of semimembranosus
Medial inferior genicular A.
Popliteus
Soleus
Posterior tibial vessels
Tibialis posterior
Flexor digitorum longus
Tibial N.
Posterior tibial vessels
Tibialis posterior
Flexor retinaculum

Fig. 18.19 Deep dissection of the back of the leg.

a short distance proximal to the attachments of the gastrocnemius (supracondylar fracture), the gastrocnemius pulls the distal fragment backwards. For this reason, these fractures are treated with the knee flexed, to relax the gastrocnemius and prevent this displacement.

The gastrocnemius and soleus play an important role as 'muscle pumps' that return venous blood from the lower limbs. Both muscles have a considerable blood supply, and the soleus contains a large venous plexus.

The plantaris can add very little to the strength of the gastrocnemius and soleus.

Tendo calcaneus

This powerful tendon is inserted into the smooth intermediate part of the posterior surface of the calcaneus. The upper part of this surface is separated from the tendon by a small bursa. ⊃ If the tendon

is ruptured, the disability in walking is severe, and running is impossible.

Dissection 18.9 continues the dissection of the back of the leg.

Tibial nerve (L. 4, 5; S. 1, 2, 3)

In the upper part of the leg, the tibial nerve lies deep to the first intermuscular septum with the posterior tibial vessels. In the lower third of the leg, it lies between the tendo calcaneus and the medial border of the tibia. Deep to the flexor retinaculum, it lies between the tendons of the flexor digitorum longus and flexor hallucis longus [Fig. 18.19]. The tibial nerve divides into medial and lateral plantar nerves, deep to the flexor retinaculum.

Branches in the leg

Muscular branches supply the tibialis posterior, flexor hallucis longus, flexor digitorum longus,

Objectives

I. To dissect and study the flexor hallucis longus, flexor digitorum longus and tibialis posterior. II. To identify and trace the tibial nerve and posterior tibial vessels and fibular artery.

Instructions

1. Separate the soleus from the tibia, and turn it laterally. Divide the blood vessels to the muscle, noting the large veins which emerge from it. Retain the nerves.

2. Look for any communications between the long saphenous vein and the deep veins. Open these, and check for valves within them.

3. The first intermuscular septum (deep to the soleus) is now exposed. Divide the septum longitudinally in the middle, and reflect it to expose the second layer of muscles and the neurovascular bundles.

4. Trace the tibial nerve as far as the ankle. Find the muscular branches arising mainly in the upper part of the leg. The small nerve to the popliteus descends over the popliteus to enter the deep surface of the muscle [Fig. 18.19].

5. Define the lower border of the popliteus, and follow it to its tendon. Do not attempt to follow it into the knee joint at this stage.

6. Remove the fascia from the lowest part of the popliteal vessels. Find the anterior and posterior tibial branches of the artery and the corresponding veins. Check the continuity of the anterior tibial vessels with the vessels in the anterior compartment. Follow the posterior tibial artery as far as the ankle. Find the fibular artery which arises from it. This artery descends posterior to the fibula, under cover of the flexor hallucis longus. Trace it.

7. Define and separate the long flexor muscles of the toes. The flexor hallucis longus is lateral to, and larger than, the flexor digitorum longus. Follow their tendons deep to the flexor retinaculum. Push the flexor hallucis longus laterally, and separate its deep surface from the second intermuscular septum and the interosseous membrane.

8. Divide the intermuscular septum covering the tibialis posterior. Trace that muscle and its tendon as far as the flexor retinaculum. Note its close association with the medial malleolus. Palpate the tendon in your own foot between the medial malleolus and the navicular, first tightening it by plantar flexing and inverting the foot.

and soleus. They arise in the upper part of the leg. The medial calcanean nerves (S. 1) arise at the ankle, pierce the flexor retinaculum, and supply the skin on the posterior and lower surfaces of the heel. Small articular branches pass to the posterior aspect of the ankle joint.

Popliteal vessels

The popliteal artery starts at the adductor hiatus and ends at the distal border of the popliteus. Here the popliteal artery divides into the anterior and posterior tibial arteries, and the anterior and posterior tibial veins unite to form the popliteal vein.

Anterior tibial artery

This vessel gives off a small posterior tibial recurrent artery to the back of the knee joint. It then passes forwards above the interosseous membrane to the anterior compartment of the leg.

Posterior tibial artery

The posterior tibial artery supplies the deep muscles of the back of the leg and is the main artery of the foot. It begins at the lower border of the popliteus and descends with the tibial nerve. It ends by dividing into the medial and lateral plantar arteries, deep to the flexor retinaculum.

Branches of the posterior tibial artery in the leg

1. The **fibular artery**: this large branch arises close to the origin of the parent artery and descends along the back of the fibula. It supplies: (a) muscular branches; (b) the **nutrient artery to the fibula**; and (c) the **perforating branch** which pierces the interosseous membrane just above the inferior tibiofibular joint and anastomoses with the lateral tarsal branch of the dorsalis pedis artery. The fibular artery gives the lateral malleolar and calcanean branches and ends by anastomosing with the posterior tibial artery on the back of the ankle joint.

2. The circumflex fibular artery runs round the neck of the fibula to supply muscles and skin.

3. A large **nutrient artery to the tibia** arises from the upper end of the posterior tibial artery. It enters the tibia a short distance below the soleal line.

Like other nutrient arteries, it is the main supply to the bone.

4. **Muscular branches** to the deep muscles of the back of the leg.
5. **Cutaneous branches** to the medial side of the leg.
6. A **communicating branch** to the fibular artery behind the ankle joint.
7. **Medial calcanean branches** that run with the corresponding nerves.

Deep muscles of the back of the leg

Popliteus

The popliteus is attached to the lateral condyle of the femur at the anterior end of the popliteal groove [see Fig. 13.21] and to the back of the lateral meniscus inside the capsule of the knee joint. It emerges through the posterior part of the capsule of the knee joint, below the **arcuate popliteal ligament**. The popliteus tendon then expands into a triangular fleshy belly which is attached to the posterior surface of the tibia above the soleal line [Fig. 18.20]. **Nerve supply**: tibial nerve. **Actions**: when the leg is free, it medially rotates the tibia on the femur at the beginning of knee flexion. When the foot is on the ground, it laterally rotates the femur on the tibia. Both movements 'unlock' the extended knee joint and allow flexion to occur. The attachment to the meniscus ensures that the meniscus moves with the femoral condyle and is not caught between the femur and the tibia.

The remaining deep muscles—flexor hallucis longus, flexor digitorum longus, and tibialis posterior—have considerable attachments to the intermuscular septa and the interosseous membrane, in addition to the bones. Note that, for muscles of the lower limb, the more distal attachments are often fixed because the foot is on the ground: The actions given for the following muscles are stated as though the distal attachment was free to move, but the reverse action occurs with equal frequency. This is especially true of muscles that stabilize the trunk on the hip joint and the femur on the tibia. The terms 'origin' and 'insertion' are used to differentiate the more proximal from the more distal attachment, rather than the more fixed from the more movable one.

Flexor hallucis longus

The flexor hallucis longus is much larger than the flexor digitorum longus—a feature determined by the relatively larger forces applied to the hallux, when compared to the other toes. It arises from the posterior surface of the fibula, below the origin of the soleus [Fig. 18.20]. Its tendon descends obliquely over the back of the ankle joint and enters the sole of the foot. In its course, the tendon lies in almost continuous bony grooves on the posterior surfaces of the tibia [Fig. 18.2] and the talus, and the inferior surface of the **sustentaculum tali**. It is inserted into the distal phalanx of the great toe. **Nerve supply**: tibial nerve. **Actions**: it flexes the metatarsophalangeal and interphalangeal joints of the great toe, and assists with plantar flexion of the ankle. These are important movements in the last phase of the 'push-off' in walking and running.

Flexor digitorum longus

The flexor digitorum longus arises from the medial part of the posterior surface of the tibia, distal to the soleal line [Fig. 18.20]. It descends behind

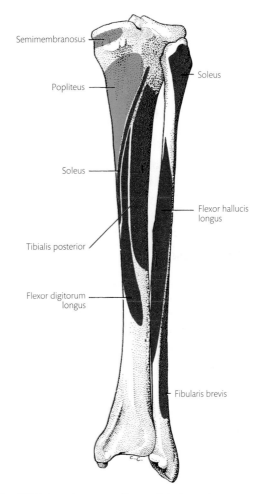

Fig. 18.20 Posterior aspect of bones of the leg to show attachments of muscles.

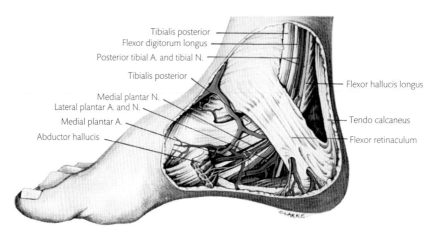

Fig. 18.21 Dissection of the medial side of the ankle, showing the structures deep to the flexor retinaculum.

the tendon of the tibialis posterior, and its tendon grooves the back of the tibia, just medial to the medial malleolus. It passes deep to the flexor retinaculum, enters the sole of the foot, and divides into four tendons, one to the terminal phalanx of each of the lateral four toes [Figs. 18.19, 18.21]. **Nerve supply**: tibial nerve. **Actions**: it flexes the metatarsophalangeal and interphalangeal joints of the lateral four toes, and assists with plantar flexion of the ankle joint. It may play a part in inversion of the foot.

Tibialis posterior

The tibialis posterior arises from the posterior surface of the interosseous membrane and the adjoining parts of the tibia and fibula [Figs. 18.19, 18.20]. Distally, its tendon grooves the posterior surface of the medial malleolus and passes deep to the flexor retinaculum. In the foot, it crosses the inferior surface of the head of the talus and is inserted mainly into the tuberosity of the navicular bone. It also sends strong slips to all the other tarsal bones (except the talus) and to the middle three metatarsals. **Nerve supply**: tibial nerve. **Actions**: it plantar flexes the foot and also inverts it because of its extensions to the lateral tarsal bones.

Flexor retinaculum

This thick band of fascia passes from the medial malleolus to the medial process of the tubercle of the calcaneus. It is continuous proximally with the deep fascia of the leg and with the septum which covers the deep muscles [Fig. 18.21]. Distally, it is

continuous with the deep fascia of the sole and gives attachment to the abductor hallucis muscle.

Beneath the retinaculum lie the tendons of the tibialis posterior, flexor digitorum longus, flexor hallucis longus, posterior tibial vessels, and the tibial nerve. The vessels and nerves lie between the tendons of the flexor digitorum longus and flexor hallucis longus. They divide into the medial and lateral plantar vessels and nerves, deep to the retinaculum [Fig. 18.21]. The position of the muscles of the leg within the fascial compartments is shown in Fig. 18.22.

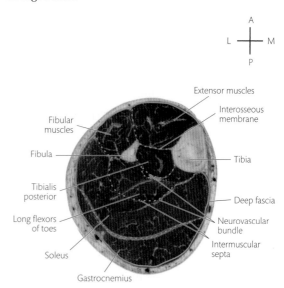

Fig. 18.22 Transverse section through the middle of the leg. A = anterior; P = posterior; M = medial; L = lateral.

Image courtesy of the Visible Human Project of the US National Library of Medicine.

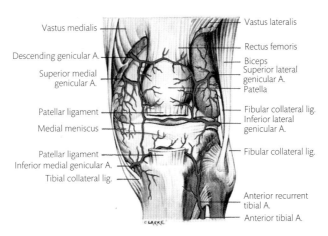

Labels on figure:
Vastus medialis — Descending genicular A. — Superior medial genicular A. — Patellar ligament — Medial meniscus — Patellar ligament — Inferior medial genicular A. — Tibial collateral lig.

Vastus lateralis — Rectus femoris — Biceps — Superior lateral genicular A. — Patella — Fibular collateral lig. — Inferior lateral genicular A. — Fibular collateral lig. — Anterior recurrent tibial A. — Anterior tibial A.

CLARKE

Fig. 18.23 Arterial anastomosis on the front and sides of the left knee joint.

Synovial sheaths

The tendons deep to the flexor retinaculum are each surrounded by a synovial sheath. The synovial sheaths begin approximately 2 cm above the tip of the medial malleolus.

Nerves and vessels of joints

Note these general features in all synovial joints: (1) the nerves which innervate the muscles that move the joint also supply the joint; and (2) all arteries in the region of the joint send branches to it. The arteries form a circular anastomosis around each bone taking part in the joint [Fig. 18.23] and supply the articular capsule and intracapsular bone.

Dissection 18.10 instructs on dissection of the nerves and vessels of the knee joint.

Nerves of the knee joint

1. The **femoral nerve** supplies the anterosuperior part of the joint through the nerves to the three vasti muscles. The nerve from the vastus medialis accompanies the descending genicular artery.
2. The **common fibular nerve** supplies the lateral part of the joint through the superior and inferior lateral genicular nerves and the recurrent genicular nerve.
3. The **tibial nerve** supplies the medial and posterior parts of the articular capsule and the central

---

DISSECTION 18.10 Nerves and vessels of the knee joint

Objective

I. To clean and trace the genicular arteries and nerves.

Instructions

1. As most of the structures around the knee joint have been dissected, it is possible to follow the various nerves and arteries to the knee.
2. Find again the genicular branches of the popliteal artery and the tibial and common fibular nerves. Follow the inferior lateral genicular artery to the fibular collateral ligament of the knee joint.
3. Cut through the tendon of the biceps above the knee, and turn it downwards to expose the fibular collateral

ligament. Follow the artery and nerve between the ligament and articular capsule.

4. Trace the inferior medial genicular artery and nerve along the upper border of the popliteus, till they disappear deep to the superficial part of the tibial collateral ligament of the knee joint.
5. Turn the tendons of the sartorius, gracilis, and semitendinosus forwards, and find the artery and nerve emerging from beneath the ligament.
6. Cut the popliteus near its tendon, and turn the muscle medially. This exposes the nerve to the popliteus.

structures within the capsule through the superior medial, middle, and inferior medial genicular nerves. They run with the corresponding arteries [Fig. 18.23].

4. The **obturator nerve** sends a branch to the posterior surface of the knee joint.

Anastomosis around the knee joint

Numerous arteries [see Figs. 15.4, 18.23] contribute to the anastomosis around the knee joint: two lateral and two medial genicular arteries from the popliteal artery; the descending genicular artery from the femoral artery; the genicular artery from the lateral circumflex femoral artery; and the anterior and posterior tibial recurrent arteries. They anastomose with each other mainly in front of the joint. (The middle genicular artery plays little part in the anastomosis, since it supplies mainly the structures that lie within the knee joint.) The anastomosis around the knee is insufficient to maintain blood flow to the distal part of the limb when the popliteal artery is blocked.

Anastomosis around the ankle joint

On the lateral side, the lateral malleolar branch of the anterior tibial artery and the lateral tarsal branch of the dorsalis pedis artery anastomose with the perforating and terminal branches of the fibular artery. On the medial side, the medial malleolar branch of the anterior tibial artery anastomoses with the medial calcanean branches of the posterior tibial artery. The posterior tibial artery also anastomoses with the fibular artery, posterior to the ankle joint.

Sole of the foot

Begin by revising the surface anatomy of the region of your own foot. Make certain that you can identify the palpable parts of the bones and the major tendons entering the foot from the leg. Note also the parts of the foot which are in contact with the ground in standing, in the various phases of walking, and in running.

The foot has many features in common with the hand. The differences are related to the function of the foot. The foot is a supporting structure carrying considerable loads in standing, and even greater loads in kicking, pushing off in running, and landing on the feet when jumping from a height. The foot is designed to be strong and resilient, unlike the hand which is designed for holding and grasping. Strength is obtained by having large tarsal and big toe bones held together by powerful ligaments. The binding of the metatarsal bone of the big toe to those of the other toes adds to the stability of the foot. Unlike in the hand, there is no opposition of the big or little toe and no muscles equivalent to the opponens muscles of the hand. Resilience is obtained by the presence of multiple joints, each of which has limited movement, and by the arrangement of the bones in an arch where tension between the components is altered in different positions of the foot. When standing, the weight of the body is supported on the heel and on the heads of the metatarsals (mainly the first metatarsal), and to a lesser extent on the lateral border of the sole of the foot. When moving forwards, the force is carried principally on the head of the first metatarsal and the big toe. (The remaining metatarsals and toes are relatively weak and can be looked upon as a stabilizing flap.) The arched shape of the foot has another advantage. It gives protection to the structures in the sole which would otherwise be subjected to the weight of the body. One special development to resist the pressure on the head of the first metatarsal is the presence of two **sesamoid bones** on its plantar surface. These transmit the pull of the small muscles of the big toe, without subjecting them to pressure, and also make a tunnel through which the tendon of the flexor hallucis longus can reach the toe.

See Dissection 18.11 for instruction on the dissection of the sole of the foot.

Superficial fascia

This fascia is dense, especially over the heel and the ball of the foot. It contains loculi of fat in dense fascial pockets. The fat make the sole firm and resilient.

The skin and superficial fascia of the sole are supplied by three sets of nerves and vessels: the **medial calcanean** nerves and vessels in the region of the heel; the branches of the **medial** and **lateral plantar** nerves and vessels in the greater part of the sole; and the **plantar digital** nerves and vessels in the toes [Fig. 18.24].

Deep fascia

In the sole, the deep fascia is extremely thick in the intermediate region (plantar aponeurosis) but

DISSECTION 18.11 Sole of the foot-1

Objectives

I. To reflect the skin.   II. To clean the superficial fascia of the sole of the foot.

Instructions

1. Cut longitudinally through the skin and superficial fascia of the sole, from the heel to the root of the middle toe. Avoid cutting into the deep fascia (plantar aponeurosis).

2. Strip the skin and superficial fascia from the deep fascia with a knife. The superficial fascia, like that of the palm, is dense and firmly bound to the deep fascia. It has fat packed tightly in its interstices, so that it forms a firm pad, especially over the weight-bearing areas. (Stripping the skin and superficial fascia in one piece removes the cutaneous vessels and nerves [Fig. 18.24], but they are difficult to follow through the dense fascia.)

3. On the lateral and medial sides, remove the fascia with care, so as to retain the digital nerves to the medial side of the big toe and the lateral side of the little toe. These become superficial further proximally, when compared with the other plantar digital nerves [Fig. 18.24].

4. Make a longitudinal incision through the skin on the plantar surface of each toe. Reflect the skin, and find the plantar digital vessels and nerves. Follow them to the ends of the toes.

5. Expose the deep fascia of the toes. This is thickened to form the fibrous flexor sheath—a dense tunnel enclosing the flexor tendons in the toes.

6. Define the plantar aponeurosis, and note the furrows at its edges. The branches of the medial and lateral plantar vessels and nerves pass through these furrows to the skin of the sole. As you approach the toes, take care not to damage the plantar metatarsal arteries and common plantar digital nerves which become superficial between the slips of the plantar aponeurosis to the toes.

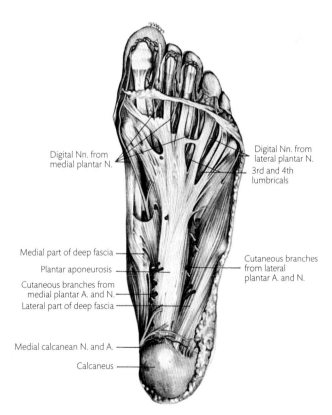

Fig. 18.24 Superficial dissection of the sole of the foot to show plantar aponeurosis. The skin and superficial fascia have been removed, and the fibrous flexor sheaths partially opened.

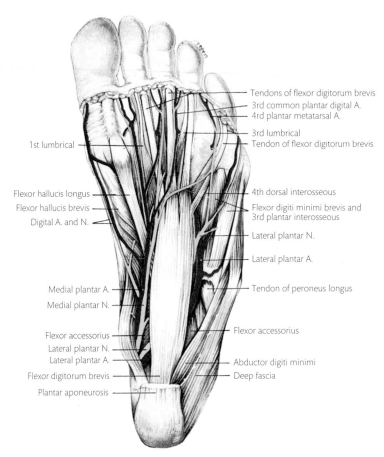

Flexor hallucis longus
Flexor hallucis brevis
Digital A. and N.
1st lumbrical

Medial plantar A.
Medial plantar N.

Flexor accessorius
Lateral plantar N.
Lateral plantar A.
Flexor digitorum brevis
Plantar aponeurosis

Tendons of flexor digitorum brevis
3rd common plantar digital A.
4rd plantar metatarsal A.
3rd lumbrical
Tendon of flexor digitorum brevis
4th dorsal interosseous
Flexor digiti minimi brevis and
3rd plantar interosseous
Lateral plantar N.
Lateral plantar A.
Tendon of peroneus longus
Flexor accessorius
Abductor digiti minimi
Deep fascia

Fig. 18.25 Superficial dissection of the sole of the foot. The plantar aponeurosis has been removed. The abductor digiti minimi and abductor hallucis have been pulled aside.

is thin medially and laterally where it covers the abductors of the big and little toes. The plantar aponeurosis is separated from the lateral and medial parts by shallow furrows, through which the cutaneous branches of the plantar vessels and nerves enter the skin of the sole [Fig. 18.25].

Plantar aponeurosis

The plantar aponeurosis is a thick layer of deep fascia attached posteriorly to the medial process on the plantar surface of the calcaneus. Anteriorly, it splits into five slips which pass to each toe. The margins of each slip curve dorsally over the sides of the flexor tendons and are attached to the plantar ligament of the metatarsophalangeal joint. The intermediate part is attached to the proximal end of the fibrous flexor sheath—the same arrangement as in the hand. Thus, each slip of the plantar aponeurosis is firmly bound to the proximal phalanx of a toe by its attachment to the plantar ligament and the fibrous flexor sheath. In being attached to the calcaneus behind and to the phalanges in front,

the plantar aponeurosis acts as a flexible connector between the ends of the longitudinal arch of the foot. It is pulled distally when the toes are forcibly extended, e.g. in pushing off with the foot. This action tightens the aponeurosis and pulls the ends of the arch together, so that it forms a rigid structure against which the push-off can be effective. Check this in your own foot by passively extending your toes with your hand. The plantar aponeurosis can then be seen and felt as a tight band which is relaxed when the toes are flexed [see Fig. 19.17].

Fibrous flexor sheaths

The fibrous flexor sheath in each toe is a thick, fibrous tunnel. It is attached to the margins of the proximal and middle phalanges (proximal only in the big toe), to the base of the distal phalanx, and to the plantar ligaments of the interphalangeal joints. It is relatively thin at the interphalangeal joints, so as not to restrict flexion. The sheath contains the long and short flexor tendons enclosed in a synovial sheath in the lateral four toes, and the

DISSECTION 18.12 Sole of the foot-2

Objective

I. To reflect the plantar aponeurosis and deep fascia.

Instructions

1. Cut across the plantar aponeurosis, 2–3 cm in front of the heel. Split the distal part longitudinally, and lift its parts away from the underlying flexor digitorum brevis. At the margins of this muscle, divide the intermuscular septa, and reflect the aponeurosis distally. Avoid injury to the plantar digital vessels and nerves lying immediately deep to the distal part of the aponeurosis.

2. Remove the deep fascia from the abductor muscles of the hallux and little toe. Retain the plantar digital nerves already found to these toes.

long flexor only in the great toe. Proximally, each sheath is continuous with the plantar aponeurosis.

Dissection 18.12 continues the dissection of the sole of the foot.

Structures in the sole of the foot are placed in a number of layers. These layers have no significance beyond that of description and are not clearly separated from one another. They represent the order in which the structures are uncovered and the general depth at which they lie.

From superficial to deep, the layers consist of:

1. Abductor hallucis, flexor digitorum brevis, abductor digiti minimi, and the plantar digital vessels and nerves distally. This is the first layer of muscles.
2. The proximal parts of the medial and lateral plantar nerves and vessels.
3. The long flexor tendons—flexor hallucis longus and flexor digitorum longus and the flexor accessorius and lumbrical muscles attached to it. This is the second layer of muscles.
4. Flexor hallucis brevis, adductor hallucis, and flexor digiti minimi brevis. This layer is the third layer of muscles.
5. The deep parts of the lateral plantar artery and nerve and their branches.
6. The bones and ligaments of the foot, the tendon of the fibularis longus, insertions of the tibialis posterior to the tarsal and metatarsal bones, the interosseous muscles, and perforating branches of the plantar metatarsal arteries. This layer is the fourth layer of muscles.

In general, the more superficial a muscle in the sole of the foot, the more likely it is to be long and to be attached to the ends of the arch, i.e. from heel to toe. Also the action of the superficial muscles helps to maintain the plantar arch. The muscles are important in drawing the bones of the arch together when the arch is subjected to powerful forces during activity. They also protect the ligaments from the more severe stresses.

Muscles in the sole of the foot–first layer

Flexor digitorum brevis

The flexor digitorum brevis takes origin from the medial process of the tubercle of the calcaneus and the plantar aponeurosis [Fig. 18.26]. It gives rise to four tendons to the lateral four toes. Each tendon enters the fibrous flexor sheath of the toe and divides into two parts which curve over the long flexor tendon to the plantar surface of the middle phalanx. **Nerve supply**: medial plantar nerve. **Actions**: it flexes the metatarsophalangeal and proximal interphalangeal joints of the lateral four toes, and helps to reinforce the longitudinal arch of the foot.

Abductor hallucis

The abductor hallucis arises from the flexor retinaculum and the medial process of the tubercle of the calcaneus [Fig. 18.26]. Part of the medial belly of the flexor hallucis brevis and the medial part of the extensor expansion formed by the extensor hallucis longus fuse with the tendon of the abductor hallucis and are inserted on the plantar aspect and adjacent medial surface of the proximal phalanx of the big toe. This plantar insertion of the abductor hallucis makes it less efficient as an abductor of the big toe (see Hallux valgus, p. 280). **Nerve supply**: medial plantar nerve. **Actions**: it moves the big toe away from the second toe, i.e. it abducts it at the metatarsophalangeal joint. It is often mainly a flexor of this joint.

Abductor digiti minimi

The abductor digiti minimi arises from both processes of the tubercle of the calcaneus [Fig. 18.26] and is inserted into the lateral side of the base of the proximal phalanx of the little toe. Part of the muscle is fused with the plantar fascia, which extends between the lateral process of the calcaneal tubercle and the base of the fifth metatarsal. **Nerve**

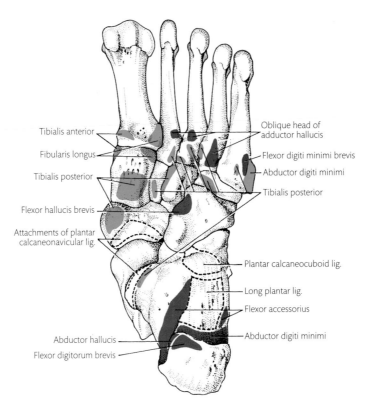

Tibialis anterior

Fibularis longus

Tibialis posterior

Flexor hallucis brevis

Attachments of plantar
calcaneonavicular lig.

Oblique head of
adductor hallucis

Flexor digiti minimi brevis

Abductor digiti minimi

Tibialis posterior

Plantar calcaneocuboid lig.

Long plantar lig.

Flexor accessorius

Abductor digiti minimi

Abductor hallucis

Flexor digitorum brevis

Fig. 18.26 Muscle attachments to the left tarsus and metatarsus (plantar aspect). Interrupted lines show areas of attachment of ligaments.

supply: lateral plantar nerve. **Action**: it abducts the little toe.

Dissection 18.13 continues the dissection of the sole of the foot.

Plantar nerves

The medial and lateral plantar nerves are terminal branches of the **tibial nerve** and arise deep to the flexor retinaculum. They enter the sole of the foot, with the corresponding branches of the posterior tibial artery deep to the abductor hallucis.

The **medial plantar nerve** gives branches to the abductor hallucis and flexor digitorum brevis, and runs forwards between them. Here it gives rise to: (1) the **proper plantar digital nerve** to the medial side of the great toe, which also

---

DISSECTION 18.13 Sole of the foot-3

Objectives

I. To identify and study the flexor digitorum brevis, abductor hallucis, abductor digiti minimi, flexor accessorius, lumbricals, and long flexor tendons.   II. To identify and trace the plantar arteries, nerves, and their branches.

Instructions

1. Find the proper plantar digital nerves in the toes [Fig. 18.27], and follow them proximally. At the metatarsals, these nerves unite to form the common plantar digital nerves. Nerves from the medial three interdigital spaces are branches of the medial plantar

nerve. The nerve from the fourth space is from the lateral plantar nerve.

2. Lift the flexor digitorum brevis, and cut across the muscle near its middle. Reflect its parts forwards and backwards, avoiding injury to the common plantar digital nerves which pass superficial to its distal part [Fig. 18.25]. Follow at least one of the tendons to its insertion. Cut the fibrous flexor sheath longitudinally to expose the tendon in the toe.

3. Turn the abductor hallucis medially, and expose the medial and lateral plantar arteries and nerves. Follow the nerves and arteries distally in the foot. Trace their

branches into continuity with the: (a) digital branches already exposed; and (b) branches to the medial side of the big toe and the lateral side of the little toe.

4. Identify the long flexor tendons and the flexor accessorius, deep to the vessels and nerves [Fig. 18.27].

5. Remove the abductor hallucis from the flexor retinaculum.

6. Cut the retinaculum, and follow the plantar nerves and arteries to their origins from the tibial nerve and the posterior tibial artery deep to the retinaculum.

7. Identify and follow the tendon of the tibialis posterior to its insertion into the navicular bone.

8. Follow the tendons of the flexor digitorum longus and flexor hallucis longus into the sole of the foot. As the tendons are separated in the foot, note the small extension from the flexor hallucis longus to the flexor digitorum longus [Fig. 18.28].

9. Note the insertion of the flexor accessorius into the tendon of the flexor digitorum longus and its origin from the calcaneus. Note the branch from the lateral plantar nerve entering the flexor accessorius.

10. Lift the superficial branch of the lateral plantar nerve, and trace its branch to the flexor digiti minimi brevis. Do the same with the medial two digital branches of the medial plantar nerve. The most medial sends a branch to the flexor hallucis brevis; the second sends a branch to the first lumbrical [Fig. 18.25].

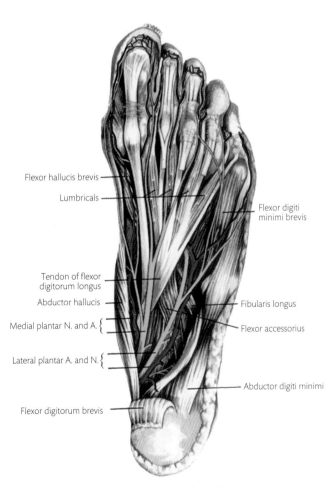

Flexor hallucis brevis

Lumbricals

Flexor digiti minimi brevis

Tendon of flexor digitorum longus

Abductor hallucis

Medial plantar N. and A. {

Fibularis longus

Flexor accessorius

Lateral plantar A. and N. {

Abductor digiti minimi

Flexor digitorum brevis

Fig. 18.27 Dissection of the sole of the foot. Most of the flexor digitorum brevis has been removed.

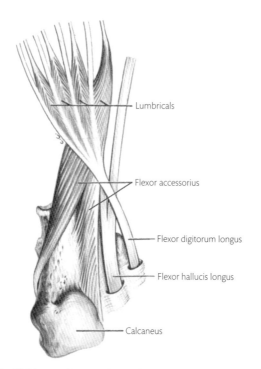

Lumbricals

Flexor accessorius

Flexor digitorum longus

Flexor hallucis longus

Calcaneus

Fig. 18.28 Long flexor tendons in the sole of the foot.

supplies the flexor hallucis brevis; and (2) cutaneous branches to the medial part of the sole of the foot. Further distally, it divides into three **common plantar digital nerves** to the medial three interdigital clefts. The proper plantar nerves to the adjacent sides of the big, second, third, and fourth toes arise from these nerves [Fig. 18.27]. The distribution in the toes is similar to that of the median nerve in the fingers. The medial common plantar digital nerve also supplies the first lumbrical.

The **lateral plantar nerve** passes between the flexor digitorum brevis and flexor accessorius, giving branches to the flexor accessorius and abductor digiti minimi. It then passes forwards and gives cutaneous branches to the lateral part of the sole. It divides into superficial and deep branches.

The **superficial branch** divides into: (1) the **proper plantar digital nerve** to the lateral side of the little toe; and (2) a **common plantar digital nerve** to the fourth interdigital cleft. The nerve to the lateral side of the little toe gives muscular branches to the flexor digiti minimi brevis, the third plantar and fourth dorsal interossei. The common plantar digital nerve gives proper digital nerves to adjacent sides of the fourth and fifth toes. These are distributed in the same manner as the corresponding branches of the medial plantar nerve. The common plantar digital nerve

of the third space (branch of the medial plantar nerve) and the common plantar digital nerve of the fourth space (branch of the lateral plantar nerve) communicate. Because of these communications, there is considerable overlap of the areas supplied by each nerve.

The **deep branch** of the lateral plantar nerve runs medially across the proximal parts of the metatarsals and supplies the remaining small muscles of the foot—adductor hallucis, flexor digiti minimi brevis, lateral three lumbrical muscles, medial two plantar interossei, and medial three dorsal interossei. The distribution of the lateral plantar nerve in the foot is very similar to that of the ulnar nerve in the hand.

Plantar arteries

The **medial** and **lateral plantar** arteries are terminal branches of the posterior tibial artery given off deep to the flexor retinaculum. The **medial plantar artery** runs with the medial plantar nerve, supplying the surrounding structures, and gives branches corresponding to those of the nerve. The medial plantar artery ends by anastomosing with the branch of the first plantar metatarsal artery to the medial side of the big toe.

The **lateral plantar artery** runs with the lateral plantar nerve. It gives branches to the surrounding skin, muscles, and bones, and forms the plantar arch beside the deep branch of the nerve. The arch gives the proper plantar digital artery to the lateral side of the little toe, and **plantar metatarsal arteries** on each intermetatarsal space. Each plantar metatarsal artery communicates with the corresponding **dorsal metatarsal artery** by a **perforating branch** in the proximal part of the space. It forms the **common plantar digital artery** which divides into **proper plantar digital arteries** to the adjacent sides of two toes [Fig. 18.29].

Dissection of the sole of the foot continues in Dissection 18.14.

Muscles in the sole of the foot—second layer

This layer consists of the long flexor tendons and associated muscles [Fig. 18.28]. Note particularly the pulley-like arrangement of the flexor hallucis longus on the plantar surface of the sustentaculum tali, and the slip which it gives to the flexor digitorum longus. Also note that the long flexor tendons cross each other, inferior to the head of the talus.

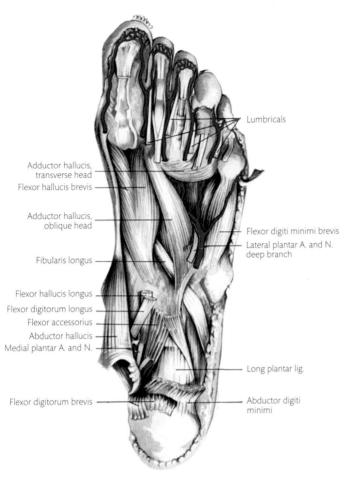

Fig. 18.29 Deep dissection of the sole of the foot.

Labels on figure:
Lumbricals
Adductor hallucis, transverse head
Flexor hallucis brevis
Adductor hallucis, oblique head
Fibularis longus
Flexor hallucis longus
Flexor digitorum longus
Flexor accessorius
Abductor hallucis
Medial plantar A. and N.
Flexor digitorum brevis
Flexor digiti minimi brevis
Lateral plantar A. and N. deep branch
Long plantar lig.
Abductor digiti minimi

DISSECTION 18.14 Sole of the foot-4

Objective

I. To dissect the long flexor tendons, flexor accessorius, and lumbricals.

Instructions

1. Reflect the abductor digiti minimi from its origin, and expose the lateral head of the flexor accessorius.

2. Remove the connective tissue from the long flexor tendons, the flexor accessorius, and the lumbrical muscles. Trace one of the tendons of the flexor digitorum longus through the fibrous flexor sheath to its insertion.

3. Trace one of the medial two lumbricals to the proximal phalanx. Attempt to find the attachment to the extensor expansion.

Flexor accessorius

The flexor accessorius takes origin from both margins of the plantar surface of the calcaneus [Fig. 18.26]. It is inserted into the tendon of the flexor digitorum longus. **Nerve supply**: lateral plantar nerve. **Action**: it assists in flexing the toes by aligning the tendon of the flexor digitorum longus to the toes.

Lumbrical muscles

These four small muscles arise from the tendons of the flexor digitorum longus [Fig. 18.28]. One tendon enters the medial side of each of the lateral four toes and is attached to the base of the proximal phalanx and to the extensor expansion. The tendons are inferior to the deep transverse metatarsal ligament and the transverse head of the adductor hallucis [Fig. 18.29]. **Nerve supply**: the first lumbrical is innervated by the medial plantar nerve, and the other three by the lateral plantar nerve. **Actions**: they are weak muscles, but they play a part in the flexion of the metatarsophalangeal joints of the lateral four toes, and they may also extend their interphalangeal joints. ➲ As in the hand, their paralysis prevents the extension of the interphalangeal joints when the metatarsophalangeal joints are fully extended by the extensor muscles. This leads to a condition known as 'hammer toe', in which the metatarsophalangeal joints of the lateral four toes are fully extended, the proximal interphalangeal joints are flexed (by the flexor digitorum brevis), and the distal interphalangeal joints are extended due to pressure on the ground.

Flexor tendons in the toes

The arrangement of the flexor tendons and the fibrous flexor sheaths of the toes are the same as in the fingers. The **synovial sheaths** begin distal to the attachment of the lumbrical muscles, and extend to the base of the distal phalanx where these tendons are inserted. The sheath of the little toe may be continuous with the synovial sheath around the main tendon of the flexor digitorum longus. The sheath of the flexor hallucis longus extends from the lower part of the leg to the insertion of the tendon into the distal phalanx of the great toe. It is incomplete where it connects with the flexor digitorum longus. The tendons within the toes have the same arrangement of **vinculae** as the tendons in the fingers.

Dissection of the sole of the foot continues in Dissection 18.15.

Muscles in the sole of the foot–third layer

Flexor hallucis brevis

This powerful muscle arises from the plantar surface of the cuboid bone [Fig. 18.26] and the adjoining fascia. It divides into two bellies which are inserted into the medial and lateral margins of the plantar surface of the proximal phalanx of the big toe. The medial belly is inserted with the tendon of the abductor hallucis, and the lateral with the adductor hallucis. Each tendon contains a sesamoid bone [see Fig. 19.14]. **Nerve supply**: medial plantar nerve. **Actions**: it flexes the metatarsophalangeal joint of the big toe and produces slight adduction because of its obliquity.

DISSECTION 18.15 Sole of the foot-5

Objective

I. To transect the muscles and tendons of the second layer—flexor accessorius, flexor digitorum longus, and flexor hallucis longus.

Instructions

1. Divide the flexor accessorius and the tendons of the flexor digitorum longus and flexor hallucis longus close to where they unite. Reflect the distal parts of the tendons to uncover the three muscles which form the fourth layer [Fig. 18.29].

2. If needed, cut across the medial plantar nerve, and reflect it distally to permit sufficient reflection of the tendons.

3. As the flexor digitorum is turned back, look for the branches of the deep branch of the lateral plantar nerve to the lateral three lumbrical muscles.

Adductor hallucis

The adductor hallucis takes origin from an oblique and a transverse head. The oblique head is from the base of the middle three metatarsals and from the tendon of the fibularis longus. The transverse head is from the deep transverse metatarsal ligament and the plantar ligaments of the lateral four metatarsophalangeal joints [Fig. 18.29]. The two heads fuse together and are inserted into the lateral margin of the proximal phalanx of the big toe, along with the lateral head of the flexor hallucis brevis. **Nerve supply**: deep branch of the lateral plantar nerve. **Actions**: the oblique head adducts and flexes the metatarsophalangeal joint of the big toe. The transverse head draws the plantar surface of the roots of the toes together and so increases the transverse metatarsal arch.

Flexor digiti minimi brevis

The flexor digiti minimi brevis arises from the base of the fifth metatarsal [Fig. 18.26] and is inserted into the lateral side of the base of the proximal phalanx of the little toe. **Nerve supply**: superficial branch of the lateral plantar nerve. **Action**: flexion of the metatarsophalangeal joint of the little toe.

See Dissection 18.16 for further instructions on dissection of the sole of the foot.

DISSECTION 18.16 Sole of the foot-6

Objectives

I. To expose and study the flexor hallucis brevis, adductor hallucis, and flexor digiti minimi brevis.

II. To identify and trace the deep branch of the lateral plantar nerve, the plantar arch, and their branches.

Instructions

1. Define the attachments of the flexor hallucis brevis, adductor hallucis, and flexor digiti minimi brevis. Avoid injury to the deep branch of the lateral plantar nerve, the plantar arch, and their branches.

2. Detach the flexor hallucis brevis and the oblique head of the adductor from their origins. Turn them forwards to expose the nerve and artery.

3. Cut across the abductor hallucis. Turn its distal part forwards with the flexor hallucis brevis. Define their common insertion, and identify the sesamoid bone in their tendon. Cut this tendon and the bone away from the articular capsule of the first metatarsophalangeal joint. Note that the sesamoid bone rests directly on the head of the first metatarsal.

4. Find the nerves to the oblique and transverse heads of the adductor. Then trace the deep branch of the lateral plantar nerve, the plantar arch, and their branches.

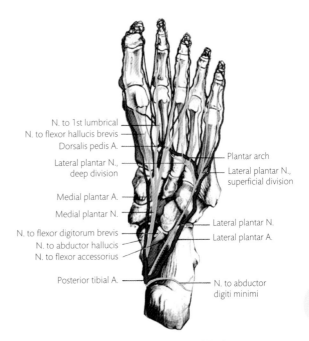

Fig. 18.30 Arteries and nerves of the sole of the foot.

N. to 1st lumbrical
N. to flexor hallucis brevis
Dorsalis pedis A.
Lateral plantar N., deep division
Medial plantar A.
Medial plantar N.
N. to flexor digitorum brevis
N. to abductor hallucis
N. to flexor accessorius
Posterior tibial A.
Plantar arch
Lateral plantar N., superficial division
Lateral plantar N.
Lateral plantar A.
N. to abductor digiti minimi

253

Sesamoid bones of the foot

There are two small sesamoid bones in each of the tendons of the flexor hallucis brevis. They extend beyond the tendons, through the plantar ligament of the metatarsophalangeal joint of the big toe, and articulate with the plantar surface of the head of the metatarsal. This arrangement increases the size of the metatarsal head of the big toe. The bones also protect against compression and devascularization of the tendons of the flexor hallucis brevis and longus. (Sesamoid bones or cartilages are also found in the tendons of the fibularis longus and tibialis posterior as they enter the sole.)

Deep branch of the lateral plantar nerve

The deep branch arises from the lateral plantar nerve at the base of the fifth metatarsal and runs medially on the proximal parts of the metatarsal bones and the interosseous muscles [Fig. 18.30]. It

is deep to the oblique head of the adductor hallucis and ends in it. It supplies the adductor hallucis, the lateral three lumbrical muscles, the medial two plantar interossei, and the medial three dorsal interossei. It sends branches to the distal intertarsal, tarsometatarsal, and intermetatarsal joints.

Plantar arch

The plantar arch is a continuation of the lateral plantar artery. It runs with the deep branch of the lateral plantar nerve to the proximal end of the first intermetatarsal space. The arch gives rise to **plantar metatarsal arteries** to each of the intermetatarsal spaces. Each of these arteries communicates with the corresponding dorsal metatarsal artery by a **perforating branch** through the space. The plantar metatarsal arteries form the **common plantar digital arteries**. In the first space, the perforating branch comes from the arcuate artery (**deep plantar branch**) and is mainly responsible for the formation of the plantar metatarsal artery of that space. Each common plantar digital artery divides into two **proper plantar digital arteries** to the adjacent sides of two toes. The proper plantar digital artery to the medial side of the big toe arises from the common plantar digital artery in the first space [Fig. 18.30]. The arch and its branches supply all the surrounding structures, including the bones and joints. The proper digital arteries anastomose with each other and with the dorsal digital arteries in the distal parts of the toes. Thus, there is a very free anastomosis between the branches of dorsalis pedis artery and the plantar arteries. This is well illustrated in the angiogram of the foot [Fig. 18.31].

See Dissection 18.17 for further investigation of the sole of the foot.

Muscles in the sole of the foot—fourth layer

Deep transverse metatarsal ligament

These strong bands of dense connective tissue unite the plantar ligaments of the metatarsophalangeal joints and are attached to the proximal phalanges through them. The ligaments help to prevent the bases of the toes from spreading out, and so maintain the transverse metatarsal arch. The interossei enter the toes, dorsal to these ligaments; the lumbricals and plantar digital nerves and vessels are on their plantar surface.

Interossei

The general arrangement of the interossei is the same as in the hand, except that the second (and not the middle) toe has two dorsal interossei. There is a plantar interosseous to each of the lateral three toes, and four dorsal interossei to the middle three toes. All the interossei are inserted into the bases of the proximal phalanges, with little attachment to the extensor expansion [Fig. 18.32]. **Nerve supply**: lateral plantar nerve. **Actions**: the plantar interossei adduct the lateral three toes to the line of the second toe—the axis of the foot. The dorsal interossei abduct the middle three toes from the axis of the foot. They also flex the metatarsophalangeal joints but usually do not extend the interphalangeal joints.

Tendon of tibialis posterior

This tendon runs over the posterior surface of the medial malleolus (which acts as a pulley for it) and beneath the medial part of the plantar calcaneonavicular ligament to the tuberosity of the navicular bone [Fig. 18.33]. It spreads out to all the other tarsal bones (except the talus) and to the bases of the middle three metatarsals. The powerful **plantar calcaneonavicular ligament** runs from the sustentaculum tali to the navicular. It supports the head of the talus which carries the weight of the body. The downward force exerted by the talus tends to separate the calcaneus and the navicular and stretch the ligament. The tibialis posterior pulls the navicular posteriorly and helps support some of the load on the ligament. Under the ligament, the tibialis posterior tendon contains a piece of fibrocartilage, which is sometimes ossified to form a sesamoid bone. The extensions of the tendon to the other bones pull the plantar surfaces of the bones together, strengthen the arches, and protect the plantar ligaments.

Tendon of fibularis longus

The tendon of the fibularis longus contains a sesamoid bone or cartilage. It turns around the lateral border of the cuboid bone and runs anteromedially in the groove on its plantar surface. The **long plantar ligament** [Fig. 18.33] converts the groove into a tunnel, in which the tendon slides in its synovial sheath. The tendon is inserted into the base of the first metatarsal and the adjacent part of the medial cuneiform bone, close to the insertion of the tibialis anterior. When the fibularis longus

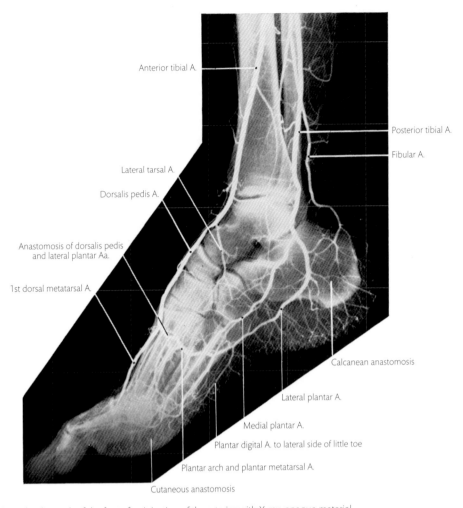

Anterior tibial A.

Posterior tibial A.

Fibular A.

Lateral tarsal A.

Dorsalis pedis A.

Anastomosis of dorsalis pedis and lateral plantar Aa.

1st dorsal metatarsal A.

Calcanean anastomosis

Lateral plantar A.

Medial plantar A.

Plantar digital A. to lateral side of little toe

Plantar arch and plantar metatarsal A.

Cutaneous anastomosis

Fig. 18.31 Lateral radiograph of the foot after injection of the arteries with X-ray-opaque material.

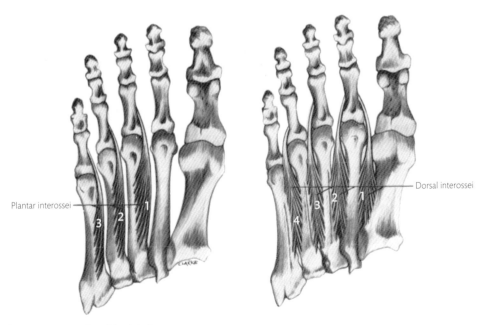

Plantar interossei

Dorsal interossei

Fig. 18.32 Interosseous muscles of the right foot.

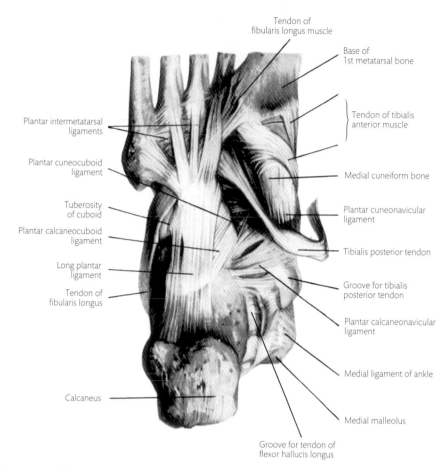

Tendon of
fibularis longus muscle

Base of
1st metatarsal bone

Tendon of tibialis
anterior muscle

Plantar intermetatarsal
ligaments

Plantar cuneocuboid
ligament

Medial cuneiform bone

Tuberosity
of cuboid

Plantar cuneonavicular
ligament

Plantar calcaneocuboid
ligament

Tibialis posterior tendon

Long plantar
ligament

Groove for tibialis
posterior tendon

Tendon of
fibularis longus

Plantar calcaneonavicular
ligament

Medial ligament of ankle

Calcaneus

Medial malleolus

Groove for tendon of
flexor hallucis longus

Fig. 18.33 Plantar aspect of the tarsal and tarsometatarsal joints.

contracts, it everts the foot. Tension developed in its tendon prevents stretching of the ligaments which maintain the transverse arch of the tarsal bones.

See Clinical Applications 18.1, 18.2, 18.3, and 18.4 for some practical implications of the anatomy discussed in this chapter.

CLINICAL APPLICATION 18.1 Varicose veins of the leg

In the long and short saphenous veins, valves ensure that the blood flows upwards towards the heart and is prevented from flowing downwards under the influence of gravity [Fig. 18.34A]. The valves in the perforators ensure that blood flows from superficial to deep, taking advantage of the fact that the deep veins (but not the superficial ones) are emptied by contraction of the surrounding muscles [Fig. 18.34B]. Commonly, one or both saphenous veins become tortuous and dilated, due to incompetency of their valves [Fig. 18.34C]. Venous blood stagnates

and pools in the superficial veins, causing discomfort and pain. As the valves in the perforators are incompetent, blood from the deep veins enters the superficial ones during muscle contraction. As the valves in the superficial veins are incompetent, blood flows distally under the influence of gravity. Varicose veins prevent proper venous return in the lower limb and dam back the entry of arterial blood to the region. This leads to poor nutrition of tissue and non-healing of injuries. Small accidental cuts into the vein wall can lead to rapid exsanguination.

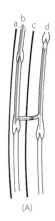 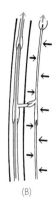 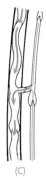

(A)   (B)   (C)

Fig. 18.34 Diagrams to show the flow of blood in the superficial and deep veins. (A) Valves in superficial and deep veins preventing downward flow of blood. (B) Deep veins are emptied by contraction of surrounding muscles. (C) Dilatation of the superficial and communicating veins makes their valves incompetent, so that blood flows distally in the superficial veins and from the deep veins to the superficial veins when the muscles contract. a. Skin. b. Superficial vein in the superficial fascia. c. Deep fascia. d. Deep vein.

Sole of the foot

257

CLINICAL APPLICATION 18.2 Intragluteal injection with damage to the common fibular nerve

A 39-year-old man developed sensory loss and foot drop after a poorly administered intragluteal injection. On examination, the patient was found to have sensory loss on the outer side of the right calf and the dorsum of the right foot. He was unable to dorsiflex the ankle and evert the foot. When he was asked to flex his knee and lift his leg, there was noticeable plantar flexion—a condition known as foot drop. He also had difficulty extending his toes.

Study question 1: of the two parts of the sciatic nerve—the tibial and common fibular—which part seems solely involved in this case? (Answer: common fibular nerve.)

Study question 2a: how do you account for the loss of sensation to the lateral side of the calf? (Answer: the lateral cutaneous nerve of the calf and the fibular communicating branch of the sural nerve arise from the common fibular nerve and are damaged.)

Study question 2b: how do you account for the loss of sensation over the dorsum of the foot? (Answer: the dorsum of the foot is supplied by the cutaneous branches of the deep fibular nerve—the first interdigital cleft and adjacent sides of the big and second toes—and by the superficial fibular nerve—the medial side of the big toe, adjacent sides of the second and third toes, adjacent sides of the third and fourth toes, and the medial side of the little toe. Deep and superficial fibular nerves are

branches of the common fibular nerve which is damaged in the gluteal region.)

Study question 3: why is the patient unable to evert his foot? Name the muscles affected and their nerve supply. (Answer: eversion is lost, because the muscles causing eversion—fibularis longus and brevis—supplied by the superficial fibular nerve are denervated.)

Study question 4: why is the patient unable to dorsiflex his foot? Name the muscles affected and their nerve supply. (Answer: dorsiflexion is lost, because the muscles causing dorsiflexion—tibialis anterior, extensor hallucis longus, extensor digitorum longus, fibularis tertius—supplied by the deep fibular nerve are denervated.)

Study question 5: if this were a case of injury to the deep fibular nerve alone, with what neurological signs would the patient present? (Answer: the patient would present with foot drop and an inability to dorsiflex his foot. Sensory loss would be confined to the first interdigital cleft. Eversion and sensation on the rest of the dorsum of the foot would be normal.)

Study question 6: explain why the patient had difficulty extending his toes. (Answer: the patient has lost the use of the extensor hallucis longus and extensor digitorum longus, so his extension is weakened. Extension is still possible, because the interossei extend the toes through their insertion into the extensor expansion.)

CLINICAL APPLICATION 18.3 Anterior compartment syndrome

During football practice, a 20-year-old student experienced severe pain over the anterolateral aspect of his right leg, which radiated down to his ankle. On examination, there was redness and swelling over the anterolateral aspect of his right leg. On palpation, the area was extremely tender and hard, and corresponded to the area of the tibialis anterior. Dorsiflexion of the foot and toes was limited. The dorsalis pedis pulse was well felt. A diagnosis of 'anterior tibial syndrome' was made. The condition is caused by impairment of blood flow to the muscles during strenuous exercise and possibly tearing of muscle fibres and microhaemorrhage. As there was no improvement with conservative treatment, surgical measures were resorted to. The fascia over the anterior aspect of the leg was incised under general anaesthesia, with good results.

Study question 1: name the bony surfaces and fascia which enclose the tibialis anterior. (Answer: the lateral surface of the shaft of the tibia, the anterior surface of the shaft of the fibula, the deep fascia of the leg, and the interosseous membrane [Fig. 18.22].)

Study question 2: name the vessels and nerves in this compartment. (Answer: deep fibular nerve and anterior tibial artery.)

Study question 3: from the given history, how do we know that the artery is not compressed? (Answer: the dorsalis pedis pulse is well felt.)

CLINICAL APPLICATION 18.4 Stress fractures

Weight-bearing bones, such as the tibia and the metatarsals, can develop 'stress fractures'. A stress fracture is a fatigue-induced fracture of the bone, caused by repeated stress over time, and may result from prolonged exercise or from repeated submaximal loading in running or jumping. Because of this mechanism, stress fractures are common overuse injuries in athletes.

CHAPTER 19
The joints of the lower limb

Hip joint

The hip joint is described in Chapter 17.

Knee joint

The massive knee joint is a synovial condylar joint between the condyles of the femur, the condyles of the tibia, and the patella. It carries severe stresses and yet has a wide range of movement. The main movements possible at the knee are flexion, which is limited only by contact between the leg and the thigh, and extension. In addition, a moderate degree of rotation is possible when the knee is flexed. In all positions of the joint, the femur articulates with the tibia and the patella. The strength of the joint depends on ligaments and muscles, rather than on the close fitting of bones. The articular surface on the femoral condyles is long and extends on the anterior, inferior, and posterior surfaces [see Figs. 13.3, 13.4]. The articular area of the tibial condyles is much smaller. As such, at any stage of movement, only a relatively small area of the convex femoral condyle articulates with the corresponding slightly concave tibial condyle. On the tibia, the periphery of the condyles are fitted with C-shaped rims of fibrocartilage—the **medial** and **lateral menisci** [Fig. 19.1]. The medial and lateral menisci extend inwards from the articular capsule between the articular surfaces of the femur and tibia. The ends of the 'C' of both menisci are attached to the median non-articular intercondylar

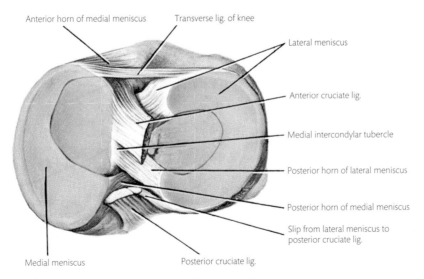

Fig. 19.1 Upper end of the tibia with menisci and portions of the cruciate ligaments.

area of the tibia. The synovial cavity extends over the thin internal edges of the menisci, and between them and the articular surfaces of the bones. The menisci are free to slide on these surfaces as far as their attachments to the articular capsule and tibia permit. The menisci deepen the articular surfaces on the tibia and help to spread the synovial fluid between the weight-bearing surfaces of the femur and tibia.

See Dissection 19.1.

Extracapsular structures of the knee joint

Articular capsule

The fibrous capsule is thin and extensive at the back, but thicker and shorter at the sides. In front, it is replaced from above downwards by the patellar tendon, the patella, and the tendon of the quadriceps. This arrangement allows full range of flexion of the knee, yet maintains necessary tension in the capsule in all positions by the contraction of the quadriceps.

Attachments of the articular capsule

Posteriorly and at the sides, the fibrous capsule is attached close to the articular margins of the tibial condyles, the femoral condyles, and the intercondylar line of the femur. Anteriorly, it follows the oblique lines on the tibia downwards to the sides of the tibial tuberosity and blends with the patellar tendon, the sides of the patella, and the tendon of the quadriceps. The fibrous capsule is perforated in two places: (1) where the tendon of the popliteus emerges from the capsule posterior to the lateral tibial condyle; and (2) where the bursa under the medial head of the gastrocnemius continues with the synovial membrane of the joint at the back of the medial femoral condyle.

Fibrous structures which strengthen the joint

Patellar tendon/patellar ligament

This powerful ligament is the continuation of the quadriceps tendon, inferior to the patella. It extends from the apex and lower parts of the patella to the smooth upper part of the tibial tuberosity. Two important structures lie deep to the ligament. The **infrapatellar pad of fat** separates the upper part of the ligament from the synovial membrane of the knee joint. The **deep infrapatellar bursa** separates the lower part of the ligament from the upper part of the tibia [Fig. 19.2].

Fibular collateral ligament

The fibular collateral ligament is cord-like and extends from the lateral epicondyle of the femur to the head of the fibula. It pierces the tendon of the biceps femoris. It is separated from the fibrous capsule of the joint by fatty tissue, in which the inferior lateral genicular vessels and nerve run. Deep to the ligament, the fibrous capsule is separated from the meniscus by the **tendon of the popliteus** [Fig. 19.3].

Tibial collateral ligament

The tibial collateral ligament is broad and flat. It arises from the medial epicondyle of the femur, in continuation with fibres from the tendon of the adductor magnus. Inferiorly, it splits into two layers. The **deep layer** fuses with the fibrous capsule and the underlying medial meniscus, and passes to the articular margin of the medial condyle of the tibia. The **superficial layer** is inserted into the medial surface of the tibia, anterior to the insertions of the sartorius, gracilis, and semitendinosus. It is separated from the medial condyle of the tibia by the inferior medial genicular vessels and nerve and by the insertion of the semimembranosus [see Fig. 18.13].

Oblique popliteal ligament

This is an extension of the semimembranosus tendon. It arises from the tendon close to its insertion, and runs upwards and laterally to fuse with the fibrous capsule [Fig. 19.4].

Patellar retinacula

These are fibrous expansions from the vastus medialis and lateralis into the fibrous capsule on the medial and lateral sides of the patellar tendon.

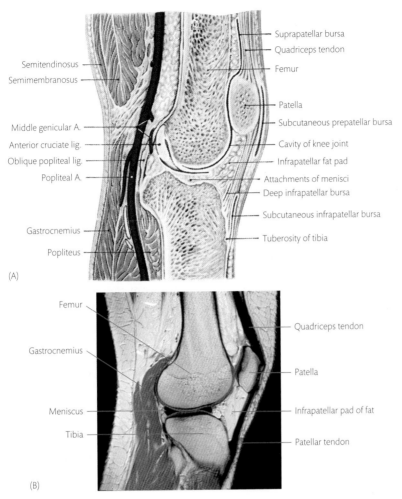

Suprapatellar bursa
Quadriceps tendon
Femur

Semitendinosus
Semimembranosus

Patella
Subcutaneous prepatellar bursa

Middle genicular A.
Anterior cruciate lig.
Oblique popliteal lig.
Popliteal A.

Cavity of knee joint
Infrapatellar fat pad
Attachments of menisci
Deep infrapatellar bursa
Subcutaneous infrapatellar bursa

Gastrocnemius
Popliteus

Tuberosity of tibia

(A)

Femur

Quadriceps tendon

Gastrocnemius

Patella

Meniscus
Tibia

Infrapatellar pad of fat

Patellar tendon

(B)

Fig. 19.2 (A) Sagittal section of the right knee joint. The popliteal vein is not shown. (B) MRI of the knee, sagittal section.

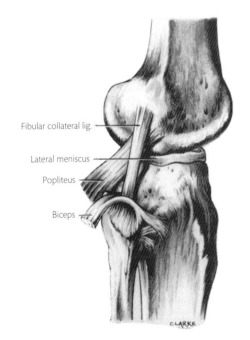

Fibular collateral lig.
Lateral meniscus
Popliteus
Biceps

CLARKE

Fig. 19.3 Fibular collateral ligament of the right knee joint.

Iliotibial tract

The iliotibial tract fuses with the fibrous capsule between the fibular collateral ligament and the patellar tendon.

See Dissection 19.2 which continues with the dissection of the knee joint.

Intracapsular structures of the knee joint

Interior of the knee joint

The cavity of the knee joint may be described as four separate communicating cavities. There is one cavity between the medial femoral and medial tibial condyles, and one between the lateral femoral and lateral tibial condyles. These are separated posteriorly by the synovial membrane which extends from the intercondylar fossa of the femur to the intercondylar area on the superior surface of the tibia. This membrane covers the front and sides of

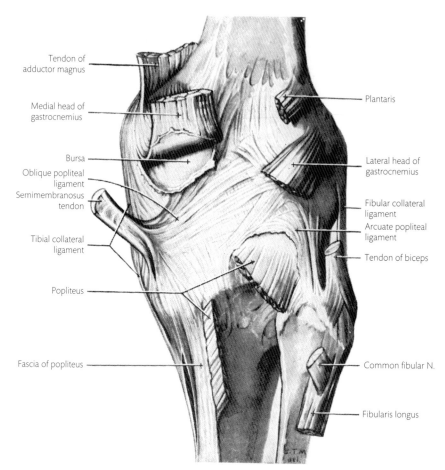

Tendon of
adductor magnus

Medial head of
gastrocnemius

Bursa

Oblique popliteal
ligament
Semimembranosus
tendon

Tibial collateral
ligament

Popliteus

Fascia of popliteus

Plantaris

Lateral head of
gastrocnemius

Fibular collateral
ligament

Arcuate popliteal
ligament

Tendon of biceps

Common fibular N.

Fibularis longus

Fig. 19.4 Posterior aspect of right knee joint.

the cruciate ligaments. The **patellofemoral cavity** lies between the anterior surface of the femur and the patella. The fourth cavity is the **suprapatellar bursa** between the quadriceps tendon and the femur [Fig. 19.2A]. The **infrapatellar fold** of the synovial membrane extends from the posterior surface of the patellar tendon to the anterior margin of the intercondylar fossa of the femur. The infrapatellar fold has a free crescentic margin directed posteriorly [Fig. 19.6].

DISSECTION 19.2 Knee joint-2

Objective

I. To open the knee joint by incising the quadriceps tendon.

Instructions

1. Cut across the quadriceps tendon, immediately proximal to the patella. Carry the ends of this incision downwards to the tibial condyles, passing 2–3 cm on either side of the patellar tendon. Turn the patella down, and expose the cavity of the knee joint [Fig. 19.5].

2. Lift the tendon of the quadriceps, and note that the cavity of the joint extends upwards, deep to it, to form the suprapatellar bursa. Split the lower part of the quadriceps longitudinally, and examine the extent of the bursa.

3. Flex and extend the joint. Note the type of movement which occurs between the tibia and femur.

4. Examine the infrapatellar fold [Fig. 19.6].

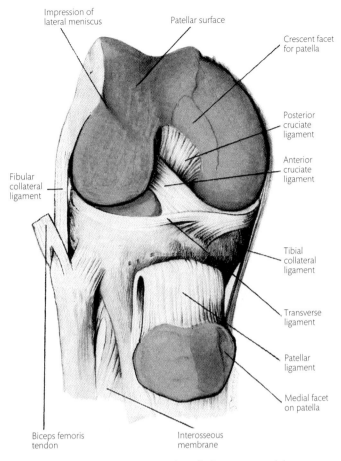

Fig. 19.5 Dissection of the right knee from the front—the patella and patellar ligament turned down.

Synovial membrane

The synovial membrane lines the capsule of the knee joint, except in the posterior part where it turns forwards to surround the cruciate ligaments [Fig. 19.6]. It also covers the non-articular structures within the fibrous capsule, i.e. the infrapatellar pad of fat and the tendon of the popliteus. It separates the popliteus tendon from the lateral condyle of the femur. The synovial membrane does not cover the articular surfaces of the bones and the menisci but lines the **suprapatellar bursa**.

See Dissection 19.3 for instructions on continuing dissection of the knee joint.

Cruciate ligaments

These ligaments cross each other like the letter 'X', which accounts for their name.

The **anterior cruciate ligament** passes from the anterior part of the intercondylar area of the tibia [Fig. 19.1] to the posterior part of the medial surface of the lateral condyle of the femur [Fig. 19.7].

The **posterior cruciate ligament** passes from the posterior part of the tibial intercondylar area [Figs. 19.1, 19.7] to the anterior part of the lateral surface of the medial condyle of the femur. It receives one or more slips from the posterior part of the lateral meniscus (**meniscofemoral ligaments**). The cruciate ligaments hold the femur to the tibia and prevent it from sliding forwards (posterior cruciate) or backwards (anterior cruciate) on the flat upper surface of the tibia. Both ligaments remain relatively tight throughout flexion and extension of the knee joint, but do not prevent these movements because their attachments to the femur are close to the axis of the movements.

However, towards the end of extension, the anterior cruciate ligament becomes tight and prevents the lateral femoral condyle from sliding back on the tibia. At this stage of extension, the medial condyle continues to slide back on the tibia, producing medial rotation of the femur on the tibia. This process screws home the joint and 'locks' it in extended position.

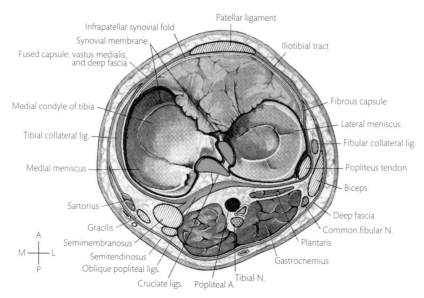

Infrapatellar synovial fold
Synovial membrane
Fused capsule, vastus medialis, and deep fascia
Patellar ligament
Iliotibial tract
Medial condyle of tibia
Tibial collateral lig.
Medial meniscus
Sartorius
Gracilis
Semimembranosus
Semitendinosus
Oblique popliteal ligs.
Cruciate ligs.
Popliteal A.
Tibial N.
Gastrocnemius
Plantaris
Common fibular N.
Deep fascia
Biceps
Popliteus tendon
Fibular collateral lig.
Lateral meniscus
Fibrous capsule

A
M — L
P

Fig. 19.6 Transverse section through the right knee joint and its surroundings, showing the synovial membrane, red; fascia and ligaments, green. A = anterior; P = posterior; M = medial; L = lateral.

DISSECTION 19.3 Knee joint-3

Objectives

I. To expose and study the tendon of the popliteus.
II. To dissect and study the cruciate ligaments.

Instructions

1. Remove the infrapatellar synovial fold and pad of fat.

2. Remove the posterior part of the fibrous capsule of the knee joint, and follow the middle genicular artery through it to the cruciate ligaments.

3. Define the posterior parts of the anterior and posterior cruciate ligaments, and then remove the synovial membrane and connective tissue from their anterior surfaces. Define their attachments to the femur and tibia [Fig. 19.7].

4. Follow the tendon of the popliteus, and note how it lies between the lateral meniscus and the fibrous capsule of the joint. The fibres of the posterior part of the fibrous capsule which arch over the aperture for the tendon of the popliteus form the **arcuate ligament**.

Menisci

The medial and lateral menisci are C-shaped plates of fibrocartilage which lie on the articular surface of a tibial condyle. They are thick at the periphery, but thin at the free concave edge internally. Both upper and lower surfaces are smooth and articular.

They are mainly attached to the tibia at the following points: (1) to the intercondylar area by their fibrous extremities (horns); and (2) to the margins of the tibial condyles close to where the peripheral part is fused with the articular capsule of the knee joint. Anteriorly, they are connected to each other by the **transverse ligament of the knee**

[Fig. 19.1]. Posterolaterally, the **tendon of the popliteus** lies between the lateral meniscus and the capsule. The **lateral meniscus** is nearly circular (in keeping with the more spherical lateral condyle of the femur). The **medial meniscus** is elongated anteroposteriorly (in keeping with the shape and movements of the medial femoral condyle). Because of the shape of the menisci, the horns of the lateral meniscus are attached closer together on the intercondylar area of the tibia, and the horns of the medial meniscus are attached further apart on the anterior and posterior parts of the tibial intercondylar area [Fig. 19.1]. The meniscofemoral

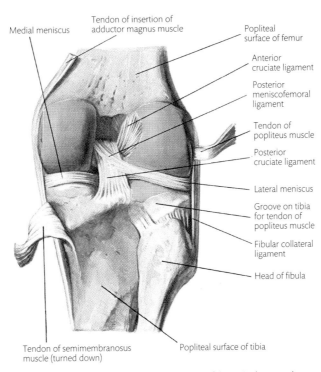

Medial meniscus

Tendon of insertion of
adductor magnus muscle

Popliteal
surface of femur

Anterior
cruciate ligament

Posterior
meniscofemoral
ligament

Tendon of
popliteus muscle

Posterior
cruciate ligament

Lateral meniscus

Groove on tibia
for tendon of
popliteus muscle

Fibular collateral
ligament

Head of fibula

Tendon of semimembranosus
muscle (turned down)

Popliteal surface of tibia

Fig. 19.7 Right knee joint opened from behind by removing the posterior part of the articular capsule.

ligaments enable the lateral meniscus to move with the femur. The medial meniscus is less free to move on the tibia than the lateral meniscus. This limited mobility and the greater anteroposterior movement of the medial condyle of the femur, make the medial meniscus more likely to be trapped and injured between the moving surfaces of the tibia and femur. ➲ Medial meniscus injury occurs especially in sudden turning movements with the foot fixed on the ground, e.g. in sudden changes of direction when running. In such movements, the medial condyle of the femur pivots around the spherical lateral condyle, slides violently on the tibia while under pressure, and may cause the medial meniscus to tear, or be torn from its attachment. If the torn piece of cartilage becomes wedged between the tibia and femur, the joint becomes 'locked' (unable to move) because the ligaments cannot stretch sufficiently to allow the bones to be forced apart. (See Clinical Application 19.1.)

Movements of the knee joint

These are mainly flexion and extension. Flexion proceeds until the calf and thigh are in contact.

Extension stops when the thigh and leg are in a straight line. In this position, the joint is firmly 'locked'. The anterior cruciate, tibial and fibular collateral ligaments, oblique popliteal ligament, and the posterior part of the capsule are taut, and the leg and thigh are converted into a rigid column. Rotation can occur at any phase of flexion. Medial rotation of the femur occurs during the end of extension, and lateral rotation during the start of flexion [Fig. 19.8].

To appreciate the movements of the knee, note that, in full flexion, the posterior surfaces of the femoral condyles articulate with the tibia. In this position, the patella articulates with the crescent-shaped facet on the medial condyle of the femur [Figs. 19.5, 19.8C]. As the knee is extended, the femoral condyles roll forwards and slide backwards on the tibial condyles. (The sliding back is essential, so that the femur can continue to articulate with the limited area for articulation on the tibia.) The points of contact of the femur with the tibia move steadily forwards on the femoral condyles [Fig. 19.8B]. When the lateral condyle reaches its maximum extension (an event which happens before the same thing happens at the medial condyle),

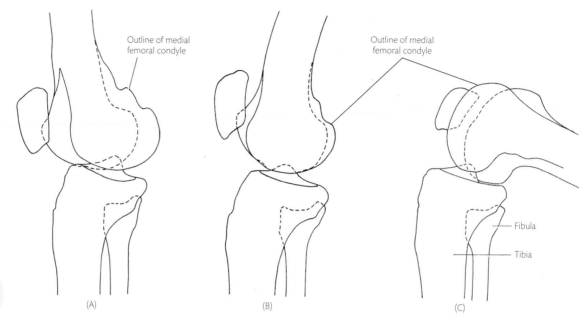

Fig. 19.8 Tracings of three positions of the right knee joint taken from radiographs, showing three phases of flexion of the knee with the foot firmly fixed on the ground. In this way, there is no movement of the tibia and fibula, and the full effects of rotation are visible in the femur. The tracings are viewed from the medial side; the parts that are hidden by the more medial structures are shown as broken lines. (A) Position of full extension with the femur fully rotated medially and the knee joint locked. (B) Slight flexion. Note that there has been considerable lateral rotation of the femur, so that the outlines of the condyles are nearly superimposed. This movement occurs at the very outset of flexion. (C) Considerable flexion of the knee with further lateral rotation of the femur on the tibia.

the groove between its patellar and tibial surfaces [Fig. 19.5] comes into contact with the lateral meniscus, and the condylar movement is stopped by the taut, fully stretched anterior cruciate ligament. Because the anteroposterior curvature of the medial femoral condyle is flatter anteriorly than the more spherical lateral condyle, the medial condyle continues to slide backwards, after the lateral condyle has stopped. Extension is completed by medial rotation of the femur [Fig. 19.8A]. This screws the femur home on the tibia, tightens the ligaments, and 'locks' the knee joint.

Flexion is produced by the same movements in the reverse order. It begins with lateral rotation of the femur because of the differences in shape of the two condyles. This 'unlocks' the knee joint, an action done by the **popliteus**. Once the knee is unlocked, flexion proceeds by the action of the knee flexors.

Rotation of the flexed joint may be produced independently of flexion and extension by the muscles at the sides of the joint. The biceps femoris is the principal lateral rotator of the tibia; the sartorius, gracilis, semitendinosus, and semimembranosus are the main medial rotators.

In addition to the movements between the femur and tibia, during extension, the patella rises to progressively higher levels on the patellar surface of the femur [Fig. 19.8]. Because the pull of the quadriceps on the patella is parallel to the obliquity of the femur, the patella tends to deviate laterally as it ascends. This lateral displacement of the patella is prevented by: (a) the greater anterior projection of the lateral femoral condyle; and (b) the lowest fibres of the vastus medialis which are inserted horizontally into the medial surface of the patella. These factors help to keep the pull of the quadriceps at right angles to the axis of flexion and extension of the knee.

In learning these many details, you should not lose sight of the fact that the knee joint is essentially a hinge joint. The axis for the movement passes through an almost straight line through the femoral attachments of the collateral and cruciate ligaments. Study the AP and lateral X-rays of the knee joint, using Fig. 19.9.

Tables 19.1 and 19.2 summarize the muscles and movements of the knee joint. The origin, insertion, nerve supply, and action of muscles acting on the knee are listed in Table 19.1. (Only details of

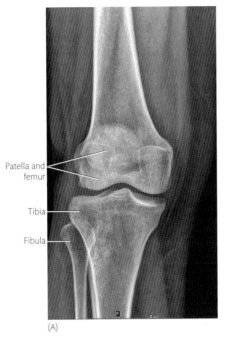
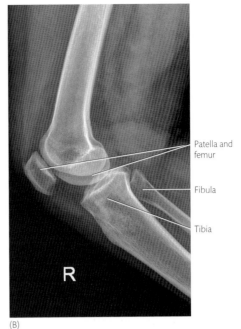

Fig. 19.9 Normal X-ray of the knee. (A) AP view. (B) Lateral view.

muscle attachments that are relevant to the understanding of the muscle actions are listed.)

Ankle joint

The ankle joint is a strong synovial hinge joint between the inferior aspect and medial malleolus of tibia, the lateral malleolus of the fibula, and the trochlea of talus. It is stable because of: (1) the powerful ligaments and tendons around it; and (2) the relatively great depth of the socket formed by the medial and lateral malleoli within which the trochlea of the talus is fitted. The socket offers flexibility because of the body of the fibula. If the talus is forced laterally, the lateral malleolus moves outwards (a movement accompanied by medial movement of the shaft of the fibula acting with the tibiofibular ligaments as a fulcrum). In extreme cases, this may lead to fracture of the fibula in the leg. The socket of the ankle joint is deepened posteriorly by the inferior part of the posterior tibiofibular ligament (transverse tibiofibular ligament [see Fig. 19.12]).

See Dissection 19.4.

Capsule of the ankle joint

As the ankle joint is a hinge joint, the main ligaments are lateral and medial. The anterior part of the fibrous capsule is thin and consists mainly of transverse fibres. It extends from the anterior margin of the distal end of the tibia to the superior surface of the neck of the talus. The posterior part of the capsule extends from the posterior margin of the distal end of the tibia and the posterior tibiofibular ligament to the posterior surface of the body of the talus.

Medial (deltoid) ligament

This very strong ligament radiates from the distal border of the medial malleolus to the medial side of the talus, the sustentaculum tali, the medial edge of the plantar calcaneonavicular (spring) ligament, the navicular bone, and the neck of the talus [see Fig. 18.10]. As such, the medial ligament not only strengthens the ankle joint, but also holds the calcaneus and the navicular against the talus.

Lateral ligament

The lateral ligament consists of three bands—the **anterior talofibular ligament**, the **posterior talofibular ligament**, and the **calcaneofibular ligament**. The anterior and posterior ligaments are thickenings of the fibrous capsule. The **anterior talofibular ligament** passes anteriorly from the anterior border of the lateral malleolus to the neck of the talus. The posterior talofibular ligament is much stronger and runs back from the fossa of

Table 19.1 Muscles acting on the knee joint

Muscle	Origin	Insertion	Action	Nerve supply
Biceps femoris long head	Ischial tuberosity	Fibula, head	Flexion Lateral rotation of leg	Sciatic, tibial part
Semimembranosus	Ischial tuberosity	Tibia, medial condyle	Flexion Medial rotation of leg	Sciatic, tibial part
Semitendinosus	Ischial tuberosity	Tibia, medial surface	Flexion Medial rotation of leg	Sciatic, tibial part
Gracilis	Pubis, body and inferior ramus	Tibia, medial surface	Flexion Medial rotation of leg	Obturator
Sartorius	Ilium, anterior superior spine	Tibia, medial surface	Flexion Medial rotation of leg	Femoral
Tensor fasciae latae	Ilium, crest	Tibia, lateral condyle	Extension Stabilizes pelvis on thigh	Superior gluteal
Gluteus maximus superficial three-quarters	Ilium, posterior to posterior gluteal line Sacrum Sacrotuberous ligament	Tibia, lateral condyle	Extension Stabilizes pelvis on thigh	Inferior gluteal
Rectus femoris	Ilium, anterior inferior spine, area above acetabulum	Patella	Extension	Femoral
Vastus medialis	Femur, intertrochanteric line, linea aspera, medial supracondylar line, tendon of adductor magnus	Patella, capsule of knee joint	Extension Medial displacement of patella	Femoral
Vastus intermedius	Femur, body anterior and lateral surfaces	Patella, suprapatellar bursa	Extension Elevates suprapatellar bursa	Femoral
Vastus lateralis	Femur, greater trochanter, linea aspera	Patella, capsule of knee joint	Extension	Femoral
Biceps femoris short head	Linea aspera	Head of fibula	Flexion Lateral rotation of leg	Sciatic, common fibular part
Popliteus	Femur, lateral condyle	Tibia, posterior surface	Medial rotation of leg Flexion	Tibial
Gastrocnemius	Femur, lateral condyle, medial condyle	Calcaneus	Flexion	Tibial
Plantaris	Femur, lateral condyle	Calcaneus	Acts with gastrocnemius	Tibial

DISSECTION 19.4 Ankle joint

Objective

I. To study the capsule and ligaments of the ankle joint.

Instructions

1. Remove the remains of the extensor and flexor retinacula.

2. Cut through, and displace, the tendons which are in contact with the joint, but do not remove them.

3. Define the anterior and posterior parts of the fibrous capsule of the joint. Both are extremely thin and easily damaged. Remove these parts of the capsule, in order to define the strong ligaments at the side of the joint.

4. Identify the medial and lateral ligaments of the ankle joint, and define their attachments [Figs. 19.10, 19.11].

Table 19.2 Movements at the knee joint

Movement	Muscles	Nerve supply
Flexion	Semimembranosus	Sciatic, tibial part
	Semitendinosus	Sciatic, tibial part
	Biceps femoris long head	Sciatic, tibial part
	Biceps femoris short head	Sciatic, common fibular part
	Gracilis	Obturator
	Sartorius	Femoral
	Popliteus	Tibial
	Gastrocnemius	Tibial
Extension	Vastus medialis	Femoral
	Vastus lateralis	Femoral
	Vastus intermedius	Femoral
	Rectus femoris	Femoral
	Gluteus maximus	Inferior gluteal
	Tensor fasciae latae	Superior gluteal
Lateral rotation of leg	Biceps femoris	Sciatic, tibial and common fibular parts
	Gluteus maximus, anterior fibres	Inferior gluteal
	Tensor fasciae latae	Superior gluteal
Medial rotation of leg when knee extended or lateral rotation of thigh when knee flexed	Popliteus	Tibial
	Semimembranosus	Sciatic, tibial part
	Semitendinosus	Sciatic, tibial part
	Gracilis	Obturator
	Sartorius	Femoral

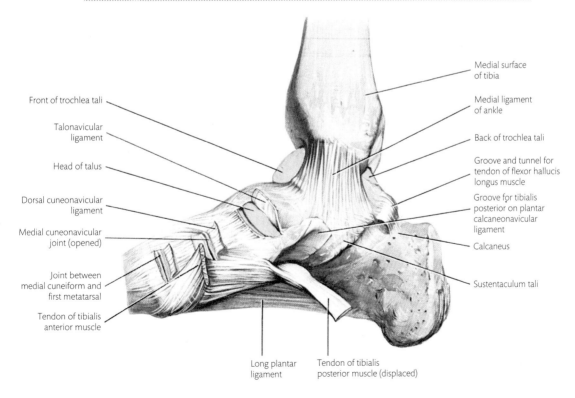

Fig. 19.10 Ankle joint and tarsal joints from the medial side.

Labels on figure:

- Front of trochlea tali
- Talonavicular ligament
- Head of talus
- Dorsal cuneonavicular ligament
- Medial cuneonavicular joint (opened)
- Joint between medial cuneiform and first metatarsal
- Tendon of tibialis anterior muscle
- Long plantar ligament
- Tendon of tibialis posterior muscle (displaced)
- Medial surface of tibia
- Medial ligament of ankle
- Back of trochlea tali
- Groove and tunnel for tendon of flexor hallucis longus muscle
- Groove for tibialis posterior on plantar calcaneonavicular ligament
- Calcaneus
- Sustentaculum tali

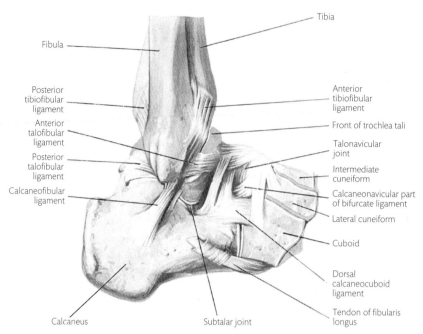

Fig. 19.11 Ligaments of the lateral side of the ankle joint and the dorsum of the tarsus.

the lateral malleolus to the **posterior tubercle of the talus** [Figs. 19.11, 19.12]. The calcaneofibular ligament is a round cord which passes inferiorly from the distal end of the lateral malleolus to the lateral surface of the calcaneus [Figs. 19.11, 19.12]. It is separate from the articular capsule of the ankle joint and functions also as a ligament of the talocalcanean or subtalar joint which it crosses.

Synovial membrane

The synovial membrane lines the fibrous capsule but is separated from it by fat pads which lie deep to the anterior and posterior parts of the capsule. There is a short extension of the synovial membrane between the tibia and fibula, inferior to the thickened lower end of the interosseous membrane.

All structures passing from the leg into the foot (except the tendo calcaneus) lie close to the ankle joint. Tendons, vessels, and nerves from the anterior compartment lie on the anterior surface; those from the posterior compartment lie on the postero-medial surface, and those from the lateral compartment (fibular tendons) lie on the posterolateral surface [Fig. 19.13].

Movements

Plantar flexion and dorsiflexion are the only significant movements at the ankle joint. The trochlea

tali is wide anteriorly, and the socket formed by the malleoli is also broader in front. Thus, the talus fits tightly into the socket when the foot is dorsiflexed. When the foot is plantar flexed, the talus is slightly loose, and some lateral movement is possible.

Tables 19.3 and 19.4 summarize the muscles and movements of the ankle joint.

Tibiofibular joints

The tibia and fibula articulate with each other at their ends and along the shaft. The superior tibiofibular joint is a synovial joint. The inferior tibiofibular joint is a fibrous joint in which the bones articulate with each other through the thickened lower end of the interosseous membrane—the interosseous tibiofibular ligament—and by the anterior and posterior tibiofibular ligaments.

See Dissection 19.5.

Interosseous membrane of the leg

The strong interosseous membrane stretches between the interosseous borders of the tibia and fibula [see Figs. 18.1, 18.2]. It consists of fibres which run downwards and laterally from the tibia to the fibula. There is an oval opening in the upper part of the membrane for the **anterior tibial vessels**,

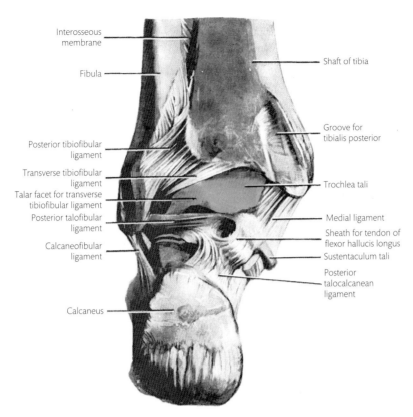

Interosseous membrane

Fibula

Posterior tibiofibular ligament

Transverse tibiofibular ligament

Talar facet for transverse tibiofibular ligament

Posterior talofibular ligament

Calcaneofibular ligament

Calcaneus

Shaft of tibia

Groove for tibialis posterior

Trochlea tali

Medial ligament

Sheath for tendon of flexor hallucis longus

Sustentaculum tali

Posterior talocalcanean ligament

Fig. 19.12 Ankle joint dissected from behind.

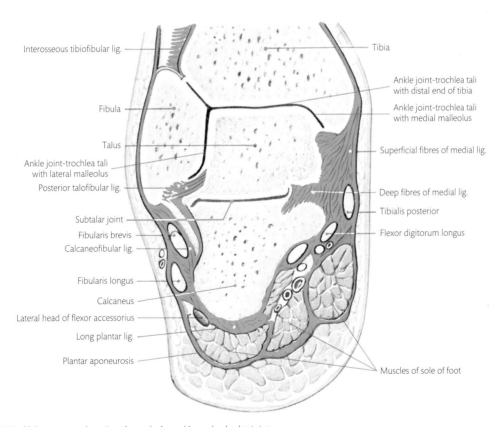

Interosseous tibiofibular lig.

Fibula

Talus

Ankle joint-trochlea tali with lateral malleolus

Posterior talofibular lig.

Subtalar joint

Fibularis brevis

Calcaneofibular lig.

Fibularis longus

Calcaneus

Lateral head of flexor accessorius

Long plantar lig.

Plantar aponeurosis

Tibia

Ankle joint-trochlea tali with distal end of tibia

Ankle joint-trochlea tali with medial malleolus

Superficial fibres of medial lig.

Deep fibres of medial lig.

Tibialis posterior

Flexor digitorum longus

Muscles of sole of foot

Fig. 19.13 Oblique coronal section through the ankle and subtalar joints.

Table 19.3 Muscles acting on the ankle joint

Muscle	Origin	Insertion	Action	Nerve supply
Gastrocnemius	Femur, lateral condyle, medial condyle	Calcaneus	Plantar flexion	Tibial
Plantaris	Femur, lateral condyle	Calcaneus	Plantar flexion	Tibial
Soleus	Tibia, soleal line and medial border Fibula, posterior surface	Calcaneus	Plantar flexion	Tibial
Fibularis longus	Fibula, lateral surface	First metatarsal, base Medial cuneiform	Plantar flexion	Superficial fibular
Fibularis brevis	Fibula, lateral surface	Fifth metatarsal, base	Plantar flexion	Superficial fibular
Tibialis anterior	Tibia, lateral surface Interosseous membrane	First metatarsal, base Medial cuneiform	Dorsiflexion	Tibial
Tibialis posterior	Interosseous membrane Adjacent parts of tibia and fibula	Navicular, tuberosity Medial cuneiform All tarsals, except talus Metatarsal bases, 2–4	Plantar flexion	Tibial
Fibularis tertius	Fibula, anterior surface	Fifth metatarsal base	Dorsiflexion	Deep fibular
Extensor hallucis longus	Fibula, anterior surface	Hallux, base of distal phalanx	Ankle, dorsiflexion Tarsal, inversion Hallux, extension	Deep fibular
Extensor digitorum longus	Fibula, anterior surface	Extensor expansion toes 2–5	Ankle, dorsiflexion Toes, extension 2–5 all joints	Deep fibular
Flexor hallucis longus	Fibula, posterior surface	Hallux, distal phalanx, base	Ankle, plantar flexion Hallux, flexion all joints	Tibial
Flexor digitorum longus	Tibia, posterior surface	Terminal phalanges toes 2–5	Ankle, plantar flexion Toes, 2–5 flexion all joints	Tibial

Table 19.4 Movements at the ankle joint

Movement	Muscles	Nerve supply
Plantar flexion	Gastrocnemius	Tibial
	Soleus	Tibial
	Plantaris	Tibial
	Tibialis posterior	Tibial
	Flexor digitorum longus	Tibial
	Flexor hallucis longus	Tibial
	Peroneus longus	Superficial fibular
	Peroneus brevis	Superficial fibular
Dorsiflexion	Tibialis anterior	Deep fibular
	Extensor hallucis longus	Deep fibular
	Extensor digitorum longus	Deep fibular
	Peroneus tertius	Deep fibular

and a small opening lower down for the **perforating branch of the fibular artery**. The tibialis posterior, the flexor hallucis longus, and all the muscles of the anterior compartment of the leg originate, in part, from the interosseous membrane.

Proximal tibiofibular joint

This joint is between the head of the fibula and the posteroinferior surface of the lateral condyle of the tibia. The articular capsule is attached at the

DISSECTION 19.5 Tibiofibular joints

Objective

I. To study the superior tibiofibular joint and the interosseous membrane.

Instructions

1. Define the anterior and posterior tibiofibular ligaments of the inferior tibiofibular joint [Fig. 19.12].

2. Strip the muscles from the front of the interosseous membrane, and define its attachments. Follow it as far inferiorly as possible. The posterior surface may also be exposed.

3. Define the fibrous capsule of the proximal tibiofibular joint. Reflect the tendon of the popliteus from its posterior surface.

4. Note that the synovial extension from the knee joint deep to the popliteus may be in continuity with the cavity of the proximal tibiofibular joint.

5. Open the joint, and confirm its synovial nature.

articular margins and is strengthened anteriorly and posteriorly by fibres running down and laterally from the tibia to the head of the fibula. The fibular collateral ligament of the knee joint and the tendon of the biceps femoris cross the lateral surface of the joint. The tendon of the popliteus with a synovial extension from the knee joint crosses the posteromedial surface. At this point, the synovial cavities of the two joints may communicate. **Nerve supply**: from the nerve to the popliteus and the recurrent genicular nerve.

Distal tibiofibular joint

At the distal tibiofibular joint, the tibia and fibula are firmly bound together by a strong **interosseous tibiofibular ligament** which extends from the longitudinal groove on the lateral side of the tibia to the rough medial side of the distal part of the fibula.

The interosseous tibiofibular ligament is strengthened and hidden by the **anterior** and **posterior tibiofibular ligaments**. These pass upwards and medially from the corresponding surfaces of the lateral malleolus to the distal end of the tibia and are continuous with the fibrous capsule of the ankle joint. The **transverse tibiofibular ligament**

passes from the malleolar fossa of the fibula to the inferior margin of the posterior surface of the tibia. It forms part of the socket for the ankle joint [Fig. 19.12] and articulates with the body of the talus.

Movements

Only a small amount of movement of the fibula on the tibia is possible. Slight medial movement of the shaft of the fibula occurs when the lateral malleolus is forced laterally by the trochlea of the talus. This movement takes place around the powerful tibiofibular ligaments and increases the stability of the ankle joint.

Joints of the foot

Numerous joints occur between the tarsal, metatarsal, and phalangeal bones. They are: (1) intertarsal joints; (2) tarsometatarsal joints; (3) intermetatarsal joints; (4) metatarsophalangeal joints; and (5) interphalangeal joints.

Arches of the foot

The tarsal and metatarsal bones of the foot together are shaped like half a dome. When the feet are placed together, the two half domes form one single dome. The rim of each half dome consists of the heel, the lateral border of the foot, and the heads of the metatarsal bones. It is these parts of the foot which imprint the ground and form the **footprint** of a bare foot. Each foot has one longitudinal and two transverse arches.

Longitudinal arch

This bony arch is higher on the medial side than on the lateral side of the foot. The talus lies at the top of the arch [Fig. 19.14]. The calcaneus forms the short, thick posterior pillar. The anterior pillar is formed by the remaining tarsal bones and the metatarsals. For descriptive purposes, the longitudinal arch can be divided into a medial column formed by the navicular, cuneiforms, and the medial three metatarsals; and a lateral column formed by the cuboid and the lateral two metatarsals.

The talus transmits the weight of the body downwards in two directions: (1) posteriorly, to the heel through the subtalar joint with the calcaneus; (2) anteriorly and medially, to the medial three metatarsals through the articulation of the head of the talus with the navicular bone; and (3) anteriorly

(A)

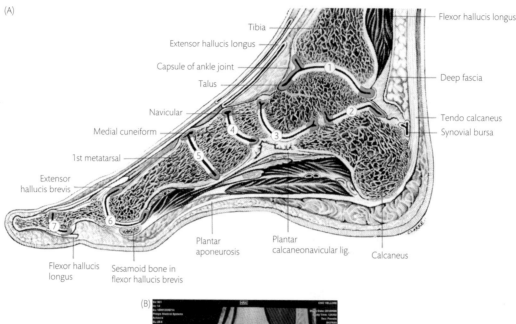

Tibia
Extensor hallucis longus
Capsule of ankle joint
Talus
Navicular
Medial cuneiform
1st metatarsal
Extensor hallucis brevis
Flexor hallucis longus
Sesamoid bone in flexor hallucis brevis
Plantar aponeurosis
Plantar calcaneonavicular lig.
Calcaneus
Synovial bursa
Tendo calcaneus
Deep fascia
Flexor hallucis longus

(B)

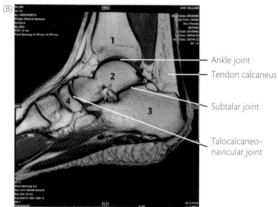

Ankle joint
Tendon calcaneus
Subtalar joint
Talocalcaneo-navicular joint

Fig. 19.14 (A) Oblique sagittal section through the middle of the heel and the middle of the big toe. Synovial membrane, blue. 1, Ankle joint; 2, subtalar joint; 3, talocalcaneonavicular joint; 4, joint between navicular and medial cuneiform; 5, first tarsometatarsal joint; 6, first metatarsophalangeal joint; 7, interphalangeal joint of big toe. (B) MRI showing ankle, subtalar, and talocalcaneonavicular joints. 1. Lower end of the tibia. 2. Talus. 3. Calcaneus. 4. Navicular.

and laterally to the lateral two metatarsals through the articulations with the calcaneus and indirectly the cuboid.

The **head of the talus** (not to be confused with the trochlea tali) fits into a deep socket between the anterior end of the calcaneus and the navicular at the **talocalcaneonavicular joint**. The **plantar calcaneonavicular** ('spring') **ligament** completes the socket for the head, as it extends from the sustentaculum tali to the navicular. The support provided by the spring ligament keeps the head of the talus from being pushed down between the calcaneus and the navicular by the weight of the body [Figs. 19.14, 19.15, 19.16]. The spring ligament and other ligaments on the plantar surfaces of the foot (**plantar ligaments**) play a part in maintaining the arches of the foot.

They are assisted by the plantar aponeurosis which holds the ends of the arch together. The plantar aponeurosis is tightened by dorsiflexion of the toes. The insertion of the **tibialis posterior** to the tarsal and metatarsal bones and the short muscles of the sole of the foot also help to maintain the arches. Fig. 19.17 illustrates the longitudinal arch of the foot in plantar flexion.

Transverse arches

The more prominent of these arches is in the region of the tarsometatarsal joints. The cuneiform bones and the base of the metatarsals are wedge-shaped, and the narrow plantar surfaces are held tightly together by plantar ligaments and by the tendon of the peroneus longus. This arrangement results in the plantar surfaces of these bones having a much

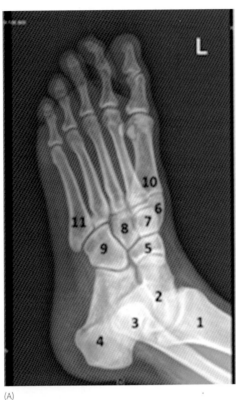

(A)

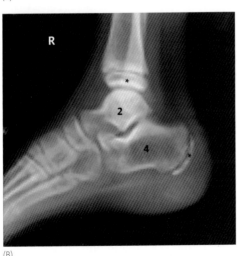

(B)

Fig. 19.15 (A) Oblique radiograph of the left foot. 1. Distal end of the tibia. 2. Talus. 3. Distal end of the fibula. 4. Calcaneus. 5. Navicular. 6. Medial cuneiform. 7. Intermediate cuneiform. 8. Lateral cuneiform. 9. Cuboid. 10. Base of the first metatarsal. 11. Base of the fifth metatarsal. (B) Ankle X-ray of a person less than 14–16 years of age. The epiphyses for the posterior aspect of the calcaneus and the distal end of the tibia (*) have not yet united.

smaller radius of curvature than their dorsal surfaces, and so forming a well-defined transverse arch. A second and lower arch exists between the heads of the metatarsals.

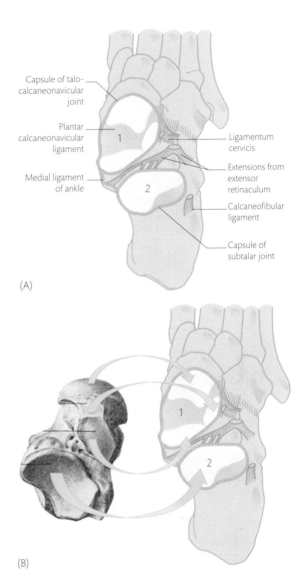

Capsule of talo-calcaneonavicular joint

Plantar calcaneonavicular ligament

Medial ligament of ankle

Ligamentum cervicis

Extensions from extensor retinaculum

Calcaneofibular ligament

Capsule of subtalar joint

(A)

(B)

Fig. 19.16 (A) The ligaments and inferior articular surfaces of the subtalar and talocalcaneonavicular joints as seen from above after removal of the talus. (B) The arrows connect articulating surfaces of the talus to articular facets of calcaneus and navicular. 1. Talocalcaneonavicular joint. 2. Subtalar joint.

Supports of the longitudinal arch of the foot

The main ligaments that maintain the longitudinal arch of the foot are the plantar calcaneonavicular, long plantar, plantar calcaneocuboid ligaments, and the plantar aponeurosis. The tibialis anterior raises the medial longitudinal arch. The tibialis posterior maintains the arch, as it holds the navicular against the head of the talus, and tightens the plantar surface of the foot through its insertion into the tarsal and metatarsal bones. The long and short flexors draw the ends of the longitudinal arches together.

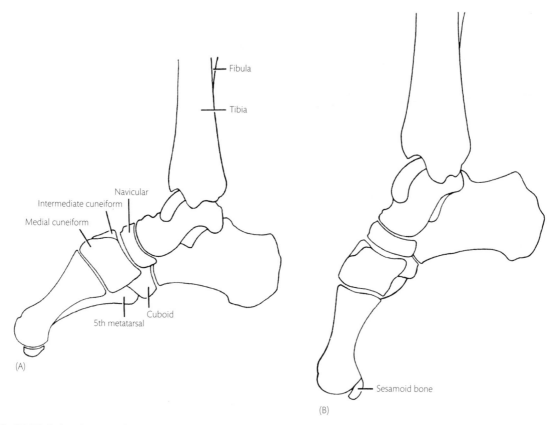

Fig. 19.17 Outline drawings of two radiographs of the same foot. In (B), the foot has been plantar flexed without any other movement. Note that virtually all of this movement takes place at the ankle joint, but that there is also slight flexion of the bones forming the medial longitudinal arch. The distance between the medial process of the tuber calcanei and the head of the first metatarsal is 7 mm less in (B) than in (A). This movement, produced by the plantar flexors, increases the height of the longitudinal arch.

⮕ The essential deformity in '**flat-foot**' is an eversion of the heel relative to the anterior part of the foot. In the reverse deformity of '**club-foot**', the heel is strongly inverted relative to the forepart of the foot, and the arch is greatly exaggerated.

The dissection of the joints of the foot is explained in Dissection 19.6.

DISSECTION 19.6 Joints of the foot-1

Objective

I. To demonstrate the ligaments and joints of the foot.

Instructions

1. Remove all muscles and tendons from the tarsal and metatarsal bones. Define the ligaments between the various bones.

2. Note that the ligaments on the plantar surfaces are much thicker than those on the dorsal surfaces.

Subtalar joint

The subtalar joint is a cylindrical joint between the lower surface of the body of the talus and the upper surface of the middle of the calcaneus [Figs. 19.13, 19.16]. The joint surface of the talus is concave, and that of the calcaneus is convex. These curvatures run transversely, allowing the calcaneus to turn around on the inferior surface of the talus in the movements of inversion and eversion. The fibrous capsule is attached near the margins of the articular surfaces [Fig. 19.16]. The deltoid ligament and calcaneofibular ligaments of the ankle joint strengthen the capsule. The **ligament of the neck of the talus (ligamentum cervicis)** passes from the neck of the talus to the calcaneus [Fig. 19.16] and strengthens the joint.

Talocalcaneonavicular joint

This is a complex 'ball-and-socket' type of synovial joint. The ball is formed by the head and adjacent part of the body of the talus. The socket is formed by the proximal surface of the navicular bone, the plantar calcaneonavicular ligament, the anteromedial part of the calcaneus, and the sustentaculum tali [Fig. 19.16]. This joint moves with the subtalar joint in inversion and eversion. The axis for these movements passes upwards, forwards, and medially through the calcaneus and the head of the talus. The talus remains stationary, while the other tarsal bones move around it. A single fibrous capsule encloses all components of the talocalcaneonavicular joint. The capsule is continuous with the plantar calcaneonavicular ligament and is strengthened by ligaments.

The dissection of the joints of the foot is continued in Dissection 19.7.

Calcaneonavicular ligaments

The **plantar calcaneonavicular** ('spring') **ligament** is a thick, triangular ligament which stretches from the sustentaculum tali to the plantar surface of the navicular bone [see Fig. 18.33]. It fills the triangular gap between these bones. Its tough, fibrocartilaginous upper surface articulates with the head of the talus [Fig. 19.16]. Medially, it is continuous with the fibrous capsule of the talocalcaneonavicular joint and the **medial ligament of the ankle joint**. Inferiorly, the tendon of the tibialis posterior supports it. This ligament plays an important part in maintaining the medial longitudinal arch of the foot and prevents the development of flat-foot.

The anterior part of the superior surface of the calcaneus, lateral to its articulation with the talus, is bound to the lateral surface of the navicular and

DISSECTION 19.7 Joints of the foot-2

Objective

I. To study the talocalcaneonavicular and subtalar joints.

Instructions

1. Cut across the ligaments which hold the talus to the calcaneus on the lateral, posterior, and anterior surfaces of the two joints. Turn the other tarsal bones away from the talus.

2. Examine the articular surfaces of the talocalcaneonavicular joint. The head and anterior part of the body of the talus has three articular surfaces, one each for the navicular, the calcaneus, and the spring ligament: (1) anteriorly, the head articulates with the navicular; (2) inferolaterally, the neck articulates with the upper surface of the calcaneus and the sustentaculum tali; and (3) inferomedially, the head articulates with the plantar calcaneonavicular ligament [Fig. 19.16].

to the dorsal surface of the cuboid by the **bifurcate ligament**. The two parts of the bifurcate ligament are the **calcaneocuboid** and **calcaneonavicular** parts [Fig. 19.11].

Tables 19.5 and 19.6 summarize the muscles and movements of the tarsal bones, mainly those occurring in the talocalcaneonavicular joint.

Calcaneocuboid joint

This is an oblique, saddle-shaped synovial joint which permits rotatory sliding of the cuboid on

Table 19.5 Muscles acting on tarsal joints, particularly the talocalcaneonavicular joint

Muscle	Origin	Insertion	Action	Nerve supply
Fibularis longus	Fibula, lateral surface	First metatarsal, base Medial cuneiform	Eversion	Superficial fibular
Fibularis brevis	Fibula, lateral surface	Fifth metatarsal, base	Eversion	Superficial fibular
Tibialis anterior	Tibia, lateral surface Interosseous membrane	First metatarsal, base Medial cuneiform	Inversion	Deep fibular
Tibialis posterior	Interosseous membrane Adjacent parts of tibia and fibula	Navicular, tuberosity Medial cuneiform All tarsals, except talus Metatarsal bases 2–4	Inversion	Tibial
Fibularis tertius	Fibula, anterior surface	Fifth metatarsal, base	Eversion	Deep fibular
Extensor hallucis longus	Fibula, anterior surface	Hallux, base distal phalanx	Inversion	Deep fibular
Extensor digitorum longus	Fibula, anterior surface	Extensor expansion, 2–5	Inversion	Deep fibular

Table 19.6 Movements at tarsal joints, particularly the talocalcaneonavicular joint

Movement	Muscles	Nerve supply
Inversion	Tibialis anterior	Deep fibular
	Extensor hallucis longus	Deep fibular
	Tibialis posterior	Tibial
Eversion	Fibularis longus	Superficial fibular
	Fibularis brevis	Superficial fibular
	Extensor digitorum longus (lateral)	Deep fibular
	Fibularis tertius	Deep fibular

the distal surface of the calcaneus. This joint lies almost in the same transverse plane as the **talonavicular joint**. The two together constitute the **transverse tarsal joint**. The movement of the transverse tarsal joint adds little to the movements of inversion and eversion.

The calcaneocuboid joint is strengthened by the dorsal calcaneocuboid ligament, and the **long plantar** and **plantar calcaneocuboid ligaments** [see Figs. 18.26, 18.33, 19.11]. The plantar calcaneocuboid ligament is attached close to the joint. The long plantar ligament lies inferior to the plantar calcaneocuboid ligament. It extends from the calcaneus to both lips of the groove for the peroneus longus tendon on the cuboid and to the bases of the middle three metatarsals. Both these ligaments are important in maintaining the lateral longitudinal arch of the foot.

Dissection of the foot is continued in Dissection 19.8.

DISSECTION 19.8 Joints of the foot-3

Objectives

I. To define the long plantar ligament.   II. To cut the long plantar ligament and expose the plantar calcaneocuboid ligament.

Instructions

1. Define the margins of the long plantar ligament [see Fig. 18.33]. Lift it from the calcaneus by passing a knife between it and the plantar calcaneocuboid ligament which projects beyond its medial edge. Detach the long plantar ligament from the calcaneus to expose the plantar calcaneocuboid ligament.

Smaller intertarsal joints

The three cuneiform bones articulate with each other and with the distal surface of the navicular bone by a single joint. The lateral cuneiform and navicular articulate with the cuboid. The articular surfaces of all these joints are flat, and all have dorsal and plantar ligaments. The intercuneiform, cuneocuboid, and cuboideonavicular joints also have interosseous ligaments. These joints give resilience to the tarsal bones, but the amount of movement at each is small.

Movements of the intertarsal joints

Acting together, the joints increase the resilience of the foot, but the main movements of inversion and eversion occur at the **subtalar** and **talocalcaneonavicular joints**. **Inversion** is the movement which raises the medial border of the foot and turns the sole medially. **Eversion** is the opposite movement which raises the lateral border of the foot and turns the sole inferolaterally. Eversion is more restricted than inversion. Inversion and eversion are important movements, while walking on uneven ground. The main evertors are the peroneus longus, brevis, and tertius. The main invertors are the tibialis anterior and posterior.

Tarsometatarsal joints

The medial three metatarsals articulate with the three cuneiform bones. The lateral two metatarsals articulate with the cuboid bone [see Figs. 18.3, 18.4]. All these joints have strong plantar and dorsal ligaments.

The joint surfaces at the base of the metatarsal bones vary. In the middle three metatarsals, the surfaces that articulate with the tarsal bones are flat. The metatarsal bases are wedge-shaped and are firmly fitted together. They have minimal mobility on the tarsus and on each other. The **second metatarsal** is the least mobile. In addition to articulating with the intermediate cuneiform, it articulates with the sides of the medial and lateral cuneiforms [see Fig. 18.3]. The base of the second metatarsal is so firmly fixed that its thin body is liable to fracture when sudden stresses are applied to the distal part of the foot. The middle three metatarsals form a relatively rigid beam in the centre of the foot. The articular surfaces of the base of the first and fifth metatarsals are slightly curved. As such, they have a greater degree of mobility than the middle three.

Intermetatarsal joints

The bases of the lateral four metatarsal bones articulate with one another. They are firmly bound together by plantar, dorsal, and interosseous ligaments.

Dissection 19.9 looks at the joints of the foot.

Metatarsophalangeal joints

In these joints, the base of the proximal phalanx articulates with the head of the metatarsal. The fibrous capsule is attached close to the articular surfaces. It is thickened at the sides to form collateral ligaments and on the plantar surface to form the plantar ligament. The dorsal part of the capsule is formed by the extensor expansion.

The thick fibrous **plantar ligament** is attached firmly to the plantar margin of the base of the proximal phalanx and loosely to the plantar surface of the neck of the metatarsal bone. The plantar ligament separates the long flexor tendon from the joint. The margins of the plantar ligaments are attached to: (1) the fibrous flexor sheath; (2) the slips of the plantar aponeurosis; (3) the deep transverse metatarsal ligament; (4) the collateral ligaments; and (5) the margins of the extensor expansions. The plantar ligament of the metatarsophalangeal joint of the big toe contains sesamoid bones which articulate superiorly with the grooves on the plantar surface of the head of the first metatarsal.

Articular surfaces

The distal surface of the head of each metatarsal has two continuous articular surfaces, one for articulation with the proximal phalanx and the other for articulation with the plantar ligament of the metatarsophalangeal joint. The articular surface for the proximal phalanx is circular and convex, and fits into the concavity of the base of the proximal phalanx to make a shallow ball-and-socket joint [Fig. 19.14A]. The articular surface for the plantar ligament is on the plantar surface. In the first metatarsal, this surface is deeply grooved on each side by a sesamoid bone.

Movements

The metatarsophalangeal joints permit flexion, extension, abduction, and adduction. Rotation is prevented by the collateral ligaments. Flexion and extension are produced by the long and short flexor and extensor muscles. The flexors are assisted by the interossei and the lumbricals. When the joints are flexed, the **plantar ligament** slides proximally towards the neck of the metatarsal, and, when they are extended, the ligament moves on to the distal surface of the head of the metatarsal. This tightens the plantar aponeurosis and the extensor expansion. When the metatarsophalangeal joints are extended, the extensor expansion is not able to act on the interphalangeal joints. The lumbricals then become the sole extensors of the interphalangeal joints if they reach the extensor expansion.

Abduction and adduction take place from the line of the second toe. These movements are produced by the interossei, the abductor of the little toe, and the abductor and adductor of the big toe.

DISSECTION 19.9 Joints of the foot-4

Objective

I. To dissect the first and second metatarsophalangeal joints.

Instructions

1. Remove the short muscles of the big toe by detaching them from the sesamoid bones. Note the connection between the tendon of the abductor hallucis and the extensor expansion, and the attachment of the abductor to the medial sesamoid bone.

2. Identify and cut through the deep transverse metatarsal ligaments on each side of the second toe. Trace the tendons of the interosseous muscles of the first two spaces to their insertions, and review the course of the lumbrical tendons.

3. Lift the extensor expansions from the dorsal surfaces of the metatarsophalangeal joints of the big and second toes. It forms the fibrous capsule on the dorsal aspect and is continuous on either side with the thickened lateral part of the capsule—the collateral ligaments.

4. Define these collateral ligaments, and then identify the plantar ligament between the long flexor tendon and the joint.

Interphalangeal joints

These are hinge-type synovial joints at which only flexion and extension take place. They are similar to the interphalangeal joints in the hand but have a smaller range of movements. The articular surfaces are sinusoidal, not circular. The single interphalangeal joint of the big toe is much larger than any of the others. It also has a flatter curvature and a smaller range of movements. This makes the joint more rigid—a necessary feature to bear the forces which are applied to it.

Movements

At rest, the interphalangeal joints are in a position of partial flexion by comparison with the extended position of the metatarsophalangeal joints. In the big toe, movements are produced by the long and short flexor, and the long and short extensor muscles. In the other toes, there is the additional action of the short flexor on the proximal interphalangeal joint.

The lumbricals extend the interphalangeal joints of the lateral four toes and are the only muscles responsible for this action when the metatarsophalangeal joints are fully extended. ◗ Thus, when the lumbricals are weakened or paralysed and the metatarsophalangeal joints are fully extended, the proximal interphalangeal joints are flexed by the long and short flexor muscles, and the distal interphalangeal joints are extended because of pressure on the ground. This position of the toes is known as 'hammer toe'.

Tables 19.7 and 19.8 summarize the muscles and movements of the joints of the toes (MP = metatarsophalangeal; IP = interphalangeal).

Hallux valgus

◗ This deformity is more common in women. It consists of a fixed adduction of the big toe at the metatarsophalangeal joint. The adduction of the big toe occurs because of the obliquity of the tendons inserted into it and because the attachment of the abductor hallucis is more to the

Table 19.7 Muscles acting on joints of toes

Muscle	Origin	Insertion	Action	Nerve supply
Extensor digitorum brevis	Calcaneus, superior surface	Hallux, proximal phalanx Extensor expansion, toes 2–4	Hallux, MP extension Toes 2–4, extension all joints	Deep fibular
Flexor digitorum brevis	Calcaneus, tuber medial process	Middle phalanx, toes 2–5	Tarsus, support Toes 2–5, MP and proximal IP flexion	Medial plantar
Flexor accessorius	Calcaneus, plantar aspect	Tendon of flexor digitorum longus	Straightens pull of flexor digitorum longus	Lateral plantar
Abductor hallucis	Calcaneus, tuber medial process Flexor retinaculum	Hallux, proximal phalanx, medial side Medial sesamoid bone	Hallux, MP abduction or flexion	Medial plantar
Abductor digiti minimi	Calcaneus, tuber both processes	Fifth toe, proximal phalanx, lateral side Fifth metatarsal, base	Fifth toe, MP abduction	Lateral plantar
Dorsal interossei	Metatarsals, adjacent sides of two	Proximal phalanx, lateral side, toes 2–4; medial side toe 2	Toes 2–4, abduction at MP	Lateral plantar
Plantar interossei	Metatarsals 3–5, medial side	Proximal phalanx, medial side, toes 3–5	Toes 3–5, adduction at MP	Lateral plantar
Lumbricals	Tendons flexor digitorum longus	Extensor expansion, toes 2–5	Toes 2–5, MP flexion, IP extension	Medial and lateral plantar
Flexor hallucis brevis	Cuboid, plantar surface, medial side	Hallux, proximal phalanx, medial and lateral sides	Hallux, MP flexion	Medial plantar
Adductor hallucis	Metatarsals 2–4, bases Plantar ligaments, MP 2–4	Hallux, proximal phalanx, lateral side	Hallux, MP adduction	Lateral plantar
Flexor digiti minimi brevis	Metatarsal 5, base	Fifth toe, proximal phalanx, lateral side	Fifth toe, MP flexion	Lateral plantar

Table 19.8 Movements of toes

Movement	Joints	Muscles	Nerve supply
Flexion	All joints	Flexor hallucis longus	Tibial
		Flexor digitorum longus	Tibial
		Flexor accessorius	Lateral plantar
	MP and proximal IP (2 –5)	Flexor digitorum brevis	Medial plantar
	MP only	Flexor hallucis brevis	Medial plantar
		Flexor digiti minimi brevis	Lateral plantar
	Toes 2–5	Lumbricals	Medial plantar, toe 2
			Lateral plantar, toes 3–5
	Toes 2–5	Interossei	Lateral plantar
Extension	All joints	Extensor digitorum longus*	Deep fibular
	Toes 2–4	Extensor digitorum brevis*	Deep fibular
	Hallux	Extensor hallucis longus	Deep fibular
	MP only	Extensor hallucis brevis	Deep fibular
	IP only toes 2–5	Lumbricals*	Lateral plantar, toes 3–5
			Medial plantar, toe 2
Abduction at MP	Toe 1	Abductor hallucis**	Medial plantar
	Toes 2–4	Dorsal interossei	Lateral plantar
	Toe 5	Abductor digiti minimi	Lateral plantar
Adduction at MP	Toe 1	Adductor hallucis	Lateral plantar
	Toes 3–5	Plantar interossei	Lateral plantar
	Toe 2	Dorsal interossei when toe 2 already abducted by other dorsal interosseous	Lateral plantar

* Full extension of MP prevents these muscles from extending IP joints which are then only extended by the lumbricals. If the lumbricals are weak or paralysed, or fail to reach the extensor expansion, 'hammer toes' result.

** This muscle is often inserted with the flexor hallucis brevis through the medial sesamoid to the plantar aspect of the proximal phalanx, so that it acts as a flexor, rather than an abductor. Thus, it may fail to prevent the tendency of the adductor hallucis and the oblique tendons of the extensor hallucis brevis and longus to cause the proximal phalanx of the great toe to deviate laterally. This condition, known as hallux valgus, exposes the medial side of the head of the metatarsal of the great toe to rubbing on the shoe. A bursa tends to form between it and the skin, and this becomes inflamed and swollen, forming a bunion.

plantar than the medial surface of the proximal phalanx—a position which makes it less efficient as an abductor.

Clinical Applications 19.1 and 19.2 look at some of the practical implications of the anatomy discussed in this chapter.

CLINICAL APPLICATION 19.1 Knee joint injury

An 18-year-old student twisted his right knee, while playing football. He experienced excruciating pain and felt as though something had torn inside his knee. On examination, he had tenderness on the medial side of the knee joint. When the knee was flexed at right angles and an attempt was made to pull the tibia forwards, there was increased mobility of the tibia. Surgical exploration under anaesthesia showed that the superficial and deep layers of the medial collateral ligament were torn. The medial meniscus was torn and detached, and was lying on the intercondylar area of the tibia. The anterior cruciate

ligament was torn from its posterior attachment on the femur.

Study question 1: name the ligaments of the knee joint which support the knee in all movements and yet prevent excessive mobility. Which ones are intracapsular? (Answer: medial and lateral collateral ligaments, anterior and posterior cruciate ligaments, patellar ligament (tendon), and oblique popliteal ligament. The cruciate ligaments are intracapsular; the others are extracapsular.)

The medial collateral ligament is frequently torn when the knee is forcefully abducted, and the tibia is laterally rotated on the femur while running. Review the attachments of the medial collateral ligament.

Study question 2: what are the normal attachments of the anterior cruciate ligament? (Answer: on the tibia, the anterior cruciate ligament is attached to the anterior intercondylar area. It runs upwards, backwards, and laterally to the medial surface of the lateral condyle of the femur.) The increased mobility observed when the tibia is pulled forwards on a flexed knee is indicative of a torn anterior cruciate ligament. It is called the 'anterior drawer sign'.

Study question 3: explain why the medial meniscus is more prone to injury than the lateral meniscus. (Answer: the medial meniscus is less mobile, when compared to the lateral meniscus, as it is fused to the medial collateral ligament. (The lateral meniscus is not attached to the capsule laterally.) Also, through the attachment of the meniscofemoral ligament, the lateral meniscus is able to move with movements of the femur. It is less likely to be trapped between the moving condyles in forceful movements of the knee. In addition, due to the larger antero-posterior diameter of the medial condyle, the medial meniscus is subject to greater movement of the medial femoral condyle on it.) Injury to the medial collateral ligament, medial meniscus, and anterior cruciate ligament is seen to occur together frequently.

CLINICAL APPLICATION 19.2 Flat-foot

A 35-year-old housewife presents with pain in her feet when standing or walking, which becomes worse as the day progresses. The pain radiates up her leg and to her back, and, by the evening, her feet are swollen. She feels her gait has changed, as she tries to minimize the pain by putting the whole foot on the ground, rather than moving her weight from the heel to the toes at every step. Prints of her feet while weight-bearing show that the entire sole of the foot leaves an imprint on the ground. The patient is diagnosed to have 'flat-foot', possibly due to chronic strain.

Study question 1: which parts of the foot normally touch the ground when a person stands? Why does the entire foot not touch the ground normally? (Answer: the heel, the lateral border of the foot, and the heads of the metatarsals imprint the ground. The medial side of the foot is raised off the ground by the longitudinal arch of the foot.)

Central to the development of flat-foot due to chronic strain is the sagging of the head of the talus. Study question 2: what structure/structures normally support the head of the talus? (Answer: the plantar calcaneonavicular ligament and the tendon of the tibialis posterior.) When the head of the talus sags under the weight of the body, the plantar calcaneonavicular ligament is stretched, and the unsupported head is displaced medially and downwards. The foot is chronically everted, and pressure on the nerves and blood vessels of the sole cause pain and discomfort.

CHAPTER 20

The nerves of the lower limb

Introduction

A **lower limb neurological examination** is part of the general neurological examination and is used to assess the integrity of motor and sensory nerves which supply the lower limb.

Sensory distribution

Fig. 20.1 shows the cutaneous distribution of the main nerves of the upper limb, and Fig. 20.2 shows the dermatomal pattern.

Motor distribution

Injury to a motor nerve will result in paralysis of the muscles supplied by it, and an inability to move the joint on which they act. Where a nerve innervates muscles in more than one segment of the limb (thigh, leg, foot), the effects of injury to the nerve depend on the level of injury. Thus, when the sciatic nerve is destroyed in the popliteal fossa, the hamstring muscles supplied by it in the thigh are not paralysed, though those in the leg and foot are. In general, the more proximal the nerve lesions, the greater will be the motor loss.

The results of lower limb nerve injuries are shown in Tables 20.1 to 20.10. (Abbreviations: the toes are numbered 1 to 5, from the medial side—1 is the big toe, and 5 the little toe. MP = metatarsophalangeal joint. IP = interphalangeal joints. PIP = proximal interphalangeal joint(s). DIP = distal interphalangeal joint(s).)

Femoral nerve

Table 20.1 shows the effects of injury on the femoral nerve.

Obturator nerve

Table 20.2 shows the effects of injury on the obturator nerve.

Superior gluteal nerve

Table 20.3 shows the effects of injury on the superior gluteal nerve.

Inferior gluteal nerve

Table 20.4 shows the effects of injury on the inferior gluteal nerve.

Sciatic nerve

Table 20.5 shows the effects of injury on the sciatic nerve.

Deep fibular nerve

Table 20.6 shows the effects of injury on the deep fibular nerve.

Superficial fibular nerve

Table 20.7 shows the effects of injury on the superficial fibular nerve.

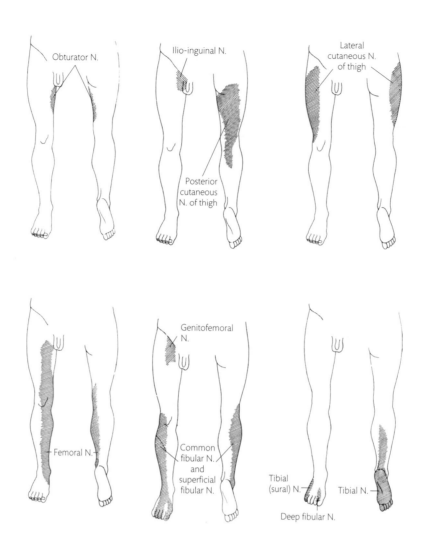

Fig. 20.1 Diagrams of the cutaneous distribution of nerves in the lower limb.

Tibial nerve

Table 20.8 shows the effects of injury on the tibial nerve.

Medial plantar nerve

Table 20.9 shows the effects of injury on the medial plantar nerve.

Lateral plantar nerve

Table 20.10 shows the effects of injury on the lateral plantar nerve.

Clinical Applications 20.1 and 20.2 look at some of the practical implications of the anatomy described in this chapter.

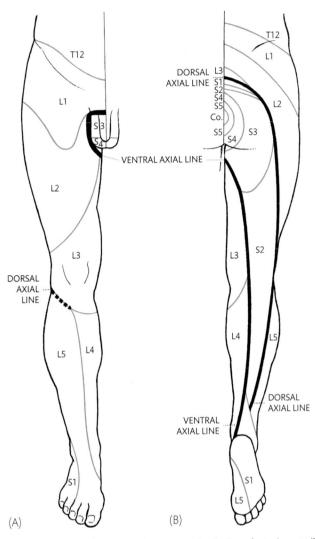

Fig. 20.2 Dermatomes of the lower limb, showing the segmental cutaneous distribution of spinal nerves (T. 12, L. I to 5, S. 1 to 5, Co.) on (A) the front and (B) the back of the limb and lower part of trunk.

After Head, 1893, and Foerster, 1933.

Table 20.1 The effects of injury to the femoral nerve

Joint involved	Movement affected	Explanation for loss/weakness of movement
Effect on hip joint	Flexion weakened	Sartorius, rectus femoris, and pectineus are paralysed. Weak flexion brought about by iliopsoas
Effect on knee joint	Extension lost or severely weakened	Quadriceps femoris is paralysed. Weak extension maintained by tensor fascia latae and gluteus maximus

Table 20.2 The effects of injury to the obturator nerve

Joint involved	Movement affected	Explanation for loss/weakness of movement
Effect on hip joint	Adduction lost	Obturator externus, adductor longus, adductor brevis, adductor magnus (adductor part), and gracilis are paralysed. Weak adduction is brought about by pectineus
	Instability in standing and walking	Due to weakness of adduction

Table 20.3 The effects of injury to the superior gluteal nerve

Joint involved	Movement affected/compensatory movement	Explanation for loss/weakness of movement
Effect on hip joint	Abduction lost. Compensatory flexion of the body to the paralysed side, to enable the opposite limb to be raised from the ground	Gluteus medius, gluteus minimus, and tensor fascia latae are paralysed

Table 20.4 The effects of injury to the inferior gluteal nerve

Joint involved	Movement affected	Explanation for loss/weakness of movement
Effect on hip joint	Extension weakened	Gluteus maximus is paralysed. Weak extension is brought about by the hamstrings

Table 20.5 The effects of injury to the sciatic nerve

Joint involved	Movement affected	Explanation for loss/weakness of movement
Effect on hip joint	Extension weakened	Adductor magnus (hamstring part), biceps femoris long head, semitendinosus, and semimembranosus are paralysed. Weak extension is brought about by gluteus maximus
Effect on knee joint	Flexion severely weakened	Biceps femoris, semitendinosus, and semimembranosus are paralysed. Sartorius and gracilis are responsible for the weak flexion
	Lateral rotation of leg on femur weakened	Biceps femoris is paralysed. Iliotibial tract is responsible for weak lateral rotation

Table 20.6 The effects of injury to the deep fibular nerve

Joint involved	Movement affected	Explanation for loss/weakness of movement
Effect on ankle joint	Dorsiflexion lost	Tibialis anterior, extensor hallucis longus, and extensor digitorum longus are paralysed
Effect on talocalcaneonavicular and calcaneocuboid joints	Inversion is weakened	Tibialis anterior and extensor hallucis longus are paralysed Weak inversion by tibialis posterior
	Eversion slightly weakened	Peroneus tertius is paralysed. Peroneus longus and brevis are responsible for eversion
Effect on first MP joint	Extension lost	Extensor hallucis longus and extensor hallucis brevis are paralysed
Effect on lateral four MP joints	Extension lost	Extensor digitorum longus and extensor digitorum brevis are paralysed
Effect on IP joint of big toe	Extension lost	Extensor hallucis longus is paralysed
Effect on IP joint of lateral four toes	Extension weakened in middle three toes Extension lost in little toe	Extensor digitorum longus and extensor digitorum brevis are paralysed. Lumbricals in the middle three toes are responsible for the weak extension

Table 20.7 The effects of injury to the superficial fibular nerve

Joint involved	Movement affected	Explanation for loss/weakness of movement
Effect on talocalcaneonavicular and calcaneocuboid joints	Eversion weakened	Peroneus longus and peroneus brevis are paralysed. Peroneus tertius and lateral part of extensor digitorum are responsible for weak eversion

Table 20.8 The effects of injury to the tibial nerve

Joint involved	Movement affected	Explanation for loss/weakness of movement
Effect on knee joint	Flexion slightly weakened	Popliteus and gastrocnemius are paralysed. Hamstrings, sartorius, and gracilis are responsible for flexion
Effect on ankle joint	Plantar flexion markedly weakened	Gastrocnemius, soleus, plantaris, flexor hallucis longus, flexor digitorum longus, and tibialis posterior are paralysed. Peroneus longus and brevis are responsible for weak flexion
Effect on first MP joint	Flexion weakened	Flexor hallucis longus and flexor hallucis brevis are paralysed. Lumbrical is responsible for weak flexion
Effect on lateral four MP joints	Flexion weakened	Flexor digitorum longus is paralysed. Lumbricals are responsible for some flexion
Effect on first IP joint	Flexion lost	Flexor digitorum longus is paralysed
Effect on lateral four PIP joints	Flexion weakened	Flexor digitorum longus is paralysed. Lumbricals are responsible for weak flexion
Effect on lateral four DIP joints	Flexion lost	Flexor digitorum longus is paralysed

Table 20.9 The effects of injury to the medial plantar nerve

Joint involved	Movement affected	Explanation for loss/weakness of movement
Effect on first MP joint	Abduction lost	Abductor hallucis is paralysed
	Flexion weakened	Flexor hallucis brevis is paralysed. Flexor hallucis longus is responsible for some flexion
Effect on MP joints of lateral four toes	Flexion weakened	Flexor hallucis brevis is paralysed. Lumbricals and interossei are responsible for some flexion

Table 20.10 The effects of injury to the lateral plantar nerve

Joint involved	Movement affected	Explanation for loss/weakness of movement
Effect on first MP joint	Adduction lost	Adductor hallucis is paralysed
Effect on MP joints 3–5 toes	Adduction lost	Plantar interossei are paralysed
Effect on MP joints 2–4 toes	Abduction lost	Dorsal interossei are paralysed
Effect on MP joint of fifth toe	Abduction lost	Abductor digiti minimi is paralysed
Effect on IP joints 2–5 toes	Extension lost if MP fully extended	Lumbricals and interossei are paralysed
Effect on IP joint of fifth toe	Flexion lost	Flexor digiti minimi brevis is paralysed

CLINICAL APPLICATION 20.1 Peripheral neuropathy (polyneuropathy)

Diseases such as diabetes, can affect nerves of the periphery, causing a condition called peripheral neuropathy where nerve functions are lost. The initial symptoms are most often sensory, and the longest nerves are affected first. Because this is a systemic disease, the condition produces symmetrical symptoms. The sensory loss on the feet has a typical 'stocking' distribution.

Study question: list all the nerves damaged in a patient who has peripheral neuropathy extending up to mid calf. (Answer: saphenous, sural, superficial fibular, deep fibular, tibial, lateral and medial plantar nerves [Fig. 20.1].)

CLINICAL APPLICATION 20.2 Motor assessment of lower limb musculature

Motor examination of the lower limb in a patient with spinal cord injury provides a reliable and quick way to localize the level of the lesion. Five muscles of the lower limb, one primarily supplied by each of the five segmental nerves L. 2 to S. 1, are tested. The integrity of each spinal segment is evaluated by the ability of a muscle supplied by it to bring about a particular movement of a joint [Table 20.11]. (The strength of the muscle is scored on a 5-point scale not included here.)

Table 20.11 Motor assessment of lower limb musculature

Spinal segment (myotome)	Primary movement	Prime muscle causing movement
L. 2	Hip flexion	Iliopsoas
L. 3	Knee extension	Quadriceps
L. 4	Ankle dorsiflexion	Tibialis anterior
L. 5	Big toe extension	Extensor hallucis longus
S. 1	Ankle plantar flexion	Gastrocnemius–soleus

Reference: *Standard neurological classification of spinal cord injury* by American Spinal Injury Association (ASIA).

CHAPTER 21
MCQs for part 3: The lower limb

The following questions have four options. You are required to choose the most correct answer.

1. **The saphenous opening**
   A. is a deficiency in the superficial fascia of the thigh
   B. is limited on the medial side by the falciform margin
   C. transmits the long saphenous vein and superficial inguinal arteries
   D. is present 4 cm inferomedial to the pubic tubercle

2. **The femoral canal contains the**
   A. femoral artery
   B. femoral branch of the genitofemoral nerve
   C. genital branch of the genitofemoral nerve
   D. lymph node

3. **All of the following statements are true regarding the sartorius, EXCEPT**
   A. it forms the lateral boundary of the femoral triangle
   B. it covers the roof of the adductor canal
   C. it is supplied by the femoral nerve
   D. it flexes the hip joint and extends the knee joint

4. **The descending genicular artery is a branch of the**
   A. femoral artery
   B. profunda femoral artery
   C. obturator artery
   D. deep external pudendal artery

5. **The nerve supply of the tensor fasciae latae is the**
   A. femoral nerve
   B. sciatic nerve
   C. superior gluteal nerve
   D. inferior gluteal nerve

6. **The articularis genu muscle is part of the**

   A. vastus medialis

   B. vastus intermedius

   C. vastus lateralis

   D. rectus femoris

7. **The pectineus is supplied by the**

   A. femoral branch of the genitofemoral nerve

   B. posterior division of the obturator nerve

   C. femoral nerve

   D. ventral rami of L. 2 and L. 3

8. **The posterior superior iliac spine lies at the level of the**

   A. fourth lumbar spine

   B. fifth lumbar spine

   C. first sacral spine

   D. second sacral spine

9. **The companion artery of the sciatic nerve arises from the**

   A. medial circumflex femoral artery

   B. lateral circumflex femoral artery

   C. inferior gluteal artery

   D. superior gluteal artery

10. **The sural nerve is the cutaneous branch arising from the**

    A. tibial nerve

    B. common fibular nerve

    C. superficial fibular nerve

    D. deep fibular nerve

11. **The structures that are attached to the anterior inferior iliac spine are the**

    A. sartorius and inguinal ligament

    B. sartorius and iliofemoral ligament

    C. rectus femoris and inguinal ligament

    D. rectus femoris and iliofemoral ligament

12. **The tendon of the peroneus longus grooves the inferior surface of the**

    A. calcaneus

    B. talus

    C. cuboid

    D. navicular

13. **The skin of the first interdigital cleft of the leg is innervated by the**

    A. deep fibular nerve

    B. superficial fibular nerve

    C. saphenous nerve

    D. sural nerve

14. The action of the tibialis posterior is

A. dorsiflexion and inversion of the foot
B. plantar flexion and inversion of the foot
C. dorsiflexion and eversion of the foot
D. plantar flexion and eversion of the foot

15. The oblique popliteal ligament is the extension of the

A. semimembranosus tendon
B. semitendinosus tendon
C. biceps femoris tendon
D. gastrocnemius tendon

Please go to the back of the book for the answers.

Answers to MCQs

Answers for part 2: The upper limb

1. C
2. D
3. A
4. B
5. C
6. D
7. C
8. B
9. D
10. A
11. A
12. B
13. B
14. A
15. A

Answers for part 3: The lower limb

1. C
2. D
3. D
4. A
5. C
6. B
7. C
8. D
9. C
10. A
11. D
12. C
13. A
14. B
15. A

Index